MAJOR SUBJECTS FOR FMGE

Dr. Kamal KV

MBBS, MS (Orthopedics)

Foreign (academic) trips (Countries and cities):

Georgia (Tbilisi, Batumi)

Russia (Nalchik, Cheboksary, Stavropol, Kazan)

Kyrgyzstan (Jalalabad, Osh, Bishkek)

Nepal (Bharatpur, Bhairahawa, Dharan)

Ukraine (Vinnytsia, Kiev)

China (Ningbo, Nanchang, Nanning, Dali, Fuzhou, Guangzhou)

Belarus (Minsk)

Kazakhstan (Almaty, Shymkent)

Uzbekistan (Fergana)

Peepee Publishers and Distributors Private Limited®

MAJOR SUBJECTS FOR FMGE

Published by
Pawaninder P. Vij and Anupam Vij

Peepee Publishers and Distributors Private Limited
Head Office: 160, Shakti Vihar, Pitam Pura, Delhi-110 034 (India)

Correspondence Address:
7/31, First Floor, Ansari Road, Daryaganj
New Delhi-110 002 (India)

Ph: 41512412, 9811156083

e-mail: peepee160@yahoo.co.in

e-mail: peepee160@gmail.com

www.peepeepub.com

join us on facebook.com/pp.publishers

First Edition: 2024

ISBN: 978-81-9720-729-7

PREFACE

We all know that Medicine, Surgery & Obstetrics-Gynecology are extremely important subjects for exams.

During early phase of preparation, when students have plenty of time, they can study these subjects in full details but as the exam approaches near and when they face time-crunch, they are not able to revise these big subjects effectively.

This was the thought behind bringing this title so that students can revise these bulky subjects in little less time and can go the examination hall with that much needed confidence.

I have tried to compile high yield topics with relevant illustrations so that student can remember the content for a longer period.

As I always say, students are the best judge of an author's work. In addition, I personally feel, there is always enough room left for further improvement. Therefore, I expect my dear students to share their valuable feedbacks regarding betterment of subsequent editions.

Despite my best efforts, some errors must have crept in. Since I have typed the entire content myself, I expect a few spelling mistakes. I request dear readers, to share the same with me (on the channels mentioned below).

Until now, students had supported all my titles. I hope the same kind of response for this title too.

Errata of this title (if any) would be updated on my **WhatsApp** group.

Please do join this group for other relevant updates as well.

Hope this title will serve its purpose.

02 June 2024

drkamalkv

Contact:

WhatsApp: **84 7000 4333**
Android App: **drkamalkvgroup**

SPECIAL THANKS

I would like to convey my heartfelt thanks to all those, who had arranged or served me during my foreign (academic) trips.

No.	Countries	College	First visit
1	**Georgia**	*i. Tbilisi*	Feb 2018
		ii. Batumi	Feb 2018
2	**Russia**	*iii. Nalchik*	Oct 2018
		iv. Cheboksary	Oct 2018
		v. Stavropol	Mar 2019
		vi. Kazan	Mar 2019
3	**Kyrgyzstan**	*vii. Jalalabad*	Dec 2018
		viii. Osh	May 2019
		ix. Bishkek	Dec 2022
4	**Nepal**	*x. Bhairahawa*	May 2019
		xi. Bharatpur	May 2019
		xii. Dharan	Sep 2019
5	**Ukraine**	*xiii. Vinnytsia*	Nov 2019
		xiv. Kiev	Nov 2019
6	**China**	*xv. Ningbo*	Oct 2018
		xvi. Nanchang	Nov 2018
		xvii. Nanning	Nov 2018
		xviii. Dali	Nov 2018
		xix. Fuzhou	June 2019
		xx. Guangzhou	June 2019
7	**Belarus**	*xxi. Minsk*	Jan 2020
8	**Kazakhstan**	*xxii. Almaty*	April 2023
		xxiii. Shymkent	March 2024
9	**Uzbekistan**	*xxiv. Fergana*	February 2024

drkamalkv

Contact:

WhatsApp: **84 7000 4333**

Facebook: **drkamalkvgroup**

CONTENTS

SECTION 1
MEDICINE

Chapter 1

Nervous System

ANATOMY OF NERVOUS SYSTEM

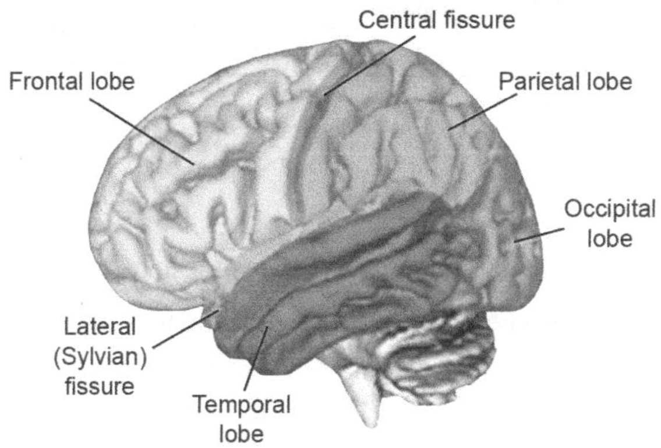

Basics

- **Sulci and Gyri:** Surface of the brain is folded into depressions (sulcus) and raised areas (gyrus)
- **Sylvian/Lateral fissure:** Separates the frontoparietal lobes (superiorly) from temporal lobes (inferiorly)
- **Central sulcus:** Runs obliquely downwards from the superior margin of the brain almost to the lateral fissure
- **White matter:** Consists mainly of myelinated fibers
- **Grey matter:** Consists of cell bodies of neurons, axons and dendrites, which are unmyelinated
- **Meninges:**
  - o Dura mater (outer)
  - o Arachnoid mater (middle)
  - o Pia mater (inner)
- **Brainstem:**
  - o Midbrain
  - o Pons
  - o Medulla
- **Thalamus:** It is the major synaptic relay station and is mainly concerned with processing of ascending sensory information to the cerebral cortex
- **Hypothalamus:** Head ganglion of the autonomic nervous system
- **Corpus callosum:** Made up of large of nerve fibers that connects the two cerebral hemispheres, which helps in coordinating activity between the cerebral hemispheres
- **Internal capsule:** Large number of nerve fibers interconnecting the cerebral cortex with the centres in the brainstem, thalamus and the spinal cord. All these fibers pass through internal capsule
- **Basal ganglia:** Main function is to modulate the motor outflow of cortex so that smooth voluntary movements occur
- **Limbic system:** Concerned with food habits, sexual and emotional behaviour

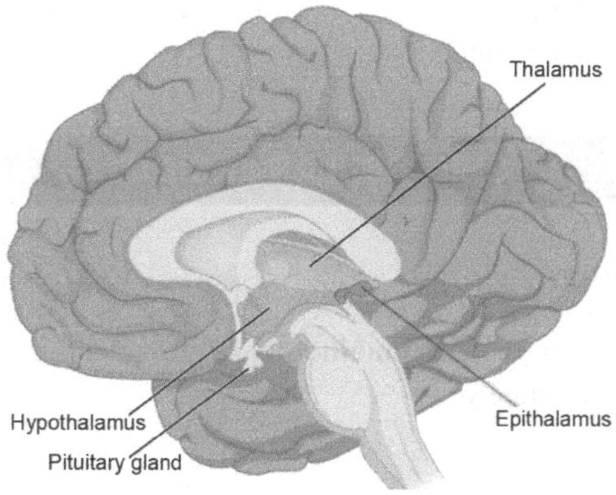

GUILLAIN-BARRÉ SYNDROME

Features

- Ascending type of motor paralysis
- Areflexia
- Flaccidity

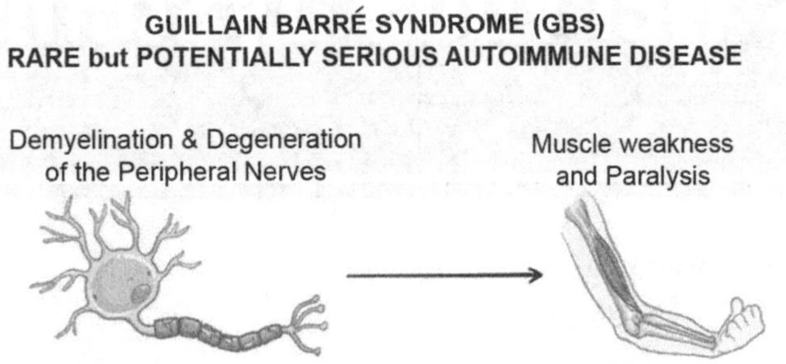

CSF examination

- Albuminocytological dissociation (increase in protein without an increase in cells)

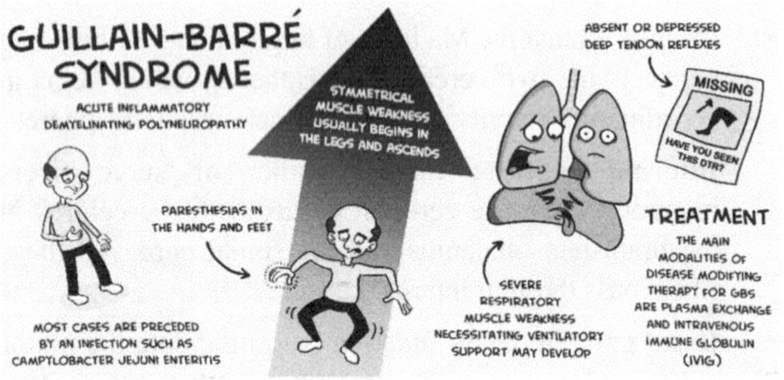

Treatment

- Plasmapheresis
- Immunoglobulin

CEREBELLAR LESION

Features

- Ataxia/asynergia (**inability** to do movements smoothly and accurately)
- Intention tremor (**NOT** resting ones)
- Head tremors/head tilt/intentional tremors
- Pendular knee jerk/decreased deep tendon reflexes

Lesion	Causes	Symptoms
Posterior lobe • Neocerebellar lesions	• Vascular, e.g., stroke • Tumours • Neurodegenerative	• **D**ysmetria, Dysdia-dochokinesia • **A**taxia • **N**ystagmus • **I**ntention tremor • **S**lurred speech • **H**ypotonia
Anterior lobe • Gait/limbic ataxia	• Alcohol • Malnutrition • > improve symptoms if stop drinking	• Drunken gait, can't walk straight • Head tremor
Midline • Truncal ataxia	• Medulloblastoma in 4th ventricle – young children • > Affect vestibular n.	• Fall towards most affected side • May involve eye movements

- Hypotonia
- Nystagmus
- Dysarthria (staccato speech)
- Ataxia with leaning towards side of lesion
- Dysdiadochokinesia (rapid alternating movements)
- Dysmetria/past pointing

MENINGITIS

	Normal	Bacterial	Viral
WBCs/μL	<5	>100-5000+	S-1000
Cell predominance	None	Neutrophils	Lymphocytes
Protein	<0.5 g/dl	Raised	Mildly raised
Glucose	2.6–4.5 mmoL	Very low	Low/normal
CSF/plasma glucose	>0.66	Very low	Low/normal

MC cause

- **Neonatal meningitis:**
  - o **Gram-negative bacilli (E. coli):** India
  - o **Group B Streptococcus:** Worldwide
- **Most common cause of meningitis in adults:** S. pneumonia

	Normal	Bacterial	Viral	Fungal/TB
Pressure (cm H_2O)	5-20	> 30	Normal or mildly increased	
Appearance	Normal	Turbid	Clear	Fibrin web
Protein (g/L)	0.18-0.45	>1	<1	0.1-0.5
Glucose (mmol/L)	2.5-3.5	< 2.2	Normal	1.6-2.5
Gram stain	Normal	60-90% Positive	Normal	
Glucose-CSF: Serum ratio	0.6	<0.4	> 0.6	< 0.4
WCC	<3	> 500	< 1000	100-500
Other		90% PMN	Monocytes 10% have >90% PMN 30% have > 50% PMN	Monocytes

Bacterial meningitis

- **CSF findings:**
  - o Purulent exudates
  - o Cloudy CSF
  - o Decreased glucose (<2.2 mmol/L)
  - o Increased protein concentration (>0.45 g/L)
- **Cells:** Neutrophils (>1000 cells)

	Bacterial	Viral	Fungal	TB
Opening pressure (N: 4-18 cm H_2O)	Elevated	Slightly elevated	Normal or high	Usually high
WBC (N: ≤ 5/mm³)	> 200/ mm³	< 200/mm³	< 50/mm³	20-30/mm³
Differential (N: ≤3 PMNs/mm³)	PMNs	Monocytes	Monocytes	Monocytes
Glucose (N: 45-80 mg/dL)	Low (< 60% serum)	Normal	Low	Low
Protein (N: 23-38 mg/dL)	Very high	Normal	High	High
RBC (N: ≤ 5/mm³)	Few	None	None	None

Viral meningitis

- **MC caused by:** Enterovirus (80-90%)
- **CSF findings:**
  - o Lymphocytic pleocytosis (>25/cubic mm)
  - o Normal glucose level
  - o Normal/mildly elevated CSF pressure

INFECTIONS

Encephalitis

- **Most common cause of sporadic viral encephalitis:** Herpes Simplex Virus
- Viral encephalitis and viral meningitis have same CSF findings

5 Stages of syphilis

Stage	Symptoms
Primary syphilis	Chancre in genitalia (often unnoticed)
Secondary syphilis	Maculopapular, Non-tender rash; Fever; Lymphadenopathy; Condyloma latum (genital)
Latent syphilis	Asymptomatic; Serum non-treponemal and Treponemal antibody tests are positive
Tertiary syphilis	Multiple organ system involvement; Nerve involvement (deafness), aortic root dilation, aortitis, gummas (liver, bone, skin, spleen)
Neurosyphilis	Any stage can progress to neurologic involvement. Most common presentation is asymptomatic pupillary afferent defect (Argyll Robertson Pupil). Focal symptoms include aphasia, paresis, blurry vision, hearing loss, seizures, ataxia, bowel or bladder incontinence, tabes dorsalis, loss of position and vibration senses, progressive ataxia, and sudden and severe pain, loss of balance, delirium, hydrocephalus, transverse myelitis, and stroke-like small vessel changes

Neurosyphilis

- **Tract involved:** Dorsal column
- **Features:**
  - o Sensory loss
  - o Argyll Robertson pupil
  - o Bladder dysfunction
- **Associated term:** Tabes dorsalis

OTHER CONDITIONS AFFECTING NERVOUS SYSTEM

Neuropathic joint disease

- **Most common cause of neuropathic joint disease:** DM
- **MC joint affected by DM:** Tarsal joints
- **Other associated conditions:**
  - o Leprosy
  - o Syringomyelia
  - o Tabes dorsalis

PARKINSONISM

Features

- 2nd **MC** neurodegenerative disease
- Intracytoplasmic proteinaceous inclusions known as Lewy bodies
- Parkinson disease is the **MC** form of parkinsonism

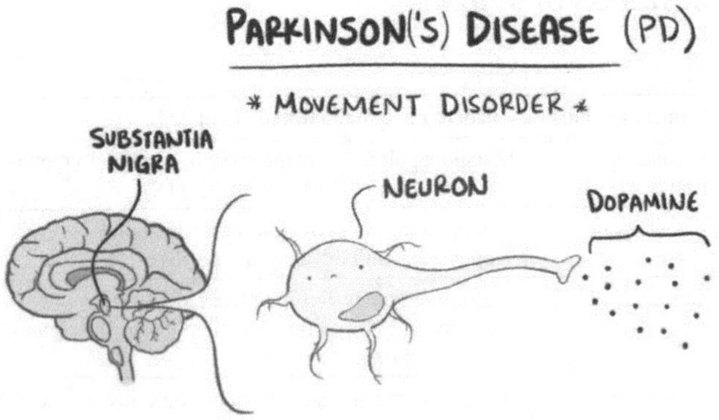

Pathology

- **Symptoms of parkinsonism are due to:** Loss of nerve cells in substantia nigra pars compacta (SNc) and the locus coeruleus (midbrain)
- **Drugs causing parkinsonism:**
  - o Methyl dopa
  - o Reserpine
  - o Metoclopramide

Features

- **Cardinal features:**
  - o Resting tremor
    - ♦ **MC** manifestation
    - ♦ Occurs at rest
    - ♦ Worsens with emotional stress
  - o Bradykinesia
  - o Rigidity, gait disturbance/postural instability (Festinating gait)
- **Other features:**
  - o Masked facies
  - o Reduced eye blink
  - o Dysphagia

Treatment

- Levodopa + peripheral decarboxylase inhibitor
- **MAO (monoamine oxidase)-B inhibitors:** Selegiline

SUBARACHNOID HEMORRHAGE

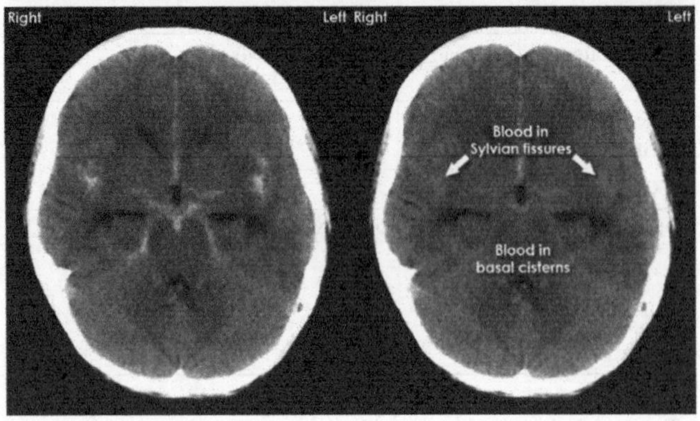

Clinical presentation

- 60 years old patient with severe headache and neck stiffness of abrupt onset
- She had never such a severe headache before
- She may have photophobia and nausea

Subarachnoid hemorrhage CSF findings

- **Pressure and proteins:** Increased
- **Colour:** Red stained
- **Cells:** RBC
- **Sugar:** Normal

PERIPHERAL NEUROPATHY

Predominantly motor loss

- Porphyria
- Lead poisoning
- Guillain-Barré syndrome
- Amyotrophic lateral sclerosis

Predominantly sensory loss

- DM
- Leprosy
- HIV

BRAIN TUMOUR

Important points

- **MC brain tumors:** Secondaries (from breast Ca, small cell Ca lung)
- **MC primary intracranial (malignant brain) tumour:** Glioma
- **MC glial tumors:** Astrocytoma
- **MC posterior fossa tumour:** Astrocytoma

Clinical features

- Nausea
- Vomiting
- Headache
- Papilledema
- Seizures

On examination

- High BP
- Low pulse

IOC

- Gadolinium enhanced MRI scan

Management

- **For cerebral edema:** Dexamethasone
- **Brain metastasis:** Radiotherapy
- **Isolated lesions in brain:** Stereotactic surgery

NEUROFIBROMA

Tumors associated with neurofibromatosis-I (Peripheral form)

- Endocrinal tumors
- Multiple cutaneous neurofibroma
- Café au lait spots
- Iris fibromas

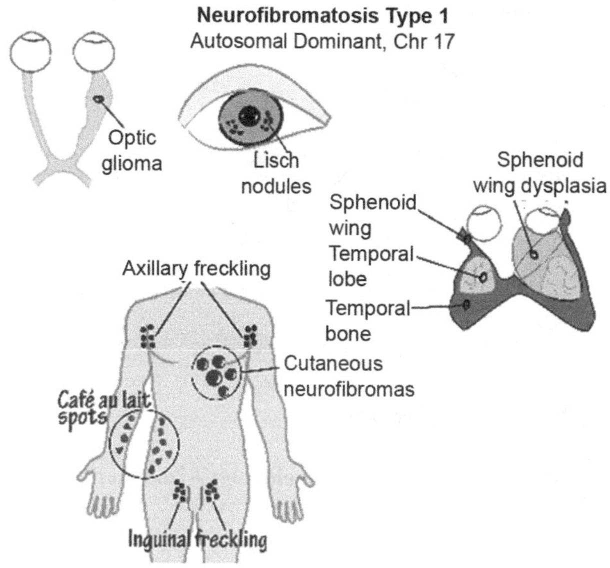

Feature of neurofibromatosis-II (Central form)

- Bilateral acoustic neuroma
- Cerebral and optic nerve gliomas
- Meningiomas

NF-1	NF-2
Common-90%	Less common-10%
Chromosome 17 mutations	Chromosome 22 mutations
Cutaneous lesions common (> 95%)	Cutaneous, eye lesions less prominent
Café au lait spots	Mild/few café au lait spots
Lisch nodules	Juvenile subcapsular opacities
Cutaneous NFs (often multiple) Plexiform NFs (pathognomonic)	
1. CNS lesions less common (15-20%)	1. CNS lesions in 1000%
2. T2/FLAIR hyperintensities (myelin vacuolization; lesions wax, then wane)	2. Bilateral vestibular schwannomas (almost all)
3. Astrocytomas (optic pathway gliomas–usually pilocytic–other gliomas)	3. Nonvestibular schwannomas (50%)
4. Sphenoid wing, dural dysplasias	4. Meningiomas (50%)
5. Moya moya	5. Cord ependymomas (often multiple)
6. Neurofibromas of spinal nerve roots	6. Schwannomas of spinal nerve roots

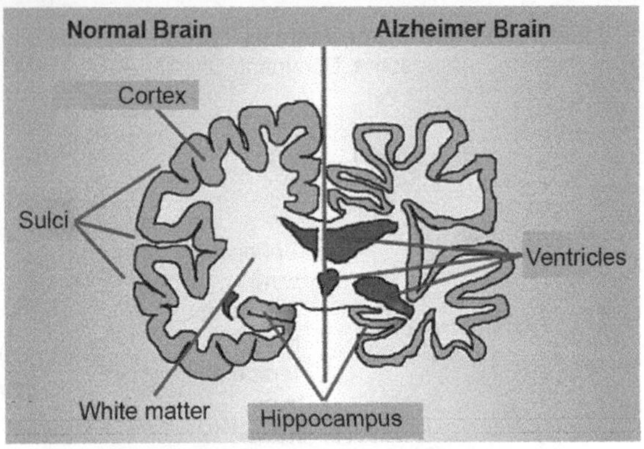

Alzheimer's disease

- **MC cause of dementia in elderly:** Alzheimer's disease
- **Presenile dementia occurs before the age of:** 60 years
- **Useful screening test for dementia:** Mini mental status examination
- **Maximum score in mini mental status examination:** 30

Creutzfeldt-Jackob disease

- **Caused by:** Prion (infectious protein)
- Neurodegenerative disease
- Rapid progression is common
- Can be transmitted by corneal implants

SECTION 1
MEDICINE

Chapter 2

Electrolyte Disorders

HYPERKALEMIA

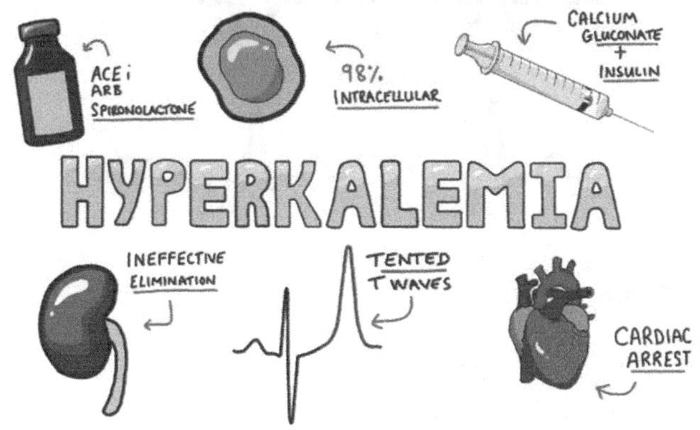

Causes

- Plasma potassium >5.5 mmol/L
- Seen in renal failure (ARF, CRF)
- Low aldosterone (hypoaldosteronism)
- **Drugs:** ACE inhibitors, heparin

Features

- Metabolic acidosis (hyperkalemia decreases net acid excretion by inhibiting renal ammonia genesis and reabsorption of ammonium)

Clinical features

- Partial depolarization of membranes results in weakness, flaccid paralysis, hypoventilation

ECG

- Tall and peaked/tentacular T waves (**Earliest**)
- Prolongation of PR interval
- Prolongation of QRS duration
- Ventricular fibrillation
- Asystole

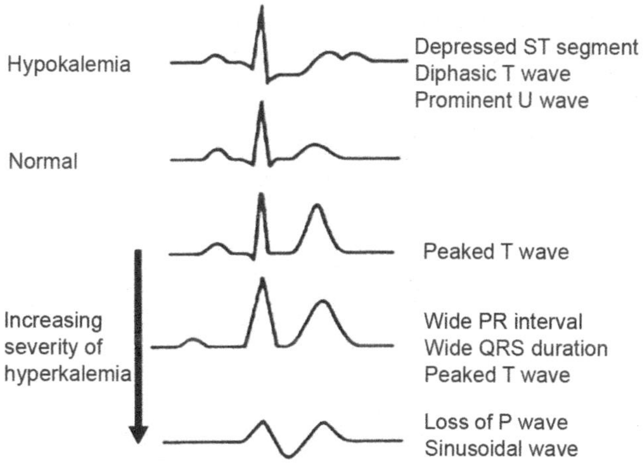

Management

- Calcium gluconate
- Insulin with dextrose
- I/V sodium bicarbonate in severe cases

HYPOCALCEMIA

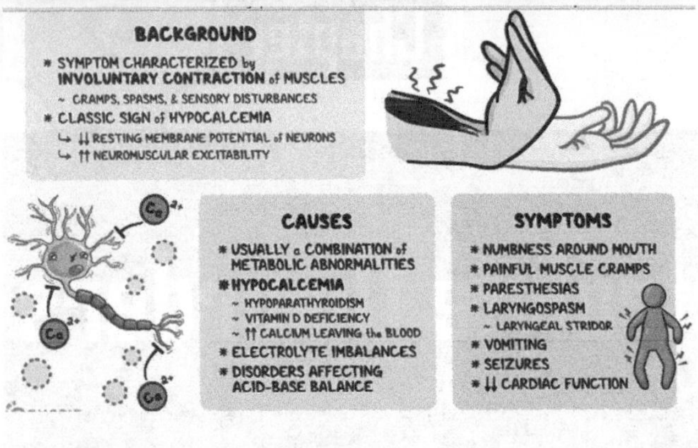

Causes

- Serum calcium <8.5 mEq/L
- Tumour lysis syndrome
- Acute pancreatitis
- Hypoparathyroidism
- CRF

Clinical features

- Increased neuromuscular irritability
- Spasm of muscles, laryngeal spasm
- Perioral tingling
- Chvostek's sign Contraction of facial muscles, elicited by light tapping of the facial nerve)
- Trousseau's sign
- Carpopedal spasm
- Hyperactive deep tendon reflexes

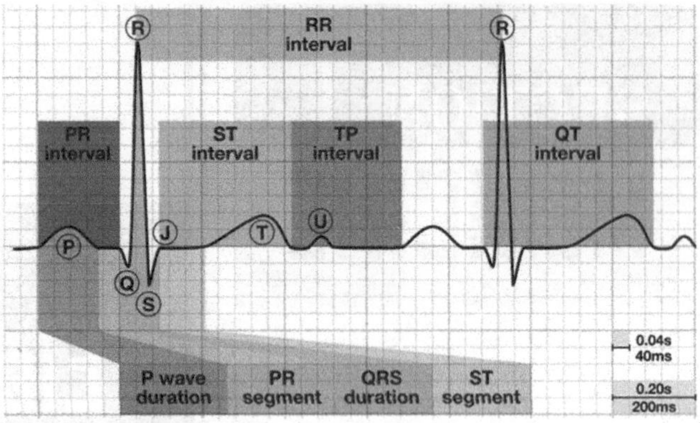

ECG changes

- Prolongation of QT interval

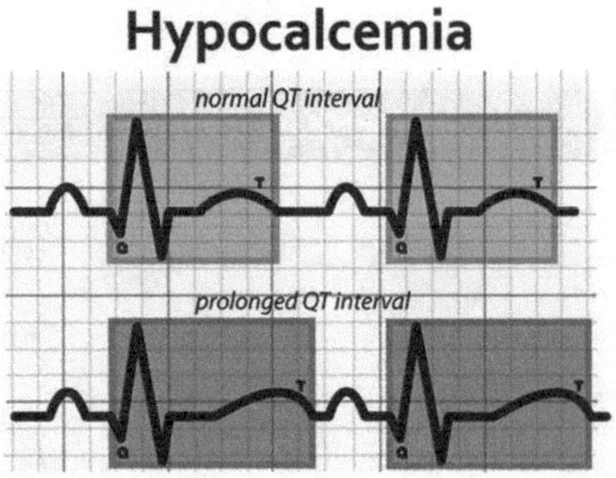

Management

- Vitamin D/calcitriol
- High oral calcium intake
- I/V calcium gluconate
- Thiazides

SECTION 1
MEDICINE

Chapter 3

Disorders Affecting Muscles

DUCHENNE MUSCULAR DYSTROPHY

Pathology

- **Inheritance:** X-linked recessive
- **Defect lies in which gene:** Dystrophin gene
- **Pathology in which protein:** Sarcolemmal protein defect

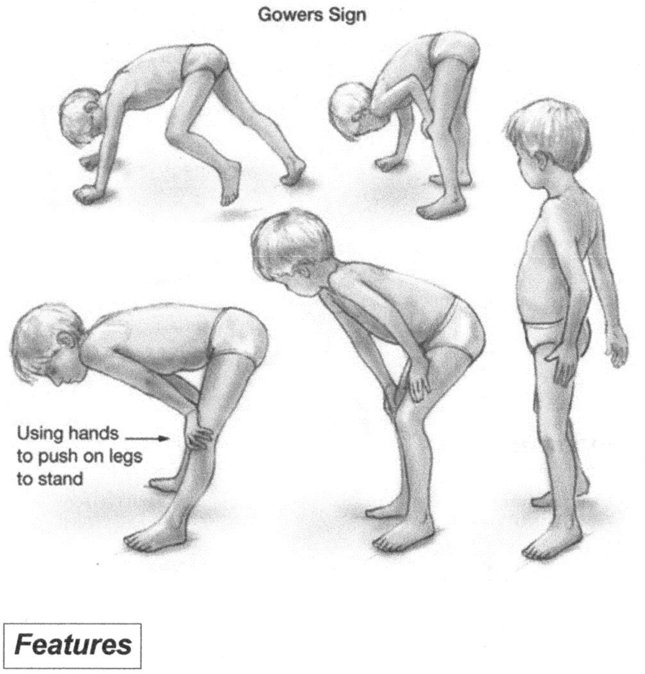

Features

- Pseudohypertrophy of muscles
- **Gowers sign:** Patient, while standing, tries to climb on himself

	Duchenne muscular dystrophy	Becker muscular dystrophy
Etiology	**X-linked recessive**, dystrophin gene mutation	
Dystrophin protein	**Absent**	**Reduced**
Age of onset	2-5 years	> 15 years
Symptoms	Rapid progression, inability to walk by approx. 12 years	Less severe, slower progression, cardiac involvement is more common
Diagnostics	↑↑ **Creatine kinase,** ↑ serum aldolase, genetic analysis (confirmatory test), muscle biopsy	
Treatment	Supportive, glucocorticoids	
Life expectancy	~30 years	~ 40 - 50 years

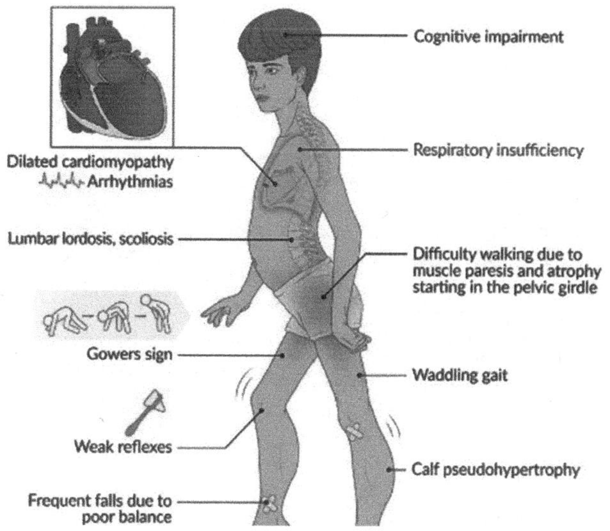

MYASTHENIA GRAVIS/MG

Pathology

- Autoimmune
- Bimodal (30-40 is women; 70-80s in men)
- Decreased myoneural junction transmission (anti-Acetylcholine receptor antibodies)

Autoantibodies Against Receptors Cause Disease by Blocking Receptor Function

Normal events at the neuromuscular junction

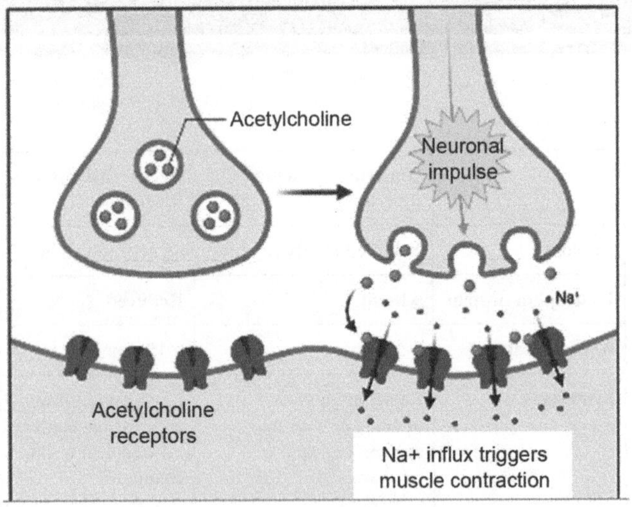

Myasthenia gravis

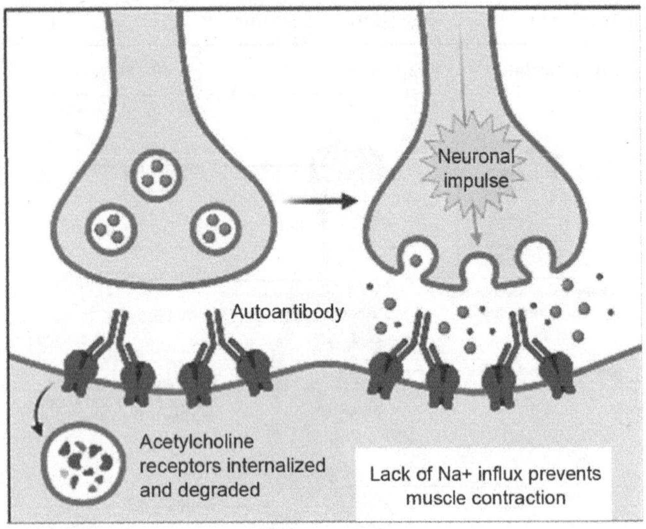

Types

- **Generalized MG:**
    - o Bulbar (Bulbar relates to medulla)
    - o Facial
- **Ocular MG:**
    - o Ptosis
    - o Diplopia

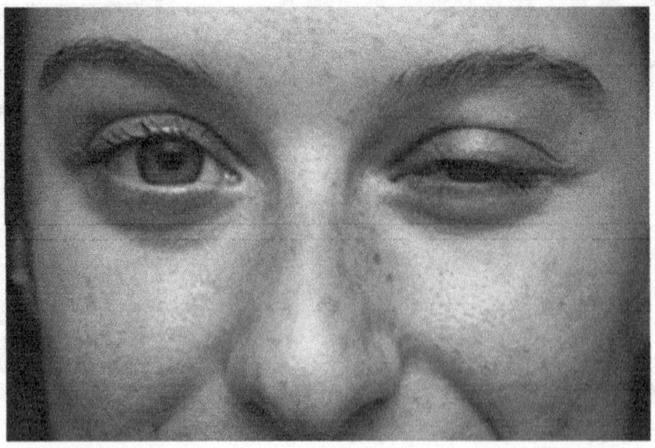

Investigation

- Edrophonium/Tensilon test (acetylcholinesterase inhibitor)
- **Single fiber EMG: Most** sensitive

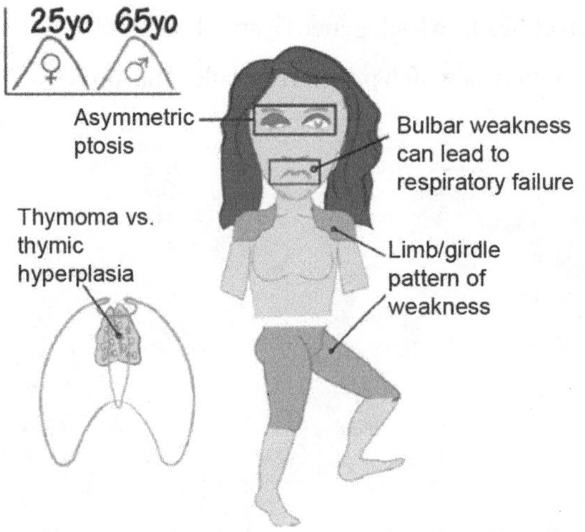

Features

- **Bulbar MG:**
    - o Dysarthria
    - o Dysphagia
    - o Fatigable chewing
- Proximal muscle weakness (muscle weakness and fatigability which **worsens** by the end of the day)
- **Normal:** Sensory modalities and deep tendon reflexes

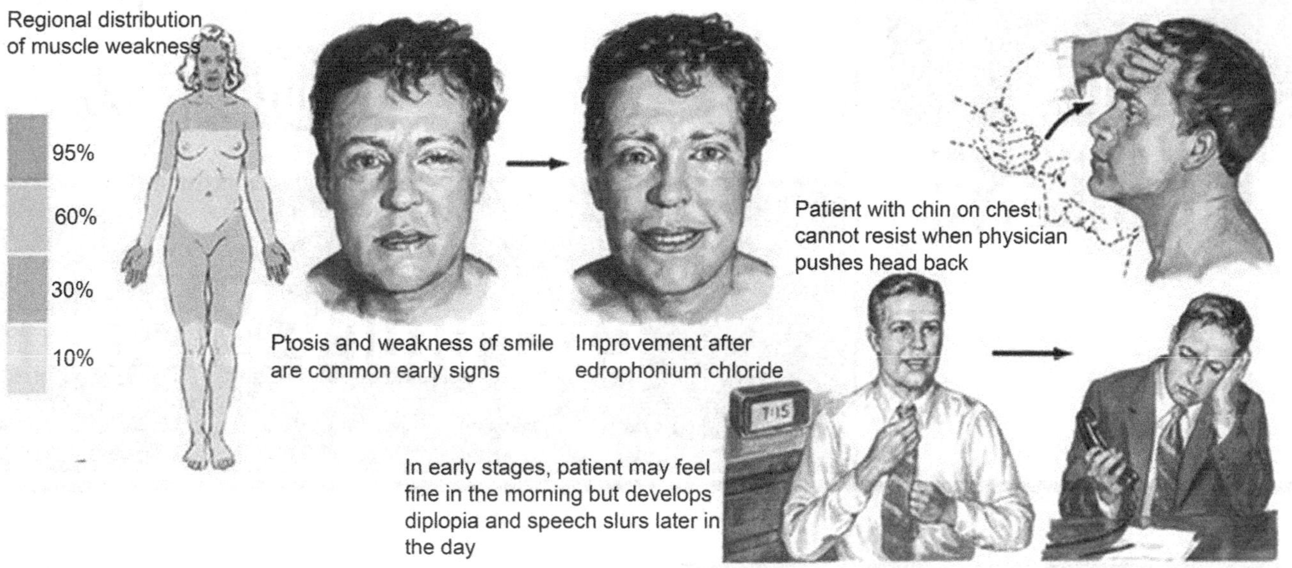

Treatment

- **MC used cholinergic drugs:** Pyridostigmine/Neostigmine (acetylcholinesterase inhibitor)
- **Surgical procedure (should be done in all cases):** Thymectomy

SECTION 1
MEDICINE

Chapter 4

Excretory System

ANATOMY

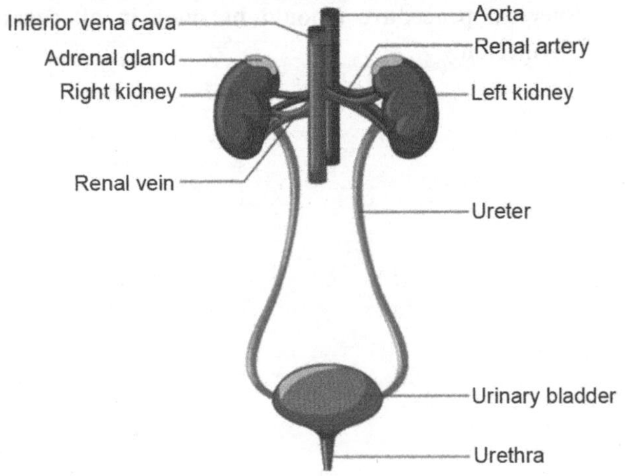

Basics

- **Kidney:**
  - o 2 parts:
    - ♦ Outer cortex
    - ♦ Inner medulla
  - o Liver on right side pushes the right kidney at a lower level than left
  - o Supplied by renal artery (from aorta)
  - o Renal vein drains into inferior vena cava
  - o Left renal vein is longer therefore left kidney is preferred for transplantation
- **Ureters:**
  - o 25 cm long
  - o Pain of the ureteric colic starts in the loin and radiates downwards and forwards to groin or up to scrotum/labium majus
- **Urinary bladder:**
  - o **Mean capacity:** 220 ml
  - o Voiding of urine (micturition) takes place when the amount of urine in urinary bladder is approx. 280 ml

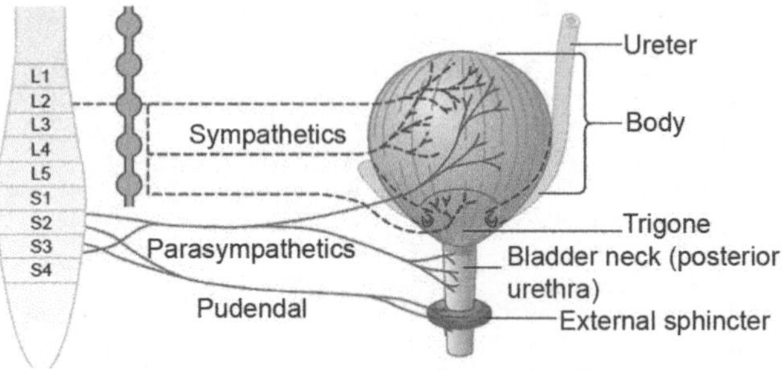

  - o Nervi erigentes (parasympathetic) is inhibitor to sphincter vesicae and motor to detrusor; promotes urination
  - o Sympathetic fibers are inhibitory to detrusor and motor to sphincter vesicae; inhibits urination
- **Urethra:**
  - o **Female urethra:**
    - ♦ 4 cm long
    - ♦ Corresponds to upper part of male prostatic urethra
  - o **Male urethra:**
    - ♦ 20 cm long
    - ♦ 4 parts

- **Prostatic:**
  - 3 cm
  - **Most** dilatable
  - **Widest**
- **Membranous:**
  - 2 cm
  - **Least** dilatable
  - Shortest
- **Bulbar**
- **Penile/Spongiosis/Cavernous:**
  - 15 cm
  - Opening of Bulbourethral glands of Cowper

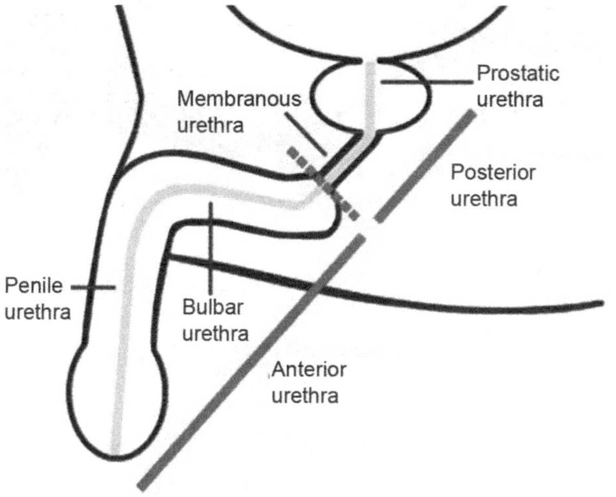

DIABETIC NEPHROPATHY

Features

- **Microalbuminuria:** 30-299 mg/d (a risk factor for CVS disease)

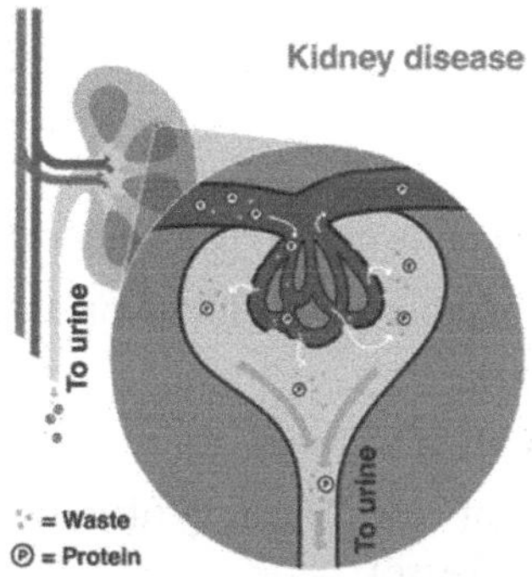

- **Macroalbuminuria:** >300 mg/d
- After macroalbuminuria, GFR starts falling and end stage renal disease sets in 8-10 years

Histology

- **Most characteristic finding:** Nodular glomerulo-sclerosis
- **Most common finding:** Diffuse glomerulosclerosis

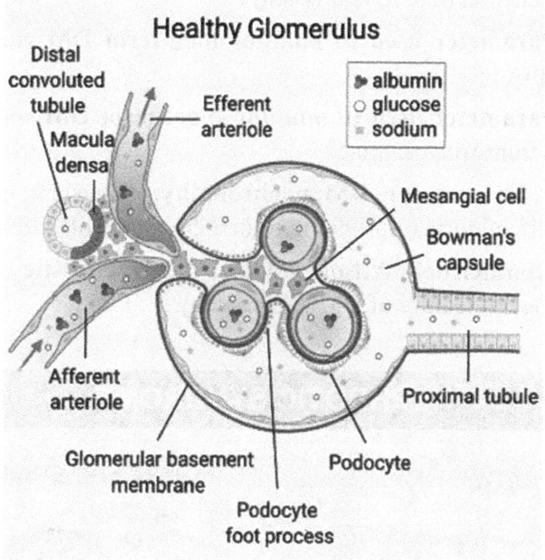

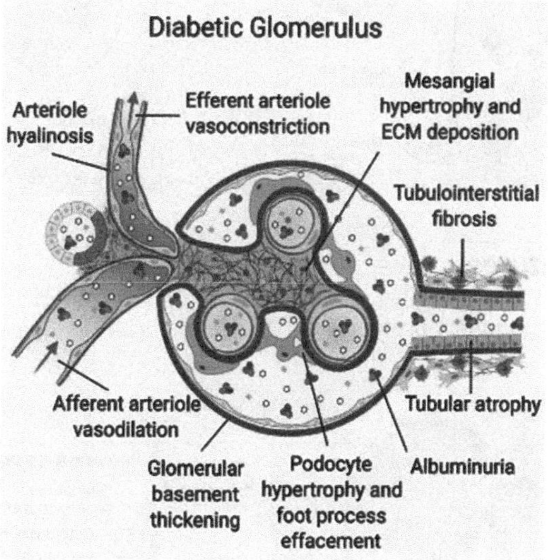

Types

- Type 1/IDDM
- **IDDM presentation:** Usually <25 years
- **Ketoacidosis commoner in:** IDDM
- Type 2/NIDDM
- **HLA link of NIDDM:** No links

Terms

- **Dawn phenomenon:** Glucose level rise in early morning
- **Somogyi effect:** Rebound hyperglycemia may appear after 1-24 hours after moderate to severe hypoglycemia

Other points

- **Absence of chest pain in DM patients is:** Silent ischemia (due to neuropathy)
- **Parameter used to monitor long-term DM control:** HbA1c
- **Parameter used to monitor short-term DM control:** Serum fructosamine
- **Early test for DM nephropathy:** Persistent micro-albuminuria (30-299 mg/d) in a 24 hours collection
- **Kimmelstiel Wilson nodule: Characteristic** histological feature of DM nephropathy

NEPHROTIC SYNDROME

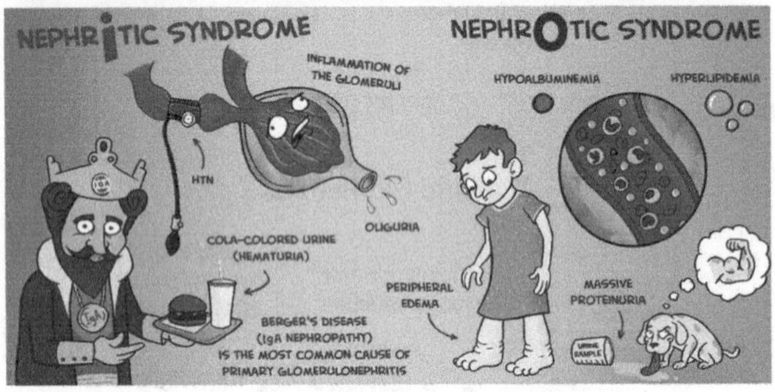

Features

- >3 gm/day proteinuria

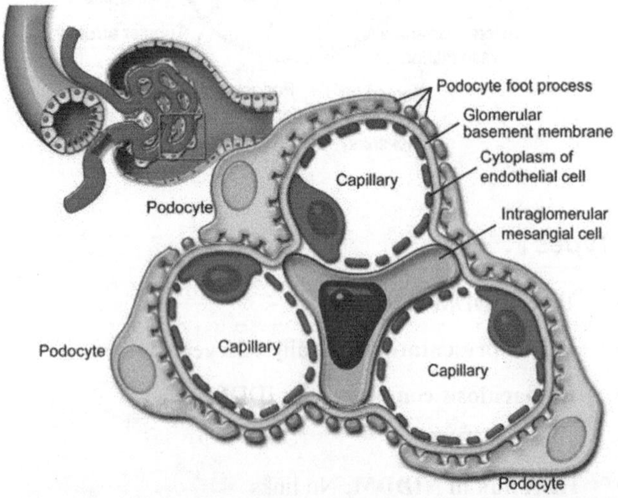

- Hypoalbuminemia
- Edema
- Hypercoagulable states
- Hyperlipidemia and lipiduria

MINIMAL CHANGE DISEASE

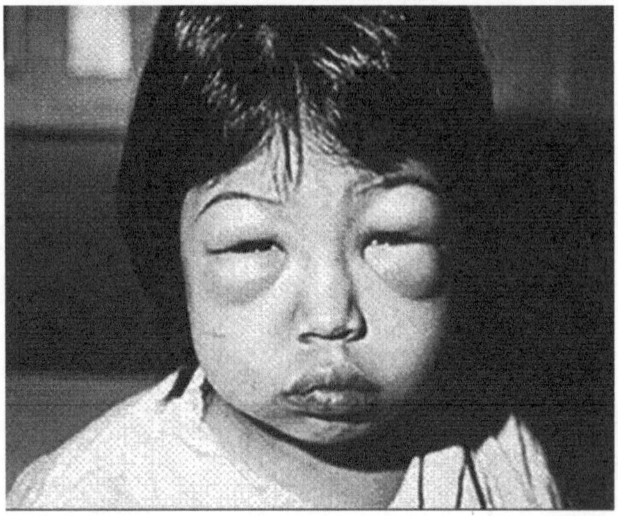

Features

- Seen in children <15 years
- 75% cases of nephrotic syndrome in children are because of MCD
- Selective proteinuria (LMW protein like albumin is excreted)
- **Normal** light microscopy

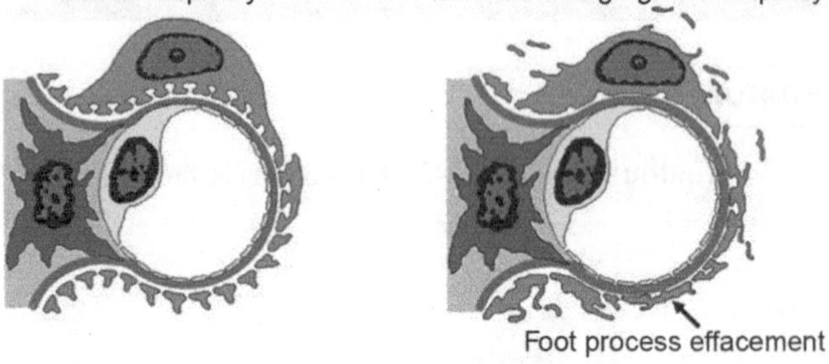

- Fusion of foot process on electron microscopy
- Remission of proteinuria with steroid therapy indicates a good prognosis
- Responds **well** to Steroids
- **No** deposits of complement/Ig (therefore also known as Nil deposit disease)

- **Electron microscopy findings:** Fusion/effacement/loss of foot process
- **Changes on light microscopy: No** change

Podocyte foot process effacement

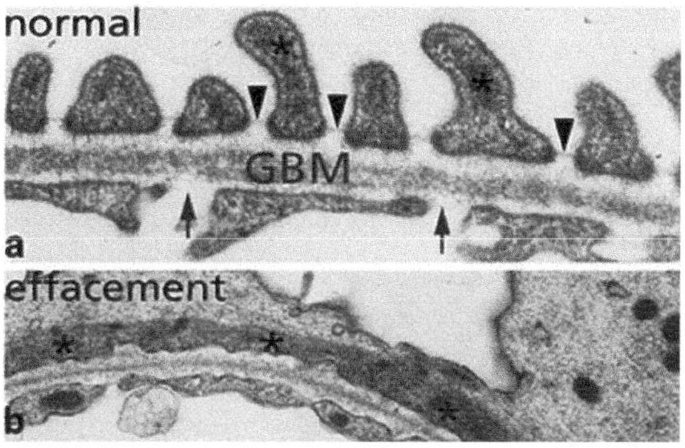

RPGN/CRESCENTIC GN

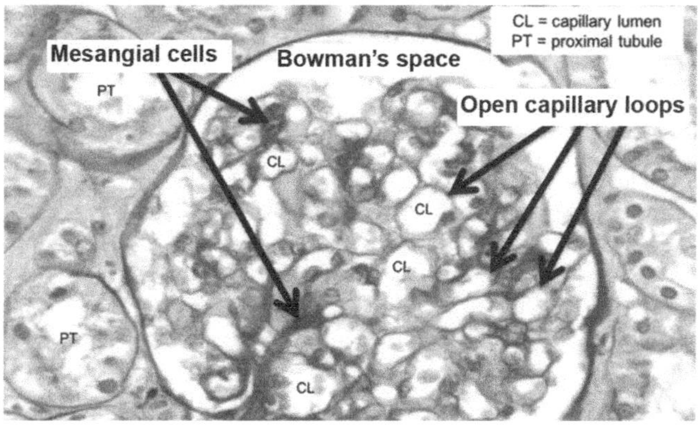

Features

- Renal failure may develop over weeks to months

Rapidly progressive glomerulonephritis is characterized by crescents in Bowman's space of the glomeruli (light microscopy) hence, RPGN may be referred to as crescentic glomerulonephritis

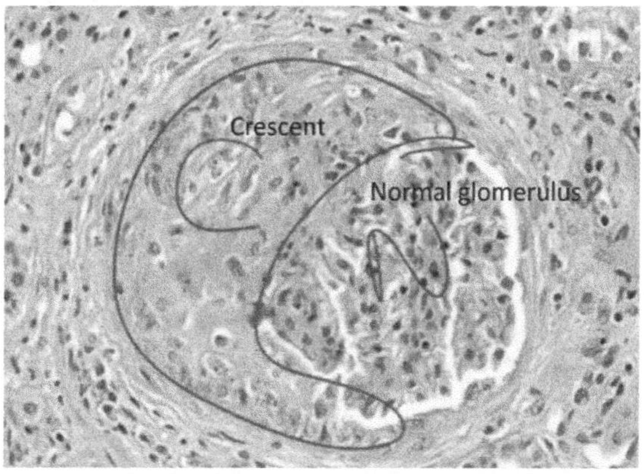

- **Classical** morphologic feature is crescentic glomerulonephritis
- Renal biopsy is the investigation of **choice**
- **Serological markers:** C3, anti-GBM antibodies, anti-neutrophil antibodies (ANA)
- Characterized by gradual onset of hematuria, proteinuria and renal failure which develops over a period of weeks to months
- 55% patient requires dialysis within 5 months of diagnosis
- Steroids + cytotoxic agents (cyclophosphamide) are used
- Rapid onset (often presents as ARF)
- Crescent formation

OTHER CONDITIONS OF KIDNEY

Hypertension

- **Benign HTN:** Hyaline arteriosclerosis
- **Malignant HTN:**
  - o Fibrinoid necrosis
  - o Hyperplastic arteriosclerosis
- **Renin dependent HTN:** Renovascular HTN
- **MC cause of paroxysmal HTN:** Phaeochromocytoma

Polycystic kidney

- **Adult PKD is:** Autosomal dominant
- **Chromosome involved in type I adult polycystic kidney disease:** 16
- **Chromosome involved in type II adult polycystic kidney disease:** 4

Polycystic Kidney

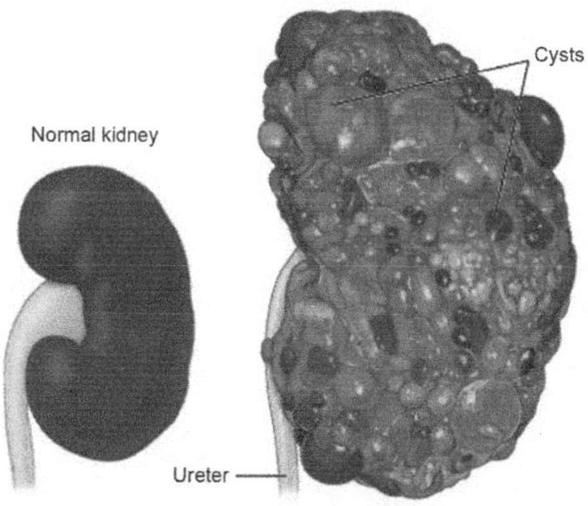

Renal artery stenosis

- **MC cause of RAS in middle age and elderly:** Atheromatous plaque (at the origin of renal artery)
- **In younger female, stenosis is due to:** Fibromuscular dysplasia
- **Most sensitive and specific modality for diagnosing RAS:** Magnetic resonance angiography/MRA

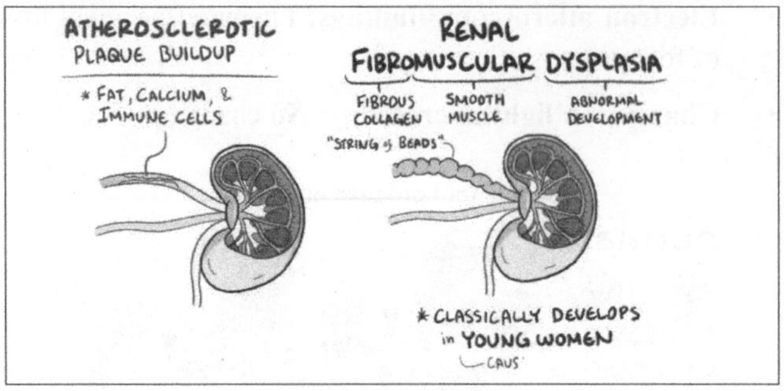

SECTION 1

MEDICINE

Chapter 5

Connective Tissue Disorders

AUTOANTIBODIES AND CONDITIONS

Antibodies/Ab

- **Anti-centromere Ab:** CREST syndrome
- **Anti-Ro and Anti-La:** Sjögren's syndrome
- **Anti-Jo1 Ab:** Polymyositis/Dermatomyositis
- **Anti-histone Ab:** Drug induced lupus
- **Anti-dsDNA and anti-Sm:** SLE

KAWASAKI DISEASE

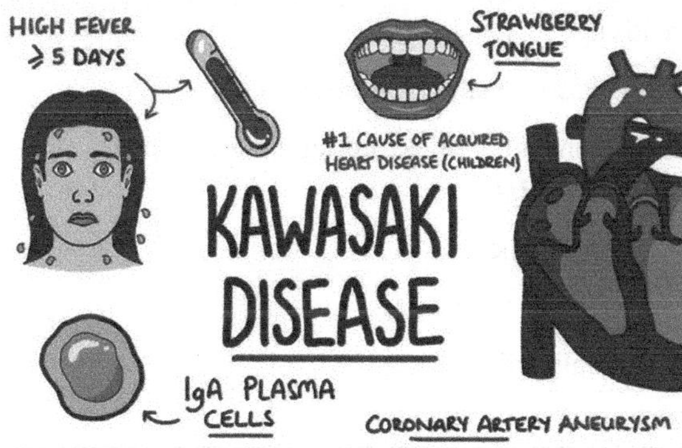

Features

- Affects medium and small vessels
- Vasculitis of arterioles, venules and capillaries in acute
- Coronary (large) arteries involvement in chronic (coronary aneurysm)
- Children affected
- Mucus membrane ulcers, conjunctivitis, lymphadenopathy, fever
- **Also known as:** Mucocutaneous lymph node disease

Standard treatment

- I/V immunoglobulin (immunotherapy)

C	Conjunctivitis (non-exudative)
R	Rash (polymorphous non-vesicular)
E	Edema (or erythema of hands or feet)
A	Adenopathy (cervical, often unilateral)
M	Mucosal involvement (erythema or fissures or crusting)

TEMPORAL/GIANT CELL ARTERITIS

Pathology

- Affects large and medium arteries (temporal and carotids)
- Segmental granulomatous inflammation of vessel

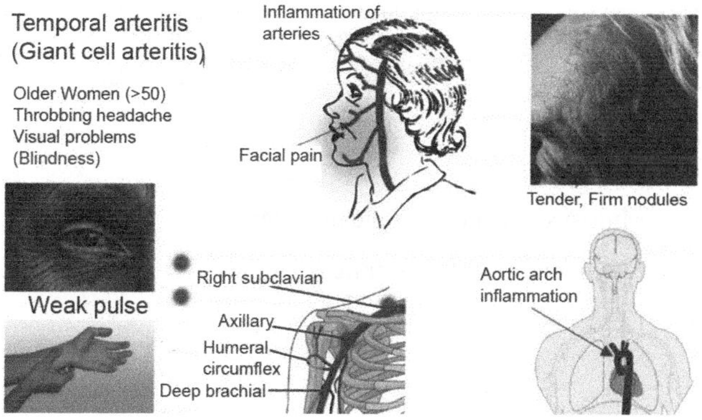

Feature

- **MC** in: Elderly females (70-80 years)
- Severe headache (temporal)
- Jaw claudication
- Polymyalgia rheumatica
- Visual disturbances
- Amaurosis fugax
- AION (inferior altitudinal visual field defect)

Clinical diagnosis should be verified by

- Temporal artery biopsy (**diagnostic**)

Raised

- ESR
- CRP
- Platelet count

Treatment

- Urgent I/V steroids needed

SLE

Epidemiology	Prevalence Age F:M sex-ratio	10-180/100000 Typically 20-40 9:1	
Clinical manifestations		Malar rash Photosensitivity Alopecia, oral ulcers, Lupus nephritis NPSLE	If present, are evocative of SLE versus DIL
Laboratory Manifestations	CRP Cytopenia	Usually normal (except with serositis) Common	
Immunological workup	ANA Anti-ENA Anti-dsDNA Anti-histone Low complement pANCA anti-MPO	> 95% Positive in up to 30% Positive in 60-80% of cases Positive in 60-80% 50-60% Negative	

Pathology

- Multisystem autoimmune disorder
- Normocytic normochromic anemia
- LE cells

Features

- Butterfly rash/malar rash (photosensitivity)
- False positive test for syphilis
- Libman-Sacks endocarditis
- **Musculoskeletal finding:** Non-erosive arthritis
- **Renal manifestations:** Wire loop lesions (diffuse proliferative lupus nephritis)
- **Pulmonary system findings:** Shrinking lung syndrome
- **MC cause of death:** Renal involvement

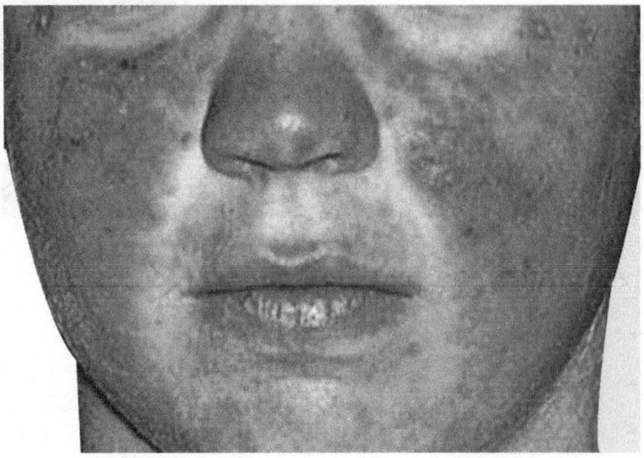

Specific antibody for SLE

- Anti-ds DNA (**very** specific and denotes **poor** prognosis)
- Anti-Sm antibodies are also **highly** specific but lack sensitivity
- ANA is 95% sensitive but **not** specific
- Anti-histone antibodies in drug induced lupus ***(Mnemonic: HIP)***:
  - o **H**ydralazine
  - o **I**NH
  - o **P**rocainamide

HENOCH-SCHÖNLEIN PURPURA

Pathology

- Affects children
- Previous history of Upper respiratory tract infection

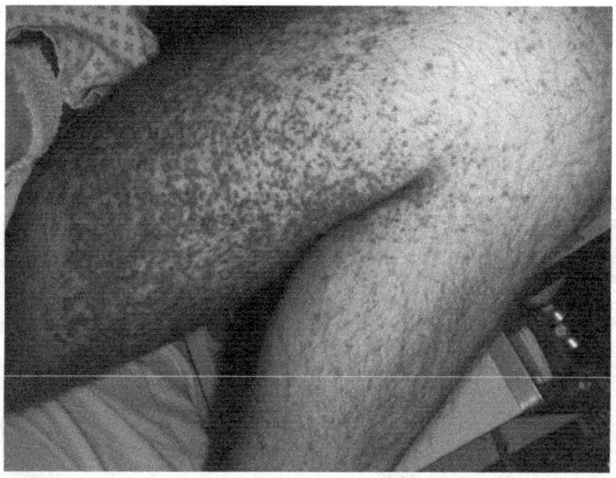

Features

- Arthralgia
- Abdominal pain
- Glomerulonephritis (hematuria)
- **Most common cause of death:** Renal failure

"Classic" Clinical Tetrad

1. Non-thrombocytopenia palpable purpura

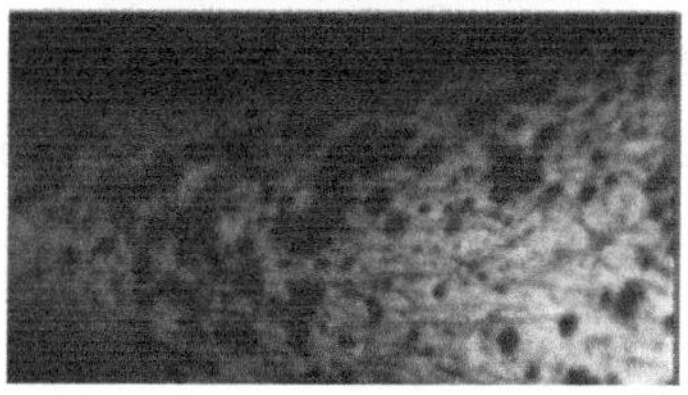

2. Abdominal pain

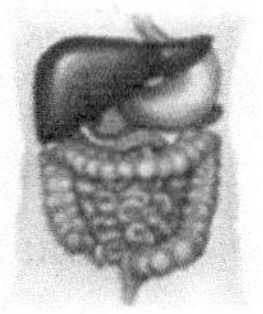

Colicky abdominal pain
Intussusception (ileoileal)
Heme positive stool

3. Hematuria

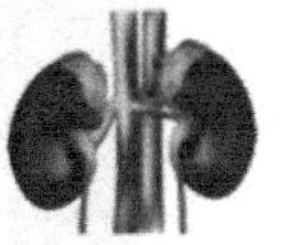

Microscopic hematuria
Proteinuria
Elevated BUN/Cr

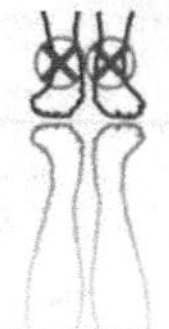

4. Arthritis

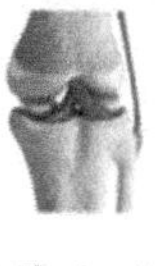

Periarticular disease of **knees** and **ankles**

Lab findings

- **IgA levels:** Elevated IgA levels
- **Normal:**
  - o RBC and platelet count
  - o Peripheral blood film
  - o Serum complements are normal

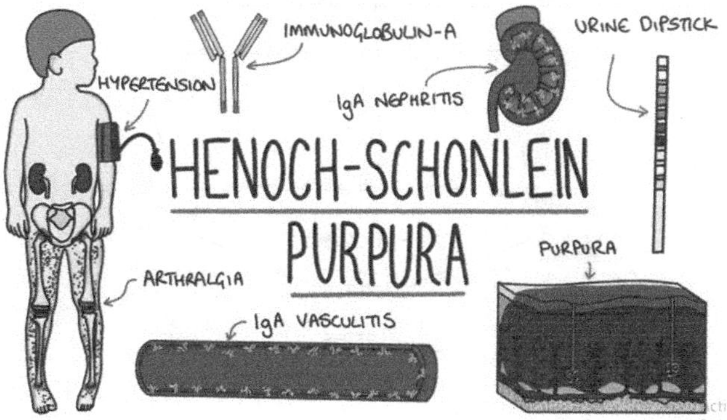

SECTION 1

MEDICINE

Chapter 6

Endocrinology

ENDOCRINE GLANDS

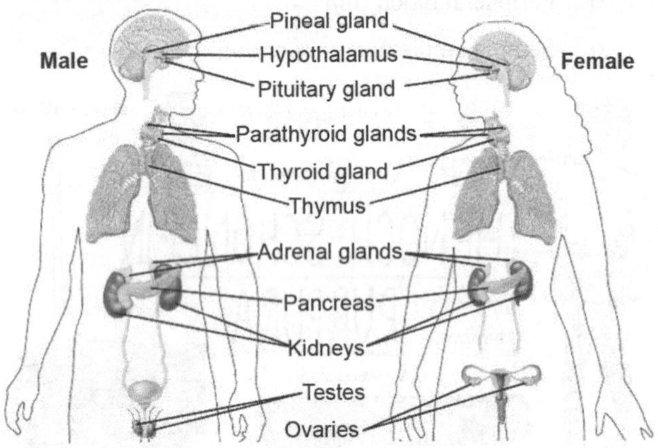

Glands and hormones

- **Pituitary gland:**
  - o **Acidophils:**
    - ♦ Growth hormone
    - ♦ Prolactin
  - o **Basophils:**
    - ♦ Follicle stimulating hormone/FSH
    - ♦ Luteinizing hormone/LH
    - ♦ Adrenocorticotropic hormone/ACTH
    - ♦ Thyroid stimulating hormone/TSH
- **Thyroid gland:**
  - o Thyroxine
  - o Tri-iodothyronine
  - o Calcitonin
- **Parathyroid gland:**
  - o Parathormone
- **Adrenal gland:**
  - o **Cortex:**
    - ♦ **Zona glomerulosa:** Aldosterone (mineralocorticoids)
    - ♦ **Zona fasciculata:** Cortisol (glucocorticoids)
    - ♦ **Zona reticularis:** Sex hormones (adrenocorticoids)
  - o **Medulla:**
    - ♦ **Catecholamines:**
      - – Epinephrine
      - – Norepinephrine
- **Pancreas:**
  - o **Alpha cells:** Glucagon
  - o **Beta cells:** Insulin
  - o **Delta cells:** Somatostatin

HYPOTHYROIDISM/HT

Types

- **Primary HT:** Defect in thyroid gland
- **Secondary HT:** Pituitary gland is at fault

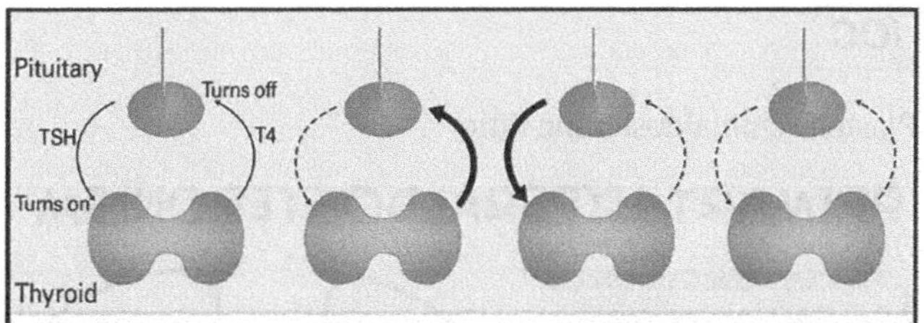

CONDITION:	Normal	Hyperthyroidism	Hypothyroidism Primary	Hypothyroidism Secondary
TSH	Normal	Low	High	Low
T4	Normal	High	Low	Low

Primary hypothyroidism

- **Parameter:**
  - o **T3:** Low
  - o **T4:** Low
  - o **TSH:** High
- **Causes:**
  - o Endemic goiter
  - o Amiodarone therapy
  - o Goitrogens (cabbage)

Secondary hypothyroidism

- **Parameters:**
  - o **T3:** Low
  - o **T4:** Low
  - o **TSH:** Low
- **Causes:**
  - o Sheehan syndrome (postpartum anterior pituitary necrosis)
  - o Empty sella syndrome

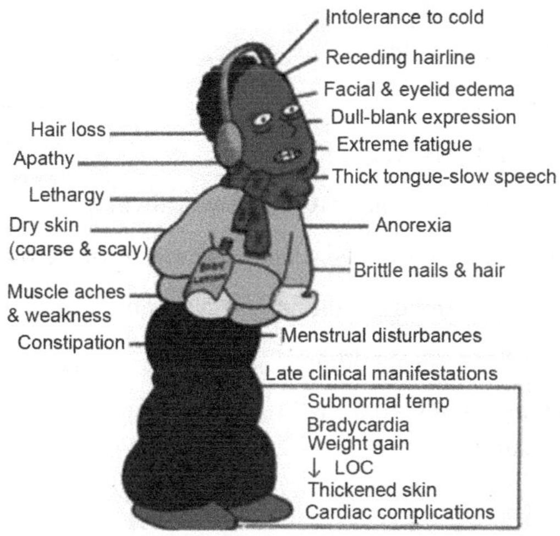

Clinical Features (Mnemonic: ABCDE)

- **A**lopecia
- **B**radycardia
- **B**ody temperature is less (subnormal)
- **C**old intolerance
- **C**onstipation
- **C**ool peripheral extremities
- **C**arpal tunnel syndrome
- **C**avity (serous) effusions
- **D**ry skin
- **D**ifficulty in concentration
- **D**yspnea
- **D**elayed relaxation of deep tendon reflexes (hung-up reflexes)
- **E**dema (peripheral)
- **E**dema (myxedema)

PRIMARY HYPERPARATHYROIDISM

MC cause

- Solitary adenoma (80%)

Features

- Bones (brown tumour)
- Stones (renal calculi)
- Abdominal groans (peptic ulcer) and
- Psychic moans (depression)

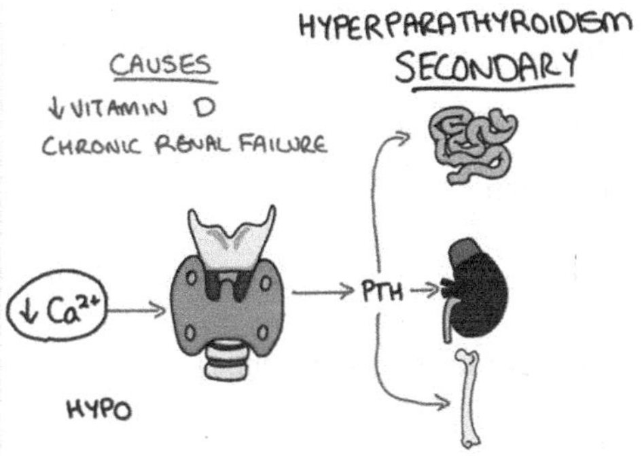

Blood chemistry

- Raised Ca
- Low phosphate
- Normal/increased alkaline phosphatase

Hyperparathyroidism	Calcium	PTH	Vitamin D	Phosphate
Primary	↑	↑→	↑	↓
Secondary	↓→	↑	↓	↑ or ↓
Tertiary	↑	↑↑	↓	↑
Key: ↑Elevated, ↓decreased, →normal				

CONN'S SYNDROME

Basic pathology

- Hyperaldosteronism

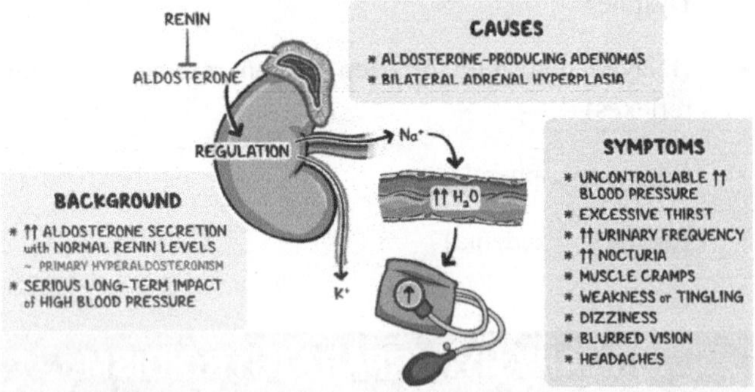

Features

- Due to adrenal adenoma or Ca
- No pedal edema
- Expansion of plasma volume
- Hypertension (diastolic)
- Decreased K^+ (muscle cramps and fatigue)
- Polyuria, polydipsia
- Proximal myopathy

Investigations

- Increased sodium
- Decreased potassium

ECG

- Prominent U waves (due to hypokalemia)

IOC

Plasma renin/aldosterone ratio

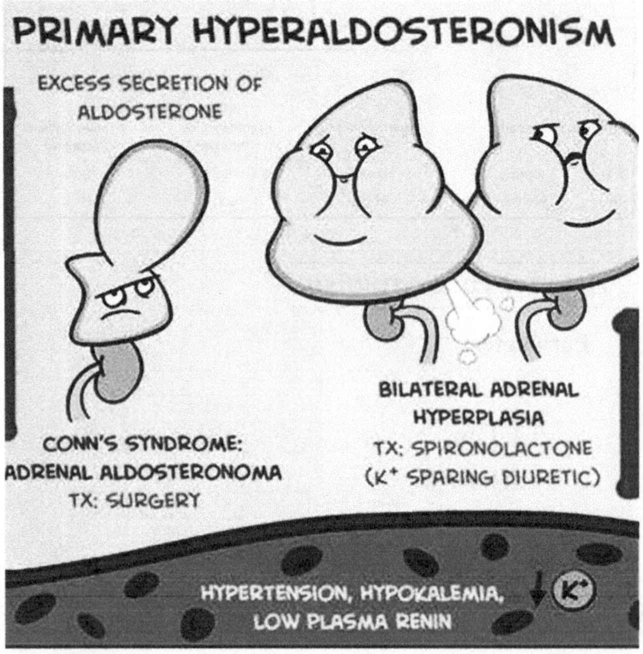

Treatment

- Surgical removal of tumour
- Spironolactone

ADDISON'S DISEASE

Pathology

- Primary adrenocortical insufficiency

Etiopathology

- Decrease in aldosterone, corticosteroids and sex steroids
- **Causes:**
  - o TB (**MC** cause in India)
  - o Autoimmune (**MC** cause worldwide)
  - o Addisonian crisis (sudden stoppage of steroid drugs)
  - o Waterhouse-Friderichsen syndrome
  - o Sheehan syndrome
- **Drug associated with addisonian like features:** Busulfan

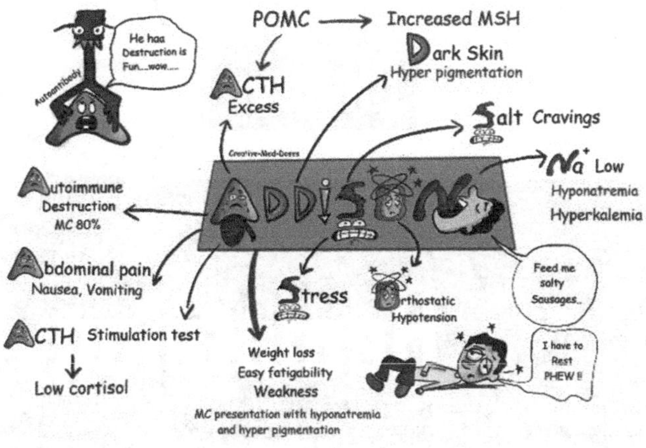

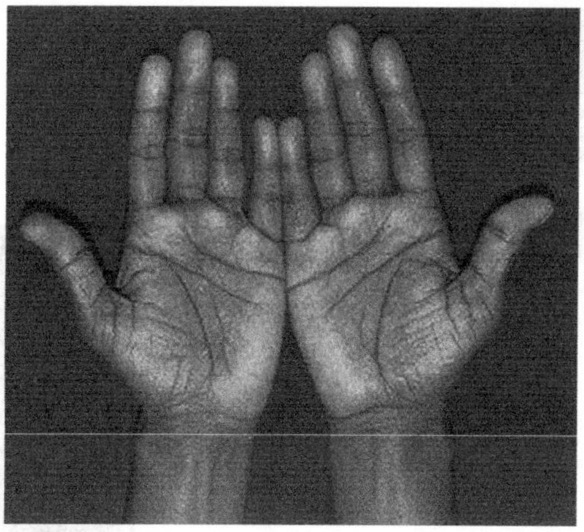

Addison's disease – hyperpigmentation involving the palms of the hand

Clinical features

- **Low:**
  - Sugar (hypoglycemia)
  - Salt (salt wasting because of loss of water and salt)
  - Mean BP
- **High:**
  - Urine output (polyuria >3L/day)
  - Potassium (hyperkalemia and metabolic acidosis)
  - ACTH (hyperpigmentation)

Metabolic effects

- Hyperkalemia
- Hyponatremia
- Increased pigmentation (increase in ACTH, which behaves like melanocyte stimulating hormone) (**EXCEPT** in secondary adrenal insufficiency due to pituitary failure)

Investigation

- Low sodium
- High potassium

ECG

- Tall peaked/tented T waves (because of hyperkalemia)

Definitive investigation

- ACTH stimulation test/cosyntropin test

Management

- **To promote salt and water retention:** Fludrocortisone
- **To reduce hypoglycemic symptoms:** Dexamethasone
- **For Addison disease:** Hydrocortisone
- **For Addisonian crisis:** Fluid resuscitation and hydrocortisone

SECTION 1

MEDICINE

Chapter 7

Hematology

RBC'S ABNORMAL MORPHOLOGY

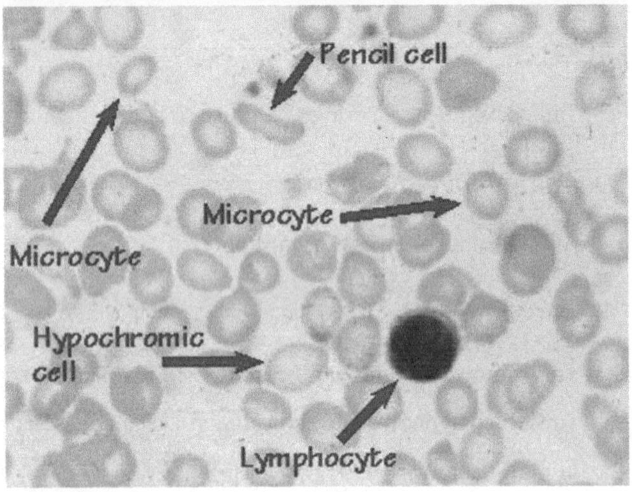

Microcytosis

- Iron deficiency anemia
- Thalassemia
- Anemia of chronic diseases
- Sideroblastic anemia
- Lead poisoning
- Copper deficiency

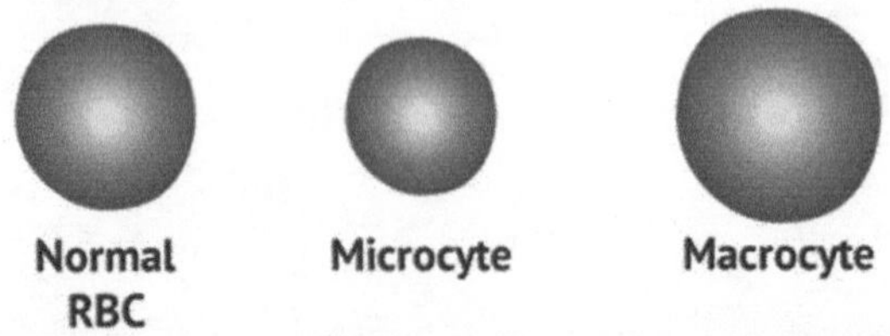

Macrocytosis

- Vitamin B12 deficiency
- Folic acid deficiency

Target cells

- Thalassemia
- Liver disease
- Post-splenectomy

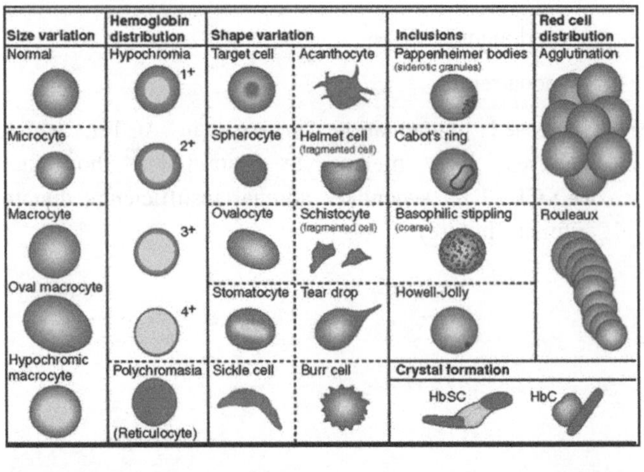

MEGALOBLASTIC ANEMIA

Types

- Vitamin B12 deficiency
- Folate deficiency

Vitamin B12 deficiency

- **Impaired vitamin B12 absorption in gut:**
  - Pancreatic insufficiency
  - Blind-loop syndrome
  - Surgical resection
- **Dietary deficiency:**
  - Pernicious anemia
  - Gastrectomy
  - Strict vegetarian

Folic acid deficiency

- **Increased requirement:**
  - Pregnancy
  - Chronic hemolytic anemia
- **Dietary deficiency:**
  - Drugs
  - Tropical sprue
  - Decreased absorption

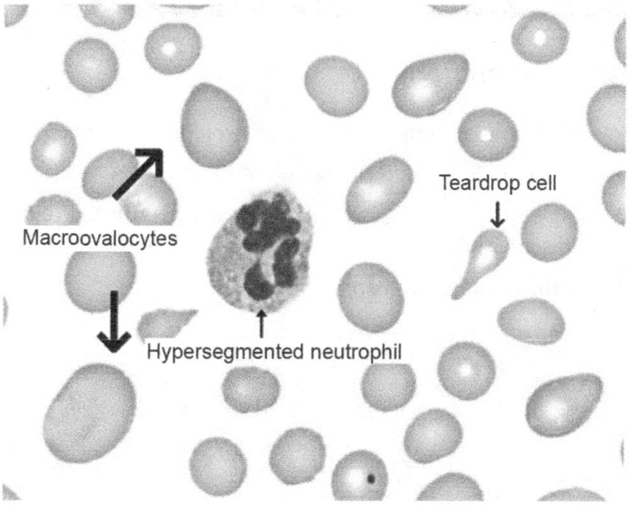

Laboratory features

- Hypersegmented neutrophils
- Increased LDH
- Giant platelets

Management

- **Associated neurological condition:** SACD of spinal cord
- It is **advised** to give vitamin B12 and folic acid concurrently because treatment with folate alone may improve anemia but leads to progression of neurological disease

HEMOLYTIC ANEMIA

Autoimmune hemolytic anemia/AIHA

- Cold agglutinin type
- Warm antibody type

Cold agglutinin type AIHA

- Acute anemia triggered by cold (<37 degree C)
- IgM mediated
- Seen in Mycoplasma infection, infectious mononucleosis, syphilis, trypanosomiasis
- Cold activated IgM and complement C3d coat RBCs and trigger hemolysis
- Hemolysis is intravascular

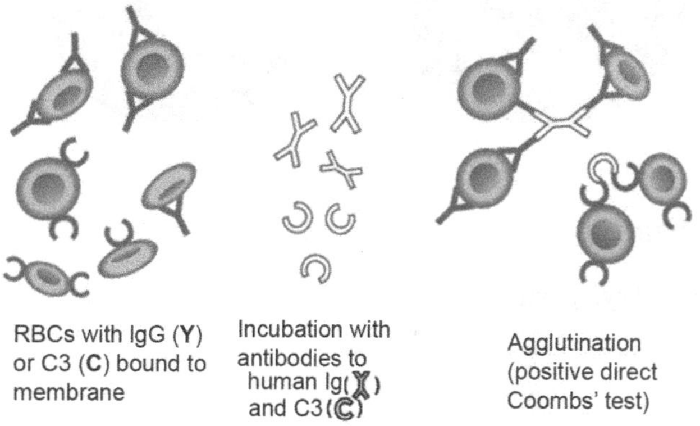

Warm antibody type

- Active at 37 degree C
- IgG mediated
- Chronic anemia seen in drugs (quinidine, penicillamine), SLE
- Autoantibody IgG attack RBCs
- Hemolysis is extravascular

SICKLE CELL ANEMIA

Pathology

- Replacement of glutamate by valine at 6 beta chain of HbA (point mutation)

- Autosomal recessive
- HbS heterozygotes are protected from malaria (falciparum)
- Thrombotic crisis/painful crisis/vaso-occlusive crisis is precipitated by:
  - o Infection
  - o Dehydration
  - o Deoxygenation
  - o Acidosis
  - o Leads to polymerization of HbS, sickling of RBCs and hemolysis

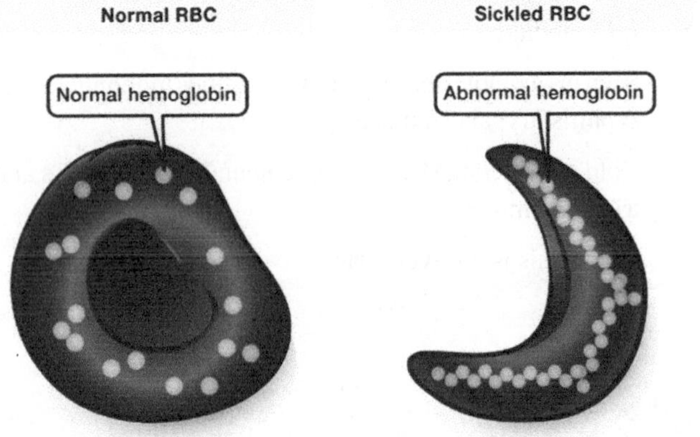

Features

- Asymptomatic
- **Sickle cell crisis:**
  - o Priapism
  - o Bone pain
  - o Chest pain
- **Features of hemolysis:**
  - o Pallor
  - o Jaundice
  - o Splenomegaly in early period

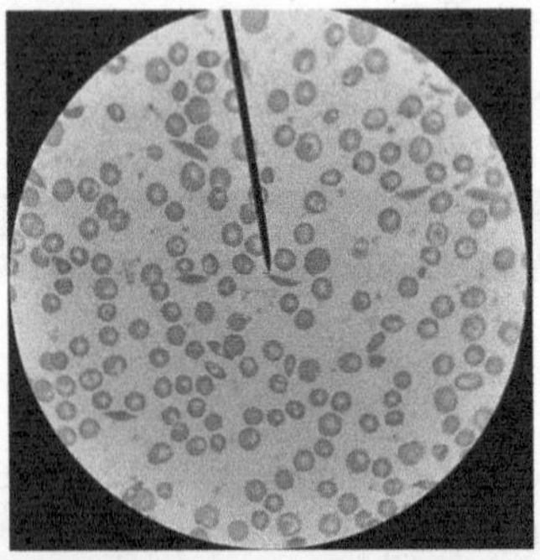

Lab findings

- Features of hemolysis
- **PBF shows:**
  - o Target cells
  - o Sickle cells
- **X-ray:**
  - o Cod-fish mouth vertebrae/H-shaped vertebrae
  - o AVN/bone infarction
  - o Periosteal reaction (bone within bone appearance)

Complications

- Salmonella osteomyelitis
- Aplastic crisis (parvovirus B19)
- Autosplenectomy
- Renal papillary necrosis (FSGN)
- Normocytic normochromic anemia

HEREDITARY SPHEROCYTOSIS

Basic pathology

- Defect in ankyrin (50%); binds protein 3 and spectrin
- Genetic defect in RBC membrane
- RBC assumes a spherical shape and hemolysed (extra-vascular hemolysis)
- **Inherited as:** Autosomal dominant

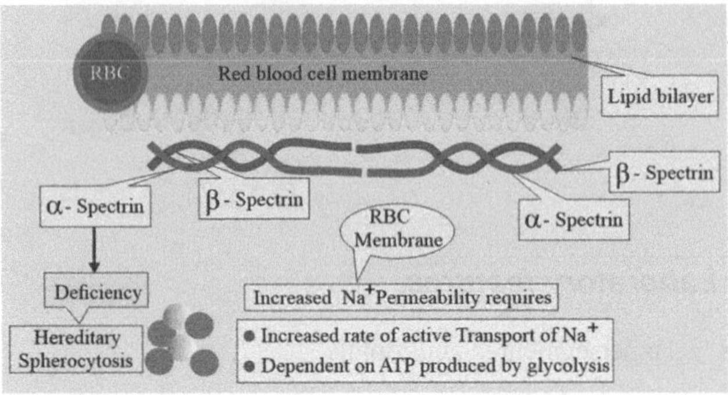

Clinical features

- Massive splenomegaly
- Anemia
- Jaundice
- Gallstones

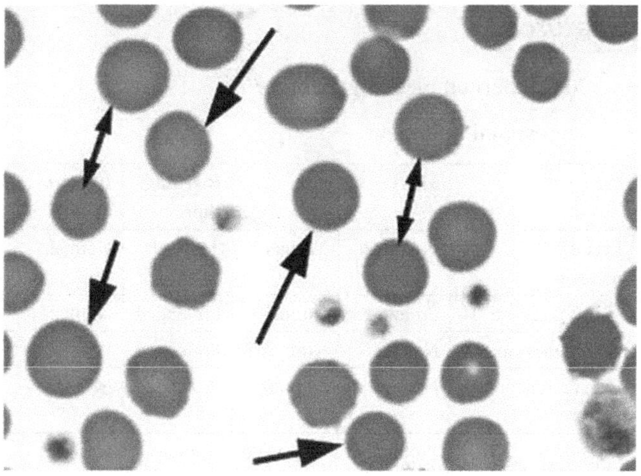

Laboratory features

- Low MCV
- Raised MCHC and osmotic fragility

Assessed by

- Raised osmotic fragility of the RBC

Management

- Splenectomy
- Howell Jolly bodies are seen after spleen removal

POLYCYTHEMIA RUBRA VERA

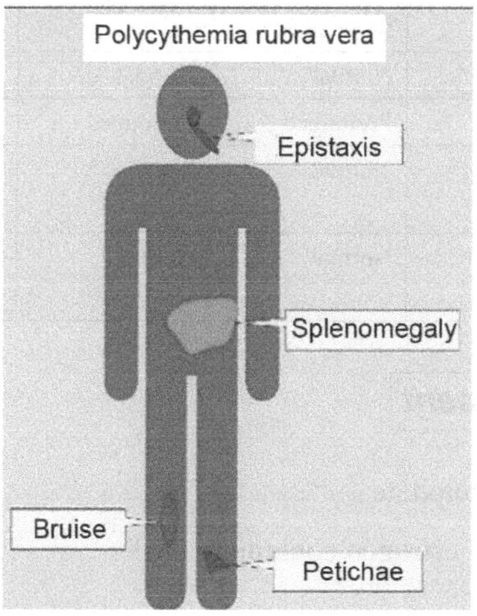

Features

- Primary type of polycythemia
- Bone marrow disorder
- Autonomous production of erythroid cells
- Independent of erythropoietin
- Low serum erythropoietin level
- JAK2V617F mutation

Clinical features

- Pruritis especially after warm bath (histamine)
- Splenomegaly
- Thrombosis

Low

- Low erythropoietin levels
- Low ESR

Raised

- LAP score
- TLC
- Platelets
- Red cell mass
- Hematocrit
- Viscosity
- Systolic BP
- Spleen size
- Increased risk of thrombosis and bleeding
- Bleeding from GIT and epistaxis

Management

- Serial phlebotomy

HEMOPHILIA

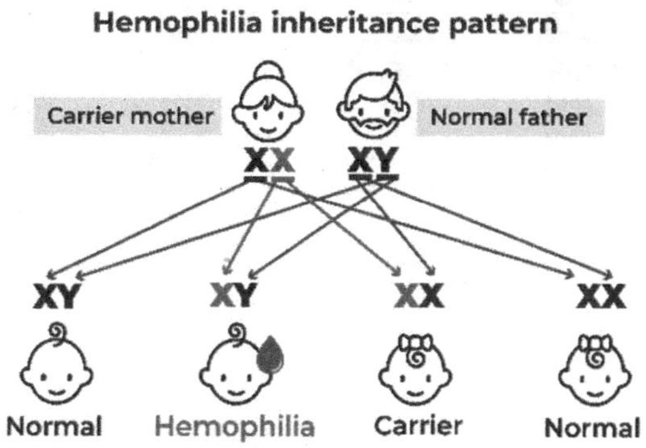

Features

- **Factor VIII deficiency/F8 gene mutation:** Hemophilia A
- **Factor IX deficiency/F9 gene mutation:** Hemophilia B/Christmas disease
- X-linked recessive (so patient is always a male)
- Recurrent bleeding into joints (hemarthroses) and muscles

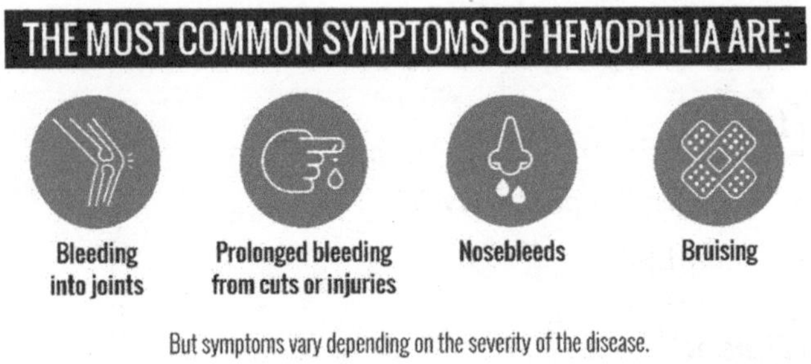

Management

- Replacement of deficient factors
- Antifibrinolytic agents (EACA, tranexamic acid)

VON WILLEBRAND DISEASE

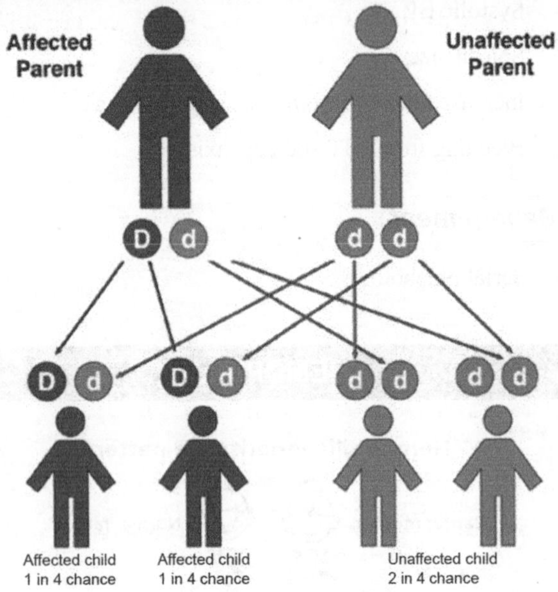

Features

- **MC** inherited bleeding disorder
- Autosomal dominant

Disorder	aPTT	PT	Bleeding time	Platelet count
Factor VIII, IX deficiency	Prolonged	Normal	Normal	Normal
Von Willebrand	Prolonged	Normal	Prolonged	Normal
Thrombocytopenia	Normal	Normal	Prolonged	Low
Platelet function defect	Normal	Normal	Prolonged	Normal
Vitamin K deficiency	Prolonged	Prolonged	Normal	Normal
DIC	Prolonged	Prolonged	Prolonged	Low

Lab findings

- Prolonged bleeding time
- aPTT is prolonged
- Normal PT
- All values normal **except** BT and aPTT

	Hemophilia A	Hemophilia B	Von Willebrand Disease
Inheritance	X-linked	X-linked	Autosomal dominant
Factor deficiency	VIII	IX	VWF
Bleeding site(s)	Muscle joint Surgical	Muscle joint	Mucous skin
Prothrombin time	Normal	Normal	Normal
Activated PTT	Prolonged	Prolonged	Prolonged
Bleeding time	Normal	Normal	Prolonged or Normal
Platelet aggregation	Normal	Normal	Normal

Management

- Cryoprecipitate
- DDAVP/estrogen containing OCPs

THROMBOTIC THROMBOCYTOPENIC PURPURA

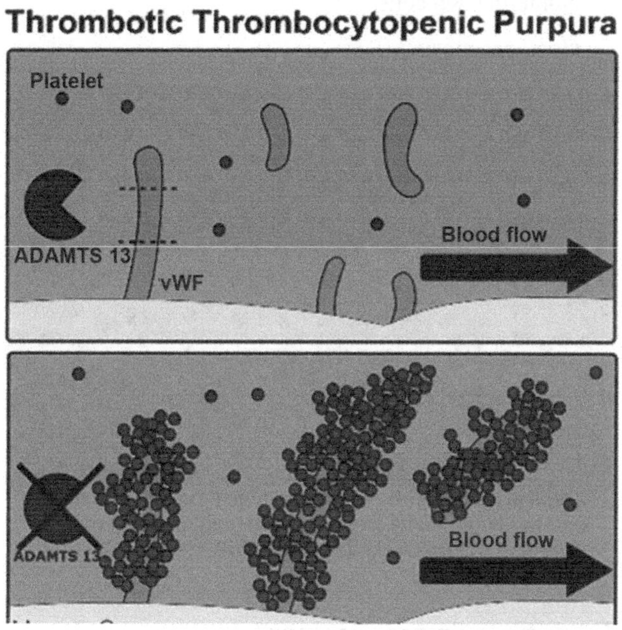

Features

- Affects young adults
- **Low:**
  - o RBC
  - o Platelet count
- Hemolysis
- **Renal:**
  - o Proteinuria
  - o Acute renal failure
- **Treat by:**
  - o Plasmapheresis
  - o Exchange transfusion
  - o NSAIDs
- Deficiency of vWf metalloprotease (ADAMTS13 beta)
- Hyaline microthrombi throughout body
- Thrombus is platelet rich
- Purpura
- Rapid onset
- Fulminant course
- Death due to intracerebral hemorrhage

Laboratory features

- Level of platelet, IgG and C normal
- Gingival biopsy positive

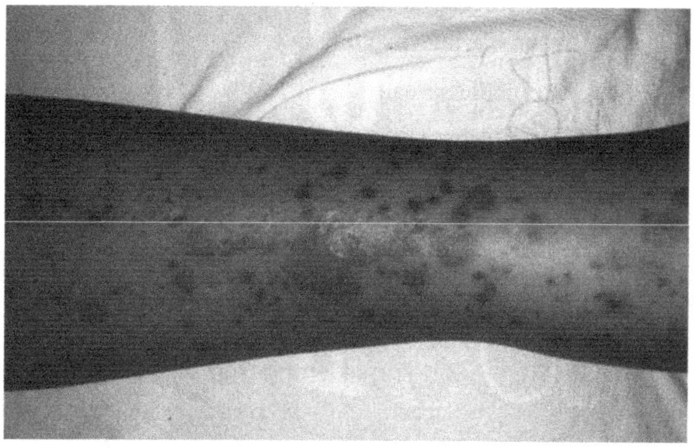

Pentad of TTP

- Fever
- Microangiopathic hemolytic anemia (MAHA)
- Thrombocytopenia
- Neurological symptoms
- Renal failure

HODGKIN'S LYMPHOMA

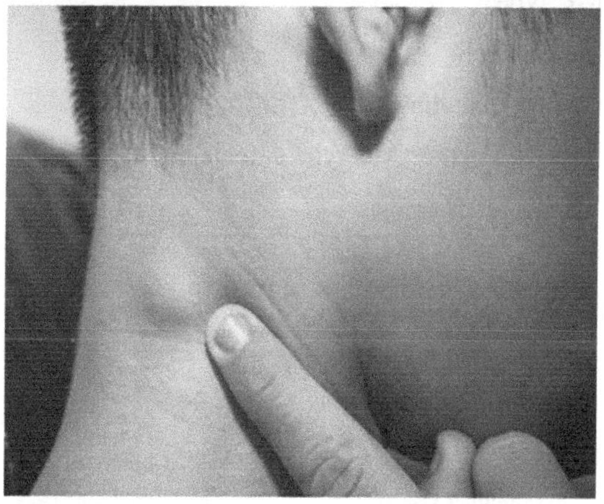

Features

- Bimodal distribution (20's and 50's)
- Cervical lymphadenopathy (localized, single group)
- Centrifugal spread
- **Constitutional features (B symptoms):**

- o Pel-Ebstein fever
- o Night sweats
- o Loss of weight
- Patients usually present in stage IIA
- Ann Arbor staging (**prognostic**)
- Less extranodal spread
- **Causative agent:** EBV
- **Malignant cell is:** Reed sternberg cell (B-cell origin, owl eye appearance)
- **RS cells are positive for:** CD 15, CD 30, **except** Lymphocytic predominant

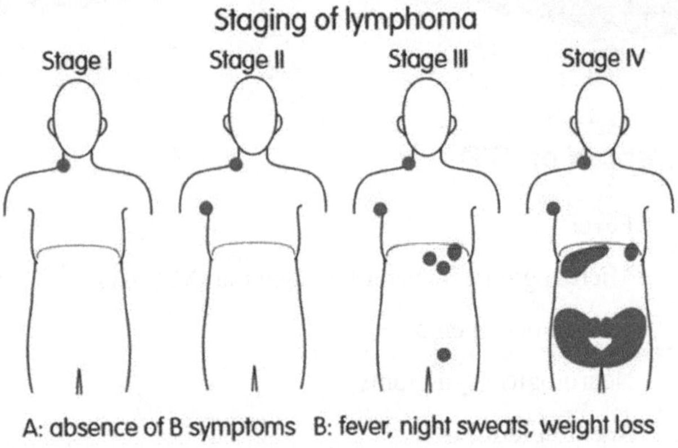

Nodular sclerosis

- **MC** type
- Lacunar cells
- Collagen banding
- Affects females (**MC** type in females)
- Very good prognosis

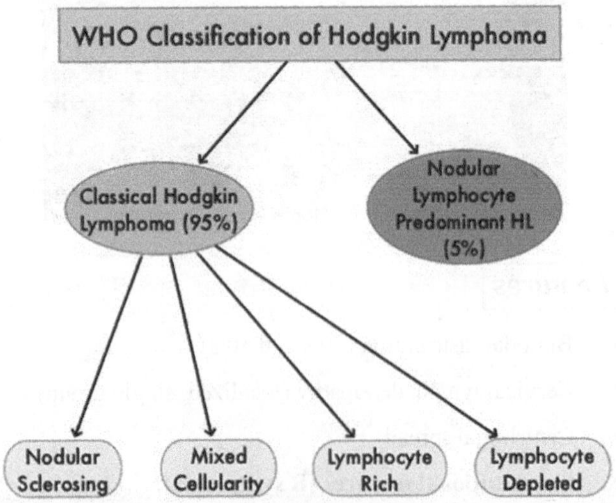

Mixed cellularity type

- **MC** type in India
- Numerous RS cells
- Good prognosis

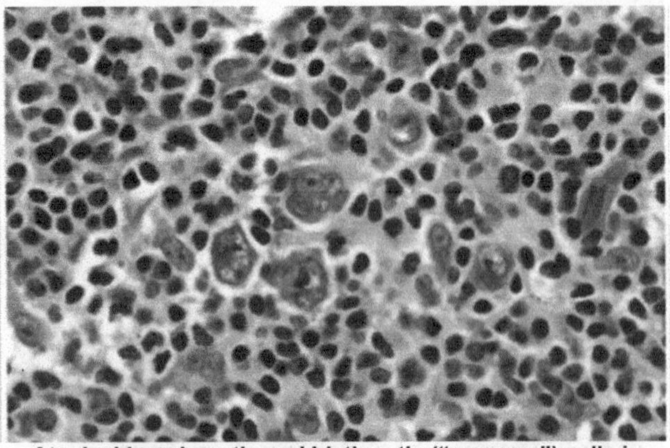

Atypical lymphocytic and histiocytic ("popcorn") cells in nodular lymphocyte-predominant Hodgkin lymphoma. Courtesy of Francisco Vega. MD, PHD

Lymphocytic predominant

- **Best** prognosis
- Popcorn cells (polypoidal)
- Histogenitically different subtype
- Lymphocytic predominant (negative for CD15, CD30) is positive for:
  - o CD20
  - o CD45

Regimes used (Stage IIB-IV)

- **ABVD:**
  - o Adriamycin
  - o Bleomycin
  - o Vincristine
  - o Dacarbazine
- **MOPP:**
  - o Mechlorethamine
  - o Vincristine
  - o Procarbazine
  - o Prednisone

Hodgkin Lymphoma	Non-Hodgkin Lymphoma
Involves Reed-Sternberg cells	No Reed-Sternberg cells
Affects only the lymphatic system (rarely extranodal)	Commonly spreads outside the lymphatic system (extranodal involvement of the gut, bone marrow, spine and liver)
Contagious spread among lymph nodes	No contagious spread among lymph nodes
Rare hepatosplenomegaly and no leukemic phase	Has a leukemic phase characterized by hepatosplenomegaly and anemia
Has a bimodal age distribution	Mostly seen in older adults
Better prognosis (more curable)	Worse prognosis (less curable)
Treated using more localized methods	Treated using more generalized methods

HAIRY CELL LEUKEMIA/HCL

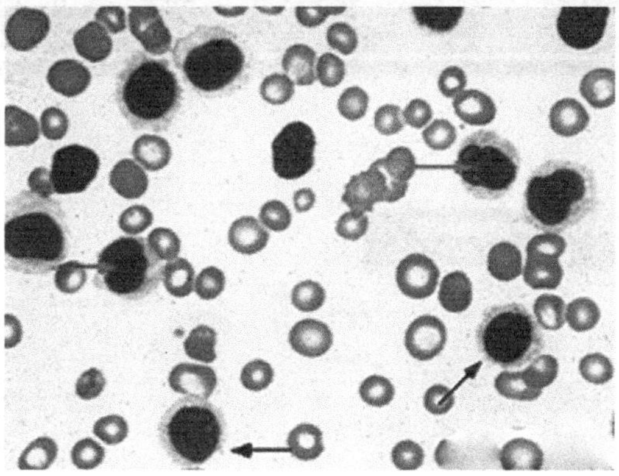

Features

- Middle age (55 years)
- Mature B-cells
- Massive splenomegaly
- Pancytopenia
- Leukemic cells with hairy cytoplasmic projections
- Dry bone marrow tap
- TRAP positive hairy cells
- **Cell of origin:** Rare malignant proliferation of B cells
- **DOC**: Cladribine

SECTION 1
MEDICINE

Chapter 8

Gastrointestinal Tract

ANATOMY OF GIT

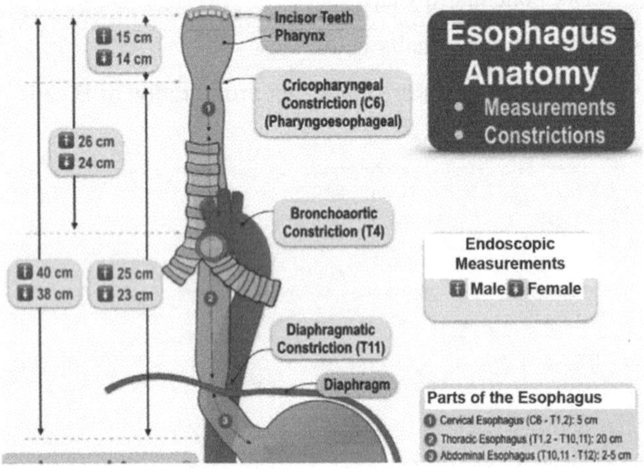

Basics

- **Esophagus:**
  - o 25 cm long
  - o Extends from cricopharyngeal junction to cardia of the stomach
  - o Lined by stratified squamous non-keratinized epithelium
- **Stomach:**
  - o **Most** dilated part of GIT
  - o **Parts:**
    - ♦ Lesser curvature
    - ♦ Greater curvature

PART OF THE STOMACH (External)

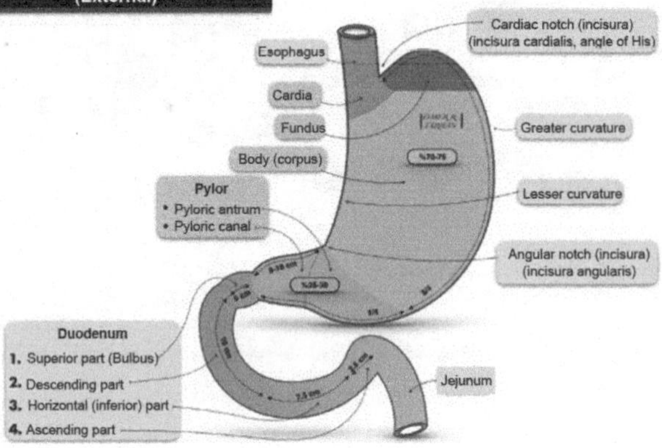

- ♦ Fundus
- ♦ Body
- ♦ Antrum
- ♦ Pylorus

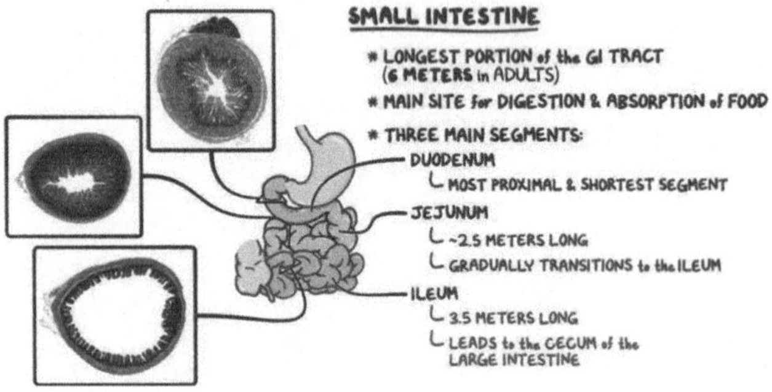

- **Small intestine:**
  - o 6 m long

- o **Duodenum:** Short, fixed and curved portion, devoid of mesentery
- o **Long mobile part attached to posterior abdominal wall by mesentery:**
  - ♦ **Proximal 40%:** Jejunum
  - ♦ **Distal 60%:** Ileum

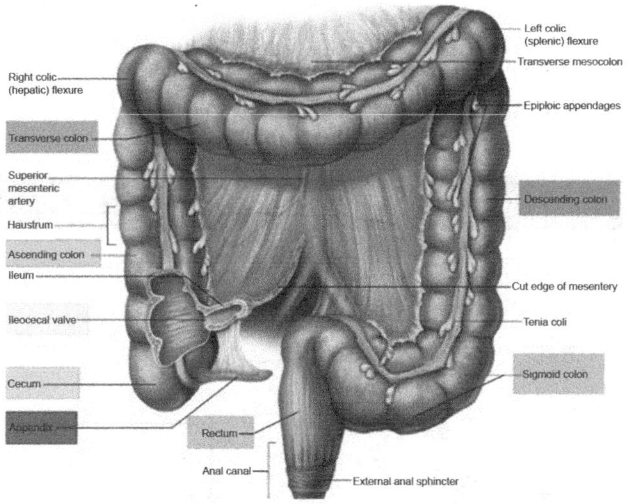

- **Large intestine:**
  - o 1.5 meters long
  - o **Parts:**
    - ♦ Caecum
    - ♦ Colon (ascending colon is the shortest part of colon)
    - ♦ Rectum
    - ♦ Anal canal

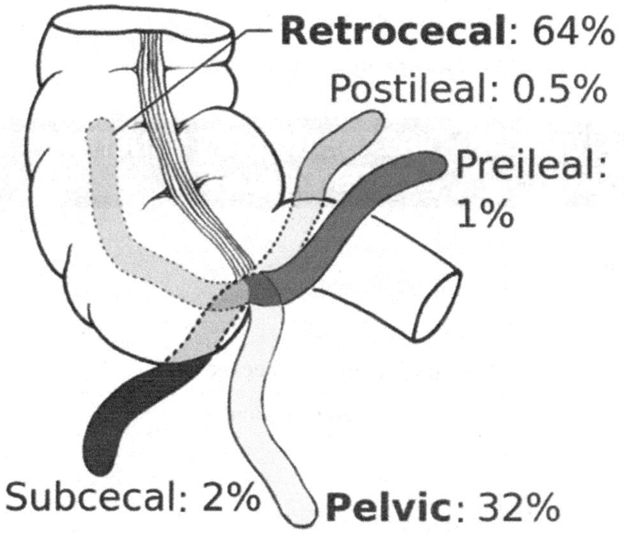

- **Vermiform appendix:**
  - o 7.5 – 10 cm long
  - o **MC** position of tip is retrocaecal
  - o Supplied by appendicular artery, branch of lower division of Ileocolic artery, which originates from superior mesenteric artery
- **Rectum:**
  - o 15 cm in length
  - o **3 lateral curvatures:**
    - ♦ **Upper and lower:** Convex to right
    - ♦ **Middle:** Convex to left
- **Anal canal:**
  - o 3.8 cm long
  - o Pectinate/dentate line is at the junction of the upper 2/3rd and lower 1/3rd of anal canal

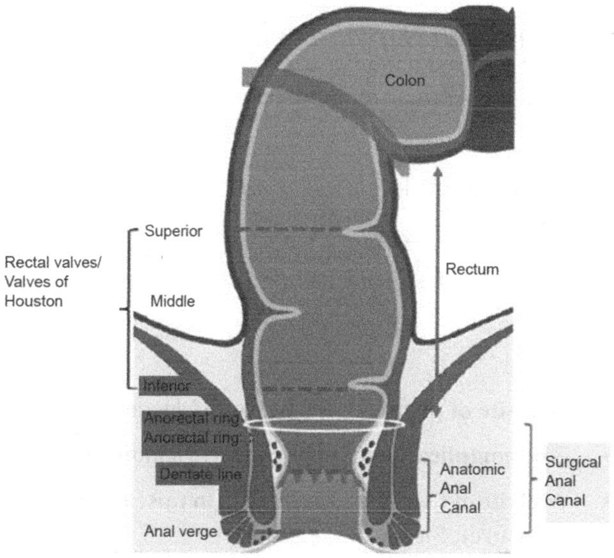

H. PYLORI

Diseases caused

- Gastritis
- Gastric Ca
- Peptic ulcer disease
- Gastric lymphoma

Test for documenting eradication

- **C^{13}/C^{14} Urea breath test:**
  - o Non-invasive

- o Simple
- o Useful for follow-up

Test for epidemiology

- Serology (**not** used for follow-up)

Tests for H. pylori

- **Non-invasive:**
  - o Urea breath test
  - o Serology
  - o Stool antigen test
- **Invasive:**
  - o Rapid urease
  - o Culture
  - o Histology

Treatment of H. pylori

- **Quadruple therapy:** (*Mnemonic:* **TOMB**)
  - o **T**etracycline
  - o **O**meprazole
  - o **M**etronidazole
  - o **B**ismuth subsalicylate

Ulcers

- **MC site of peptic ulcer:** 1st part of duodenum
- **MC complication of peptic ulcer:** Hemorrhage
- **MC site of Cushing's ulcer (seen in raised intracranial pressure):** Stomach
- **Curling's ulcer:** Stress ulcer after burns

DUODENAL ULCER

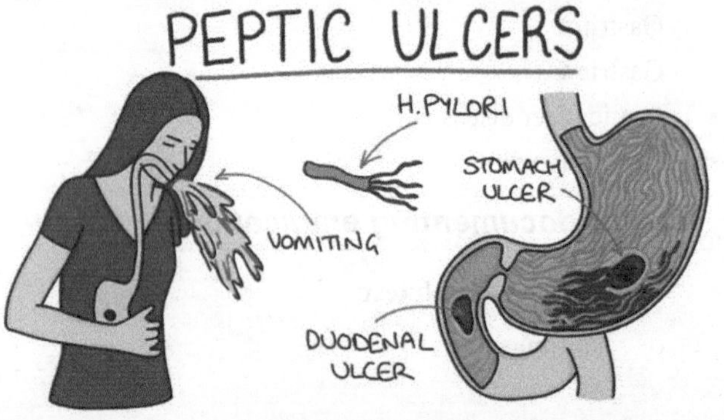

Features

- Blood group O
- Caused by H. pylori
- More common than gastric ulcer
- Pain 2-4 hours after eating/night pain/empty stomach
- Pain relieved by eating
- Normal gastrin levels
- **MC** in: 1st portion of duodenum

WHIPPLE'S DISEASE

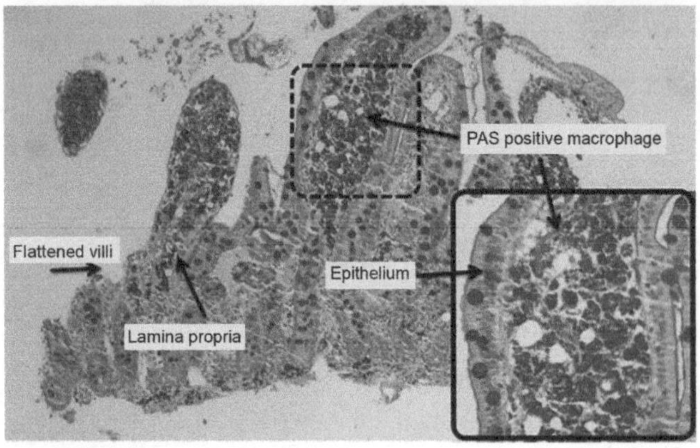

Features

- Common in older men
- Arthralgia, neurologic and cardiac symptoms
- **Specific test:** Biopsy (PAS positive foamy macrophages in lamina propria of intestine)
- **Caused by:** Tropheryma whipplei
- Management by Co-trimoxazole/ceftriaxone

COELIAC DISEASE/GLUTEN SENSITIVE ENTEROPATHY

Features

- HLA-DQ2
- Manifest within 1st year/3rd decade
- Sensitivity to protein gluten, found in:
  - o Wheat
  - o Barley
  - o Rye

- Associated with dermatitis herpetiformis
- **Antibodies:**
  - o IgA anti endomysial
  - o Anti-tissue transglutaminase/tTGA (for screen-ing)
  - o Anti-gliadin
- **Diagnosed by:**
  - o Immunology
  - o Jejunal biopsy

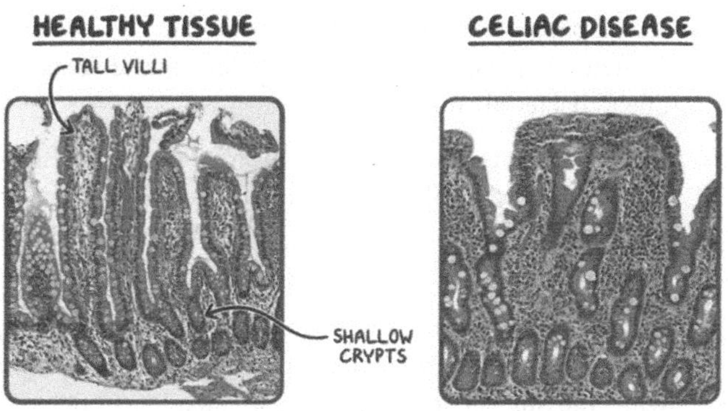

- **Findings on jejunal biopsy:**
  - o Total Villous atrophy (duodenal and jejunal villi)
  - o Crypt hyperplasia BUT thickness of mucosa unaltered
- Gluten free diet is **recommended**

CROHN'S DISEASE

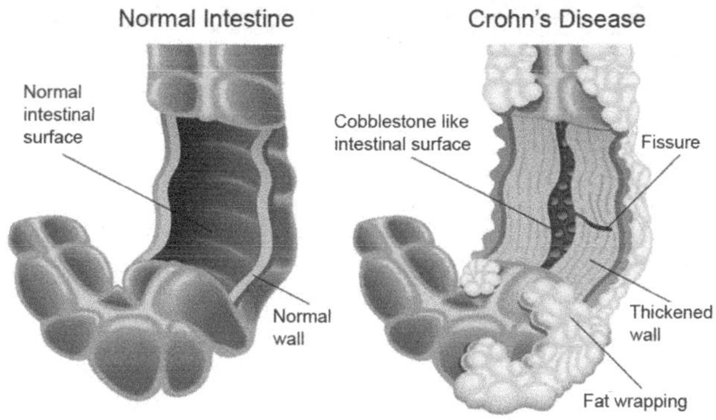

Features

- Skip lesions
- Creeping fat
- Anti saccharomyces cerevisiae antibodies/ASCA
- Usually discontinuous involvement of bowel (skip areas)
- Transmural disease
- Granulomas are sometimes seen
- May affects small and large bowel
- Mass felt in right lower quadrant
- Constant pain

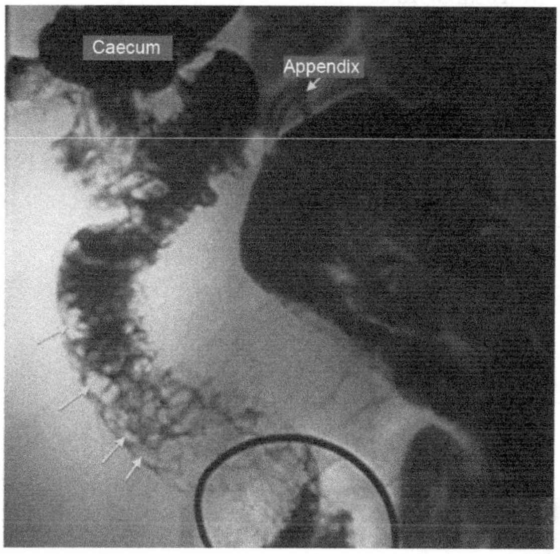

Radiography

- Narrowing of bowel lumen

Barium enema

- Skip lesions
- Rose thorn appearance
- String sign
- Cobblestone

ULCERATIVE COLITIS

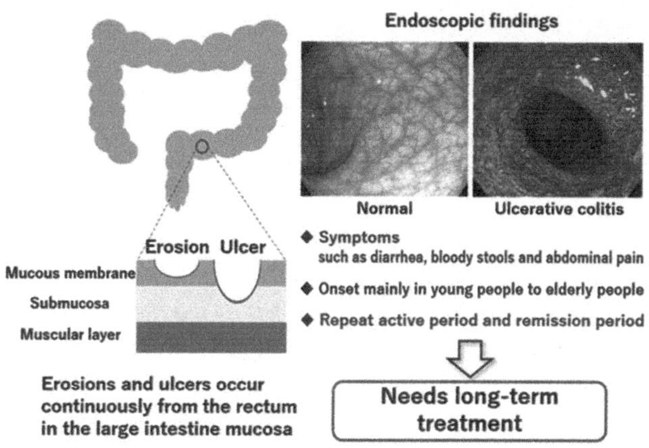

Features

- Toxic megacolon
- Pseudopolyps
- Involvement of bowel continuous from rectum
- Mucosal disease
- Affects colon only
- Usually, bloody stool
- Crampy lower abdominal pain

Radiography

- Loss of haustrations
- Shortening of bowel

Barium enema

- Loss of haustrations (pipe stem colon)
- Pseudopolyps
- Shortening of bowel

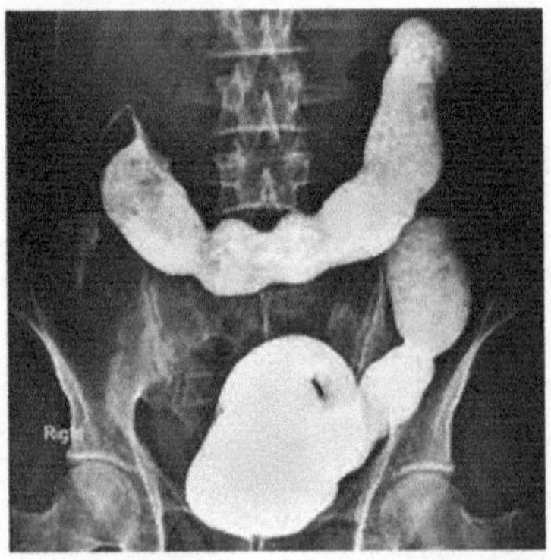

ENTERIC FEVER

Features

- **Incubation period:** 1-3 weeks
- **Classic** signs of enteric fever include malaise, headache, stepladder rise of fever, abdominal cramps, nausea, vomiting, delirium, constipation, hepatosplenomegaly and relative bradycardia
- Rose **spots** appear at the end of 1st week over the trunk – pink papule 2-3 mm in diameter that fades on pressure – often <5 spots, disappears in 3-5 days – rose spots are due to bacterial emboli
- Constipation is likely due to obstruction at the ileo-cecal valve by swollen Peyer's patches, it may last for the entire duration of illness or '**pea**-soup' diarrhoea in between
- In the 3rd week patient is toxic, tachypnea, meningism, psychosis, 'muttering delirium' or 'coma vigil' with picking at bed clothes or imaginary objects, polyneuropathy, cerebellar signs, fits, coma

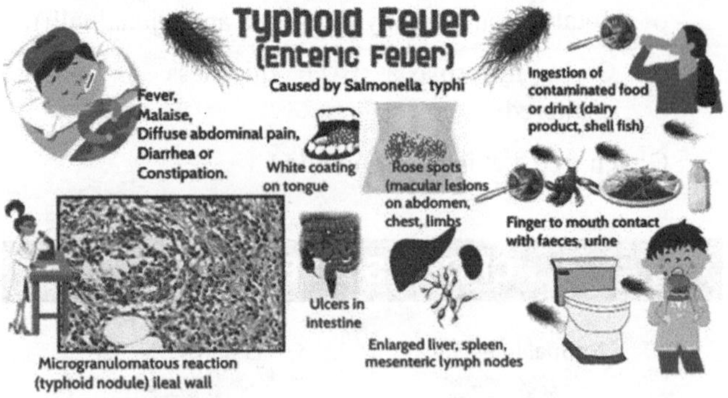

SECTION 1
MEDICINE

Chapter 9

Hepatology

ANATOMY OF LIVER

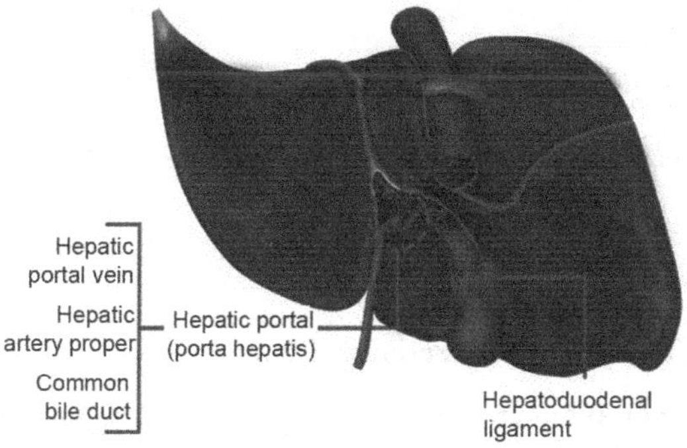

Basics

- **Weight:** 1500 grams
- **Blood flow:** 1500 ml/minute
- **Porta hepatis:**
  - o Portal vein
  - o Hepatic duct (right and left duct)
  - o Hepatic artery (right and left branches)
- **Lobes:**
  - o **Anatomical:** 4
    - ♦ Right
    - ♦ Left
    - ♦ Caudate
    - ♦ Quadrate
  - o **Surgical:** 2 (by a plane connecting gallbladder and Inferior vena cava)
    - ♦ Right
    - ♦ Left
  - o **Couinaud's segments:** 8
    - ♦ Demarcated by the vascular supply and biliary drainage

HEPATITIS

Hepatitis

- **Spreading by feco-oral route:**
  - o HAV
  - o HEV
- **MC cause of sporadic hepatitis in adults:** HEV
- **Worst prognosis in pregnancy:** HEV
- **Most prone to chronicity:** HCV

Interpretation of Hepatitis B serological markers				
HBsAg	**Anti-HBc**	**IgM anti-HBc**	**Anti-HBs**	**Interpretation**
Negative	Negative		Negative	No HBV infection, susceptible
Negative	Negative		≥ 10 IU/L	Immune, due to HBV vaccination
Negative	Positive		≥ 10 IU/L	Past/resolved infection
Negative	Positive		<10 IU/L	Isolated anti-HBc*, probably past infection
Positive**	Negative			Probably false-positive HBsAg or early infection^
Positive**	Positive	++		Acute infection
Positive**	Positive	+/–		Chronic infection***

Markers of HBV

- **First viral marker to appear after HBV infection:** HBsAg
- Indicator of intrahepatic viral replication/presence of which marker indicates **high** infectivity:
  - o HBeAg
  - o HBV DNA
- **Recent infection of HBV is indicated by:** IgM anti-HBcAg
- HBsAg appears **first** (declines by 3-6 months)
- HBeAg, HBV-DNA and DNA polymerase are markers of **active** viral replication
- **Persistence of HBeAg:** Continued viral replication and infectivity and progression to chronicity
- **IgM anti-HBc: First** antibody to appear followed by anti-Hbe
- **Anti-HBe:** Suggests recovery (good prognosis)
- **IgG anti-HBc:** Slowly replaces the IgM over months

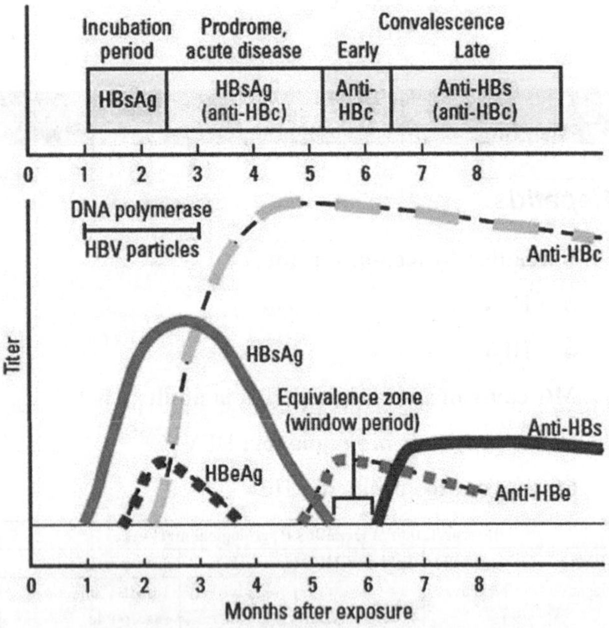

WILSON'S DISEASE

Pathology

- **AR** inheritance
- Genetic defect on chromosome 13
- Neuropsychiatric disorder
- Sunflower cataract

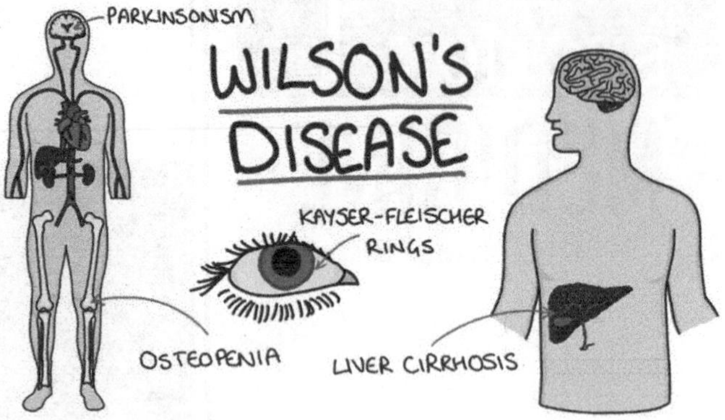

Features

- Hepatic dysfunction
- Eye changes (KF rings in Descemet's membrane of cornea)
- Neurologic manifestations (**NO** sensory changes)

Investigations

- **Serum ceruloplasmin:** Low
- **Total serum copper:** Low
- **Free copper:** High
- **Urine copper excretion:** >1.6 mmol/day
- **Liver biopsy:** Copper concentration >250 microgram/gm of dry tissue
- **KF rings:** Present in all patients

Treatment

- **Drug used as alternative to zinc:** Trientine (**2nd** DOC)
- **Drug of choice/DOC for maintenance therapy:** Zinc acetate/gluconate (**1st** DOC)

IDIOPATHIC HEMOCHROMATOSIS

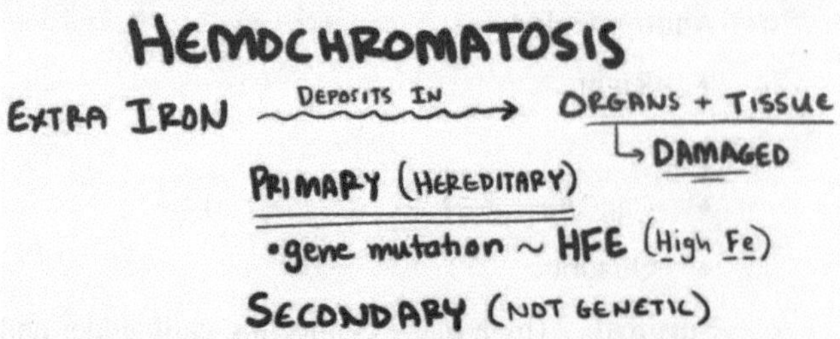

Pathology

- AR inheritance
- Abnormal gene on HLA A6 on short arm of chromosome 6

Associated with

- DM
- Arthropathy (MCP joints)
- Cardiac involvement (Congestive heart failure)

Investigation

- **Serum iron:** High (180-300 microgram/dL)
- **TIBC:** High (250-370 microg/dL)
- **Serum ferritin:** High (600-900 microgram/L)
- **Transferrin saturation:** High (50-100%)
- **Liver biopsy:** >1000 microgram/100 mg of dry weight
- Hepatocellular carcinoma may develop despite management

Treatment

- Venesection
- Phlebotomy (treatment of **choice**)
  - o Weekly phlebotomy of 500 ml of blood for 2-3 years to achieve a Hb of 11 and serum ferritin of 10
- Desferrioxamine (chelating agent)

SECTION 1
MEDICINE

Chapter 10
Cardiovascular System

ARTERIAL SUPPLY OF HEART

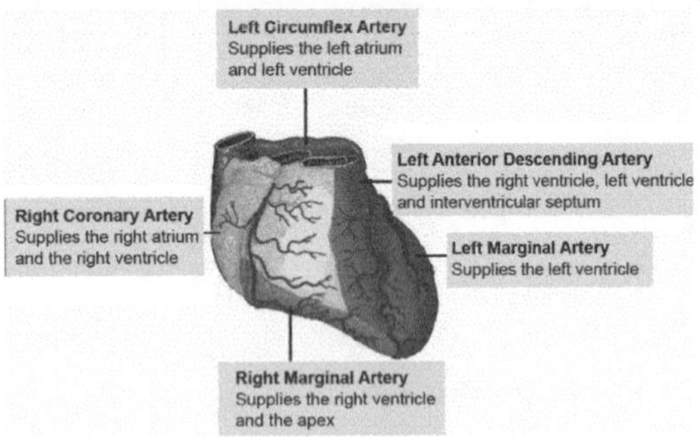

Left coronary artery

- **2 main branches:**
  - o Left anterior descending artery
  - o Circumflex artery
- **Supplies:**
  - o Anterior 2/3rd of interventricular septum
  - o Anterior part of left and right ventricle
  - o Lateral wall of left ventricle
  - o A-V groove
  - o SA node in 40% of cases

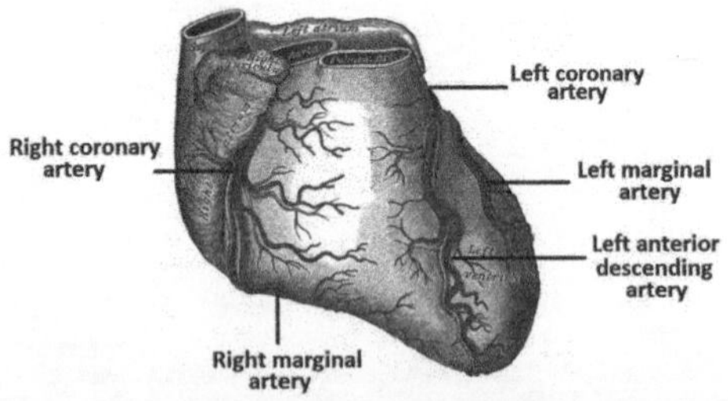

Right coronary artery

- **2 main branches:**
  - o Posterior descending artery
  - o Marginal artery
- **Supplies:**
  - o Posterior 1/3rd of interventricular septum
  - o Right atrium
  - o Right ventricle
  - o SA node (60% cases)
  - o AV node

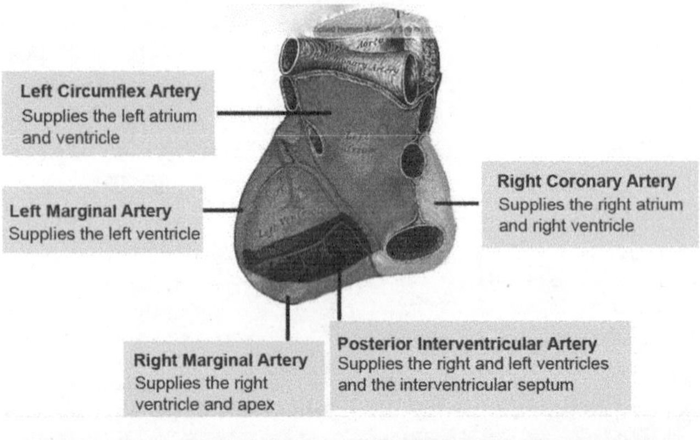

PULSE

Pulsus bisferiens (rapid rising and twice beating)

- Mild aortic stenosis with severe aortic regurgitation
- HOCM

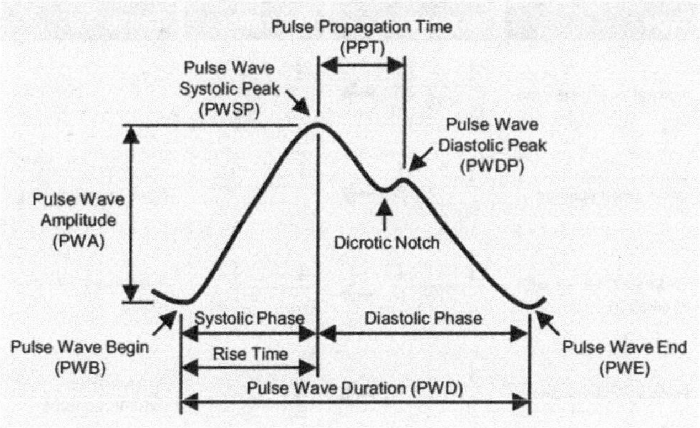

Dicrotic pulse

- Has 2 palpable waves
- One in systole and one in diastole
- Seen in dilated cardiomyopathy

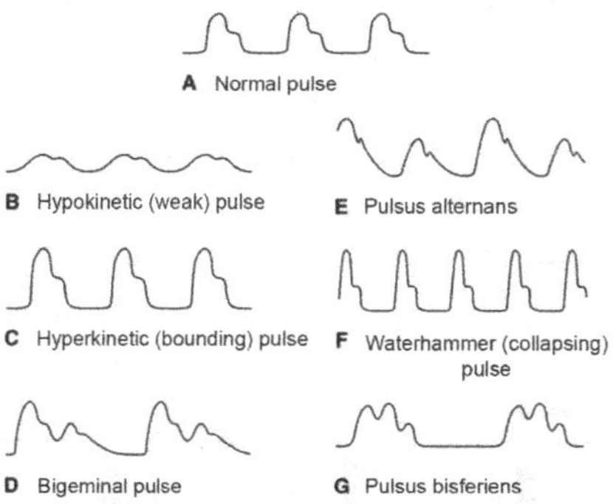

Water hammer/collapsing pulse

- Large bounding pulse
- Aortic regurgitation
- PDA
- Hyperdynamic circulation

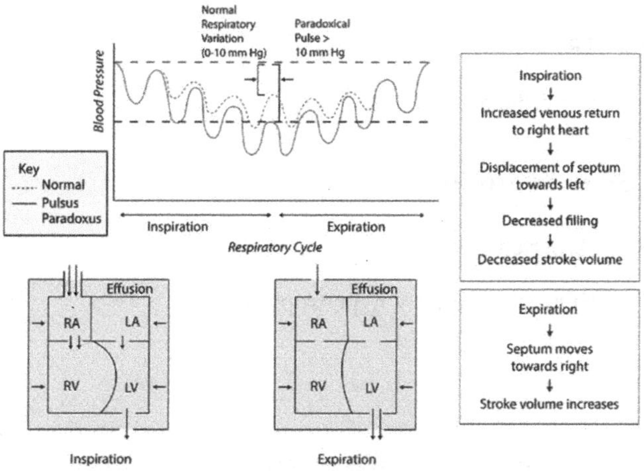

Pulsus paradoxus

- Exaggeration of normal; fall in systolic BP of >10 mm Hg on inspiration
- **Lungs:**
  - o Asthma (COPD)
  - o Emphysema
- **Heart** (***Mnemonic:*** **CC**):
  - o **C**onstrictive pericarditis
  - o **C**ardiac tamponade/pericardial effusion

JUGULAR VENOUS PULSE

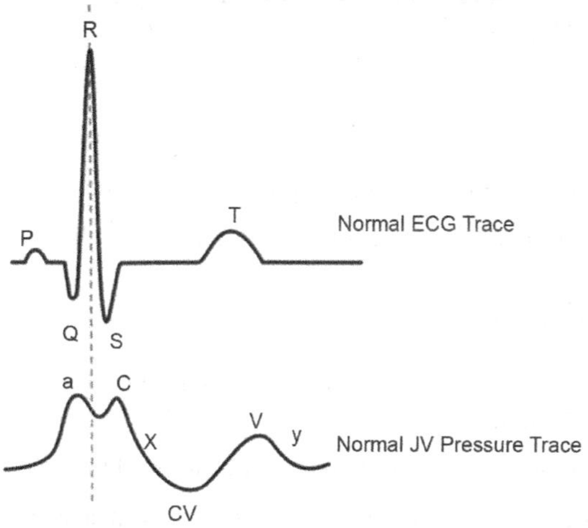

Positive waves and events of cardiac cycle

- **'a' wave is due to:** Atrial systole
- **'c' wave is due to:** Isometric ventricular contraction phase causing bulging of AV valves into atrium/tricuspid closure
- **'v' wave is due to:** Atrial filling

Abnormalities of JVP

- **Large 'a' wave:** TS/PS/pulmonary hypertension
- **Cannon 'a' wave:**
  - o CHB
  - o AV dissociation with ventricular tachycardia
- **Slow 'y' descent:** TS
- **Deep 'x' and 'y' descent:**
  - o Constrictive pericarditis
  - o Pericardial tamponade

HEART SOUNDS

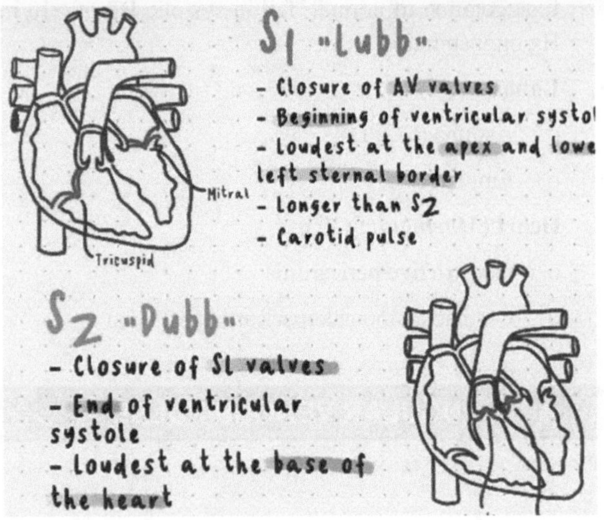

Soft S1

- Mitral stenosis (long standing, calcified and rigid)
- Poor conduction of sound through chest wall

2nd heart sound

- Produced because of closure of Semilunar valves (aortic and pulmonary)
- **Sequence of valve closure:** A2 followed by P2
- **Effect of respiration:** Split increases in inspiration as in inspiration blood increases in RV but decreases in LV (reverse in expiration)

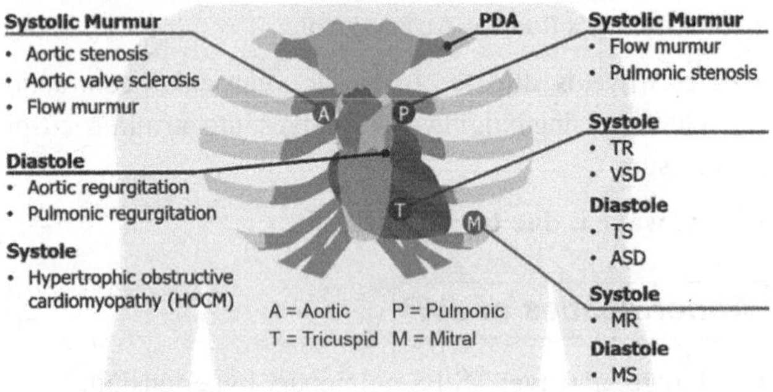

Wide split S2

- Pulmonary stenosis
- RBBB

Type	Inspiration	Expiration	Cause
Normal or physiologic	S_1 S_2 (A P) →	S_1 S_2 (AP)	
Wide, fixed splitting	S_1 S_2 (A P) →	S_1 S_2 (A P)	Atrial septal defect
Wide split, varies with inspiration	S_1 S_2 (A P) →	S_1 S_2 (A P)	Pulmonary stenosis, RBBB
Paradoxical splitting	S_1 S_2 (PA) →	S_1 S_2 (P A)	Hypertrophic cardiomyopathy

Reverse splitting of S2

- Left bundle branch block
- Aortic stenosis

Wide, fixed splitting

- ASD

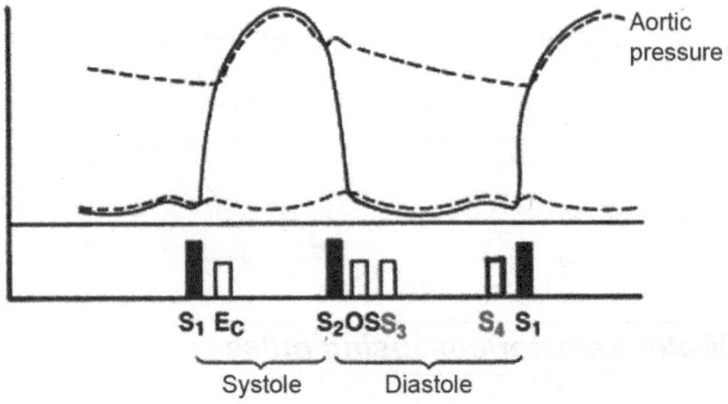

S3 is heard in

- Young people (< 30 years)
- MR
- TR
- Hyperdynamic states

S4 is heard in

- Hypertension
- HOCM (severe LV hypertrophy)

ECG

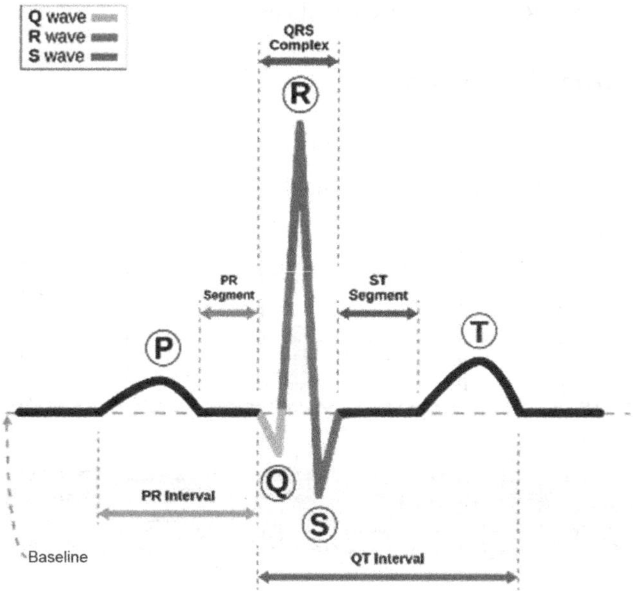

Waves and events of cardiac cycle

- **P wave is due to:** Atrial depolarization
- **PR interval (beginning of P to beginning of R):** Conduction through AV node
- **QRS complex (End of P-wave and beginning of ST segment):** Ventricular depolarization
- **Duration of QRS complex:** 0.08-0.10 seconds
- **QT interval (beginning of Q to end of T):** Mechanical contraction of ventricles
- **ST segment (end of S to the beginning of T):** Isoelectric ventricular contraction
- **T wave:** Ventricular repolarization

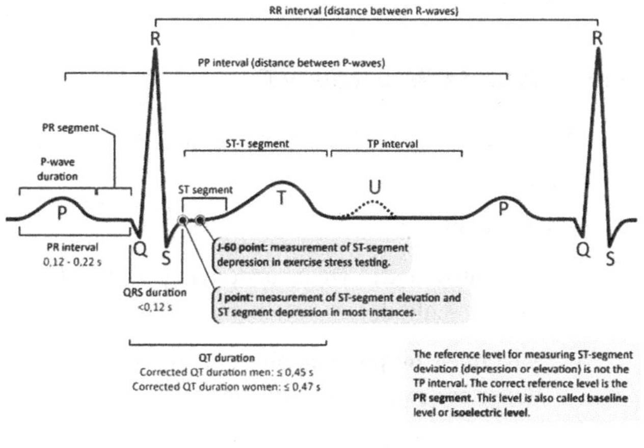

PR interval

- **Measured from:** Beginning of P wave to beginning of R wave
- Includes Atrial depolarization and conduction through AV node, Bundle of His and Purkinje fibers
- **Represents conduction time through:** AV node
- **Shortened in:** WPW syndrome
- **Prolonged in:** Acute rheumatic fever

Abnormalities in ECG

- **Tall tented T waves, decreased p wave amplitude, widening of QRS complex:** Hyperkalemia
- **Prominent U waves, small T waves:** Hypokalemia
- **Shortening of QT interval:** Hypercalcemia
- **Widening of QT interval:** Hypocalcemia
- **Convex elevation of J point/J waves/Osborne waves:** Hypothermia
- **SIQIIITIII:** Pulmonary embolism

WOLF-PARKINSON-WHITE SYNDROME

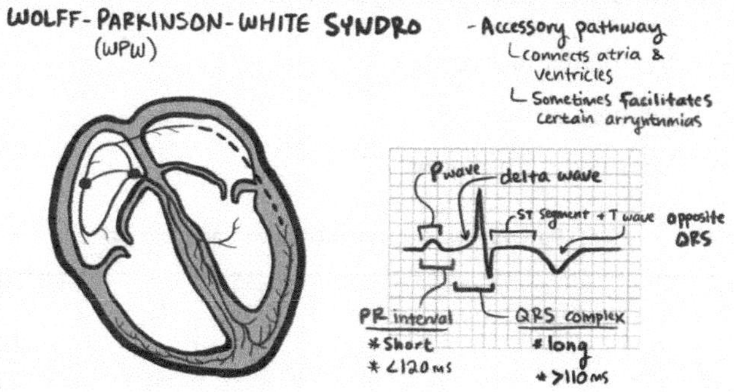

Pathology

- Abnormal band of atrial tissue which connects atria and ventricles (bundle of Kent)
- AV node is electrically bypassed and A-V conduction is abnormally rapid (short PR interval <0.12 sec)
- Verapamil and digoxin is avoided as they reduce refractory period and increased conduction in the bypass tract

ECG changes

- Delta wave

- Short PR interval
- Wide QRS

Management

- Procainamide/Amiodarone/Flecainide
- Radiofrequency ablation

CARDIAC ARRHYTHMIAS

Types

- Atrial tachyarrhythmias
- Supraventricular tachyarrhythmias (QRS complex duration and morphology normal)
- PSVT (Paroxysmal Supraventricular Tachycardia)

Atrial tachyarrhythmias

- Atrial tachycardia
- Atrial fibrillation
- Atrial flutter

Ventricular tachyarrhythmias

- Ventricular tachycardia
- Ventricular flutter
- Ventricular fibrillation

PSVT: Paroxysmal Supraventricular Tachycardia

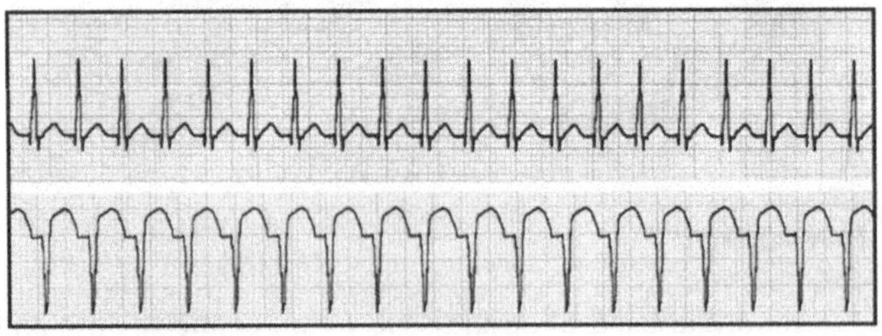

Stable Vital Signs:
Carotid Massage→ Adenosine (6, 12, 12mg) IVP → Verapmil (2.5mg→ 5mg) IV slow

Unstable Vital signs:
Synchonized Cardioversion 50 Joules

PSVT

- Normal wave is followed by QRS complex, but no p wave because p wave s p wave is merged with QRS complex

- **ECG:**
  - o P wave absent
  - o R-R interval decreased/constant

Atrial fibrillation

- Heart rate is >350 beats/minute
- QRS morphology is normal

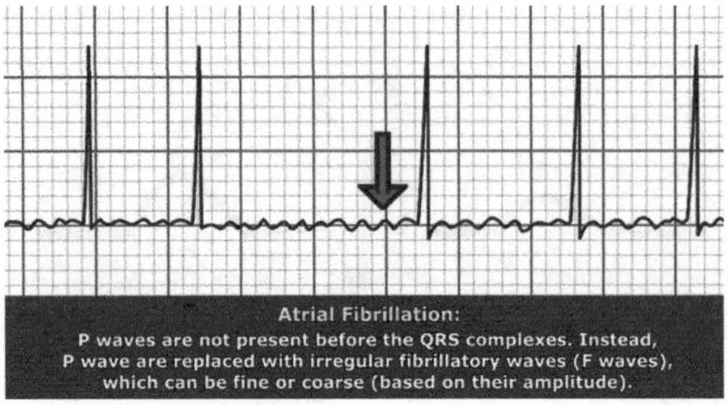

- R-R interval variable and irregular
- **Management of AF:**
  - o Control fast ventricular rate by blocking AV node (beta blocker, Calcium channel blocker)
  - o Convert AF into sinus rhythm (DC cardioversion)
  - o Maintenance of sinus rhythm (Amiodarone, Sotalol)

Normal ECG

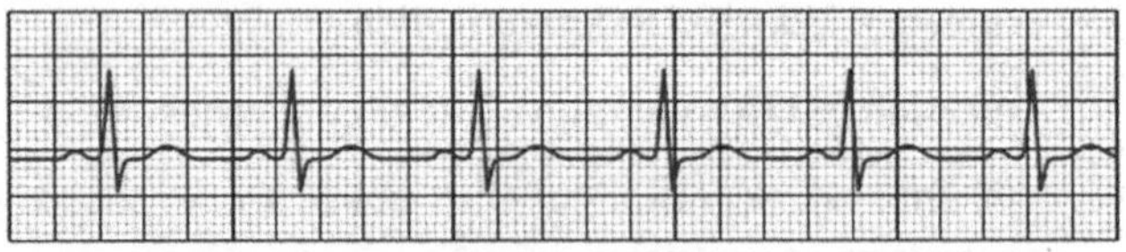

Monomorphic ventricular tachycardia

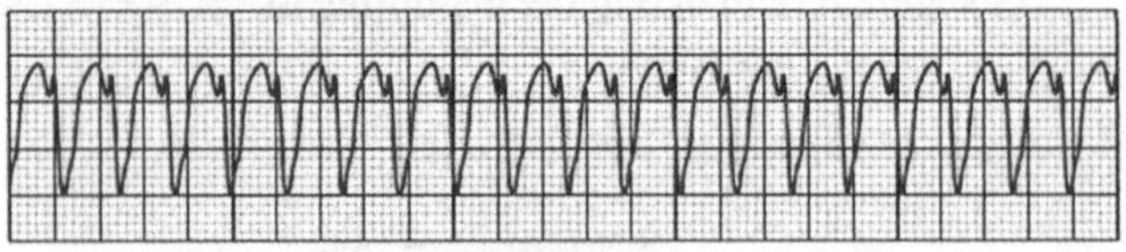

Ventricular tachycardia/VT

- >3 consecutive ventricular ectopic at HR >100 beats/minute
- **Management of VT:**
  - o **Non-sustained:** Treat underlying cause (amiodarone, ibulitide)
  - o **Sustained or polymorphic:** Treat like ventricular flutter or ventricular fibrillation

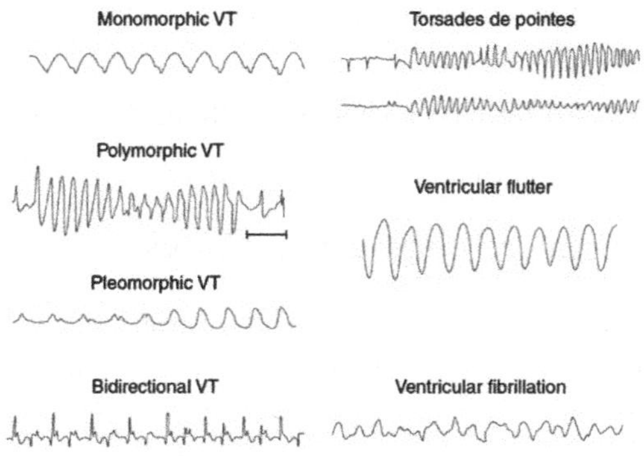

Polymorphic VT

- Also known as Torsade de pointes
- Chiefly due to drugs (terfenadine, sevoflurane) and electrolyte imbalance (hypomagnesemia and hypokalemia)
- **ECG:**
  - o Prolonged QTc (>460-480 ms)
  - o Resting bradycardia (<60 beats/min)
- Can result in ventricular fibrillation and sudden death

Congenital long QT syndrome

- Known as Romano Ward syndrome
- It is because of recurrent bouts of rapid polymorphic ventricular tachycardia known as Torsade de pointes

Ventricular flutter/VF

- Heart rate >250/min
- Only QRS, no other wave seen on ECG
- DC cardioversion and I/V lignocaine followed by amiodarone maintenance

Ventricular fibrillation

- Chaotic pattern on ECG
- DC cardioversion and I/V lignocaine followed by amiodarone maintenance

HEART BLOCK

Types

- SA node block
- AV node block
- Bundle branch block (right and left)

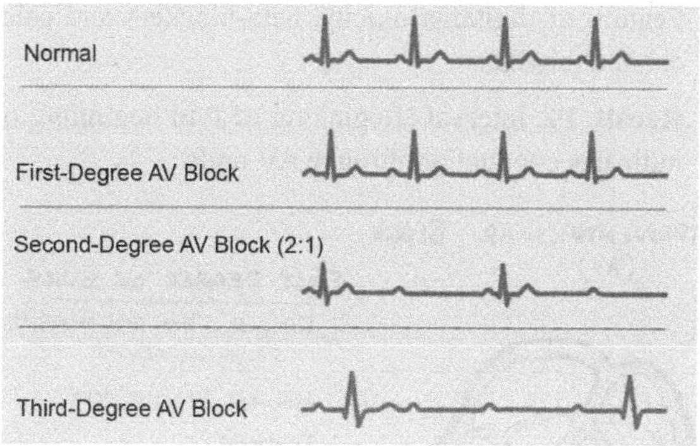

AV block

- Conduction from atria to ventricles is lost
- **Types:**
  - o **Incomplete AV block:**
    - ♦ Partial disturbances in conduction (1st and 2nd degree)
  - o **Complete AV block:**
    - ♦ Complete loss of conduction between atria and ventricles (3rd degree)
- **2nd degree AV block/intermittent AV block:**
  - o All impulses do **not** reach ventricles
    - ♦ Mobitz type I
    - ♦ Mobitz type II

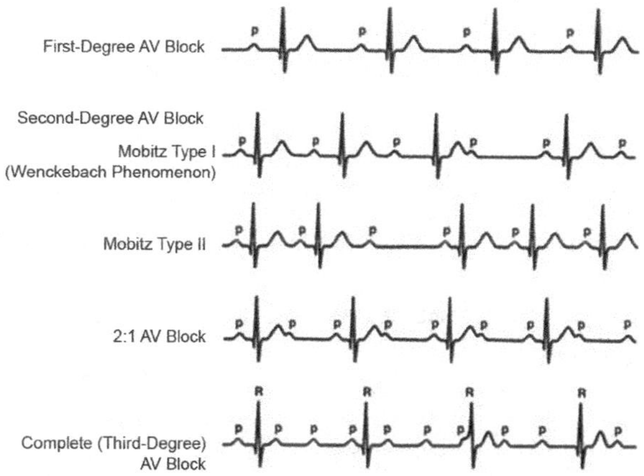

1st degree AV block

- All atrial impulses reach the ventricles but PR interval is abnormally prolonged

- **Atria:** Ventricle ratio is 1:1
- Abnormally prolonged PR interval (>0.20 seconds)
- Feature of digitalis toxicity, beta-blockers and calcium channel blocker
- **Recall:** PR interval (Beginning of P to beginning of R) indicates conduction through AV node

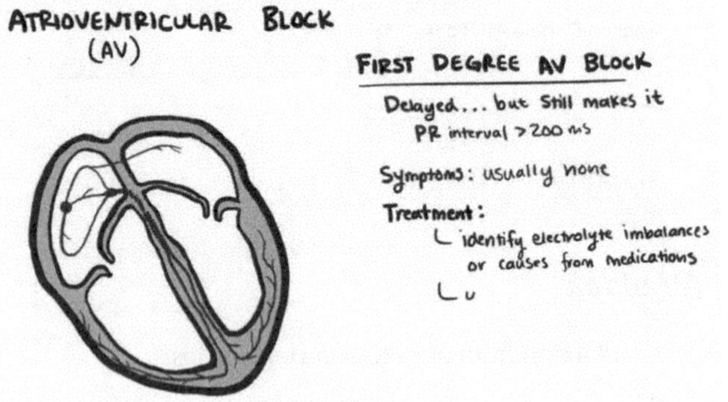

Second degree AV block

- All impulses do **not** reach ventricles
- **Atria:** Ventricle ratio is 2:1 or 3:1
- Abnormally prolonged PR interval (>0.2 seconds)
- **Two types:**
  - o Mobitz type I (Wenckebach block)
  - o Mobitz type II

Mobitz type I block

- Normal QRS, but gradual lengthening of PR interval (Wenckebach phenomenon)
- Seen with digitalis toxicity and beta blockers use
- May be seen transiently in inferior wall MI

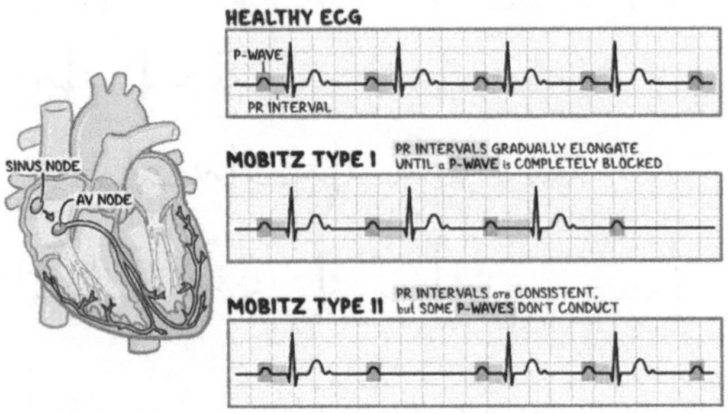

Mobitz type II

- PR interval is normal but QRS widened
- Seen in conduction defects of Bundle of His and Purkinje fibers
- Sudden drop in beat without any PR interval prolongation
- Require pacemaker

Complete/3rd degree heart block

- Complete loss of conduction between atria and ventricles so ventricles beat at a much slower rate (idioventricular rhythm)
- **Stokes Adams syndrome:**
  - o If 3rd degree heart block develops suddenly, dizziness and fainting may occur
- Seen in digitalis toxicity or myocardial infarction
- Requires pacemaker

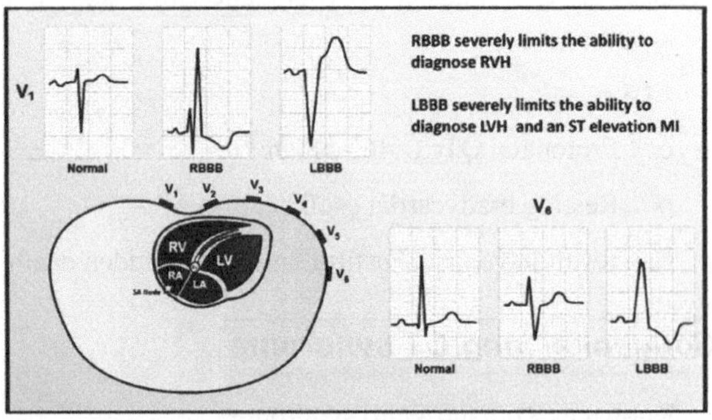

Bundle branch block

- **LBBB:** Left ventricle contracts after right ventricle
- **RBBB:** Right ventricle contracts after left ventricle
- Left anterior hemiblock/fascicular block
- Left posterior hemiblock/fascicular block

RHEUMATIC HEART DISEASE

Features

- Caused by GABHS (group A beta-hemolytic streptococci)
- Follows pharyngeal infection
- Type II hypersensitivity reaction

Minor criteria

- **Clinical:** Arthralgia, fever, previous rheumatic fever, RHD

- **Laboratory:** Prolonged PR interval on ECG, increased acute phase reactants (ESR, CRP, leucocytes)

Major criteria

- Subcutaneous nodule
- Erythema marginatum
- Sydenham's chorea
- Carditis
- Migratory polyarthritis

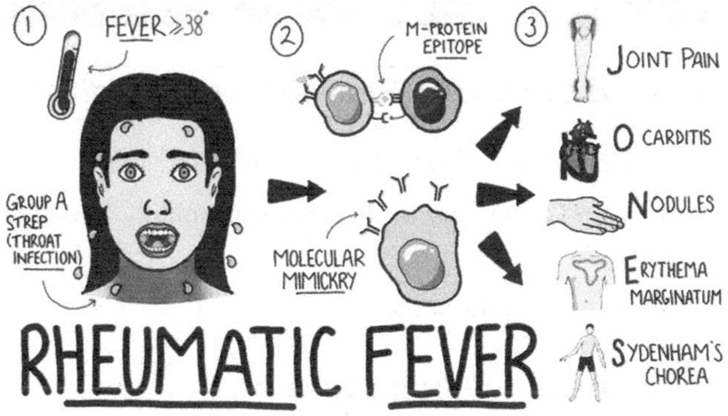

Associated terms

- **Aschoff bodies:**
  - Focal inflammatory nodules
  - Pathognomonic
- Anitschkow cells/Caterpillar cells (large activated histiocytes)
- Pancarditis
- McCallum patch (Subendocardial collection of Aschoff nodules in left atrium)

MITRAL STENOSIS/MS

Features

- **MC cause:** RHD
- Initially asymptomatic (up to 10 years)
- **Later features of heart failure:**
  - Dyspnea on exertion
  - Orthopnea
  - **Atrial fibrillation:** 400 ± 50 heartbeats/minute)
  - Hemoptysis
  - Pulmonary hypertension
  - Hoarseness of voice (Ortner syndrome)

Auscultatory findings

- Opening snap after S2
- Rumbling late mid-diastolic murmur, which is best heard at apex
- Loud S1

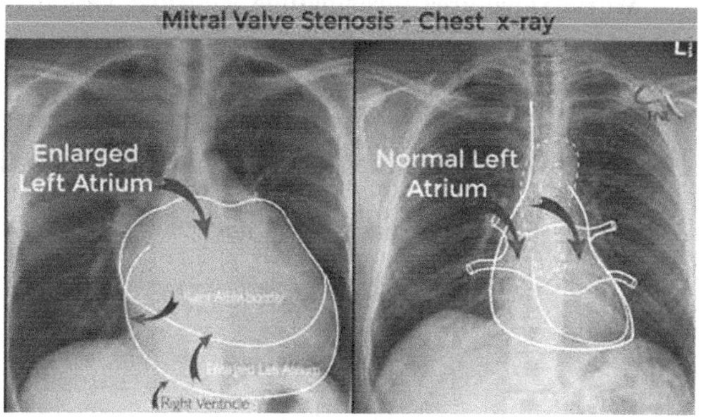

X-ray of chest

- Straightening of left border
- Left atrial enlargement
- Double atrial shadow
- Right ventricular hypertrophy

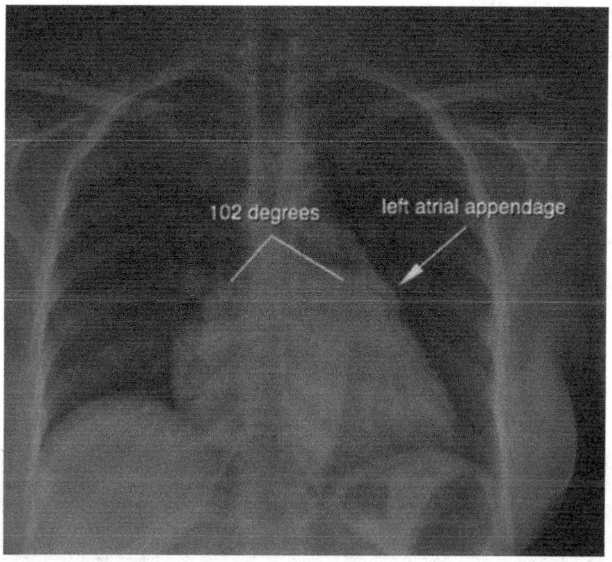

IOC for MS

- Echocardiography

Treatment

- **Most important differential diagnosis:** Left atrial myxoma
- Diuretics (for reducing preload)
- Antiarrhythmics (for atrial fibrillation)
- Balloon valvuloplasty
- Valve replacement
- **Mitral valve area incompatible with life:** Less than 0.6 cm^2

HOCM

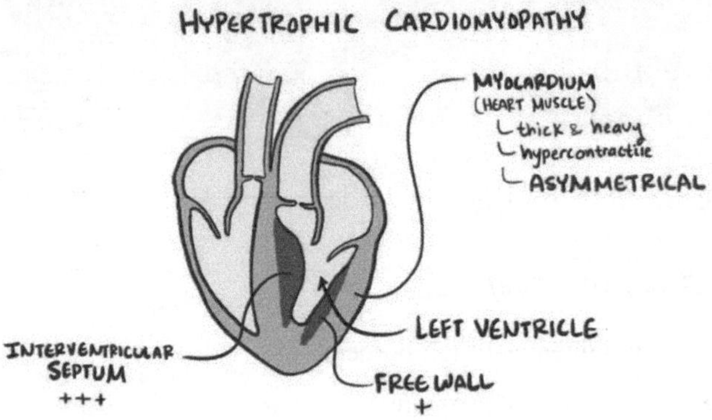

Features

- Diastolic dysfunction
- Dyspnea
- Syncope
- Double/triple apical pulse
- Loud S4
- Bisferiens carotid pulse
- **Systolic ejection murmur:**
  - o Increases with decrease in preload (Valsalva maneuver, nitrates, diuretics)
  - o Decrease in afterload (vasodilator)

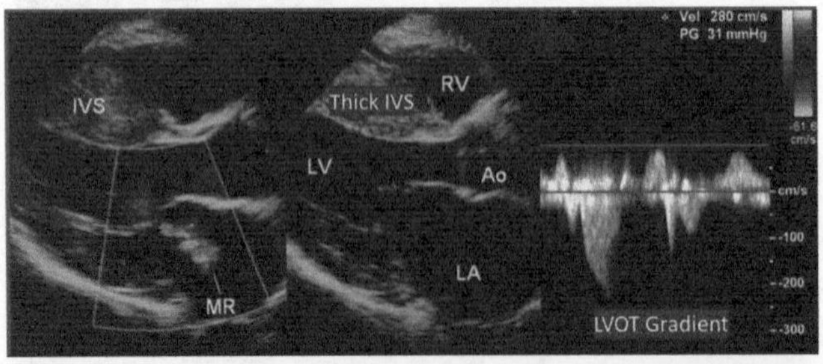

ECHO

- Thickened septum and ventricular wall
- Mitral regurgitation

Management

- Avoid strenuous work, digoxin, diuretics, nitrates
- Cardiac workload decreased by beta-blockers and CCBs

INFECTIVE ENDOCARDITIS

MC cause of SABE (Subacute endocarditis)

- Streptococcus viridans (low virulence)
- Smaller vegetations in diseased/congenitally abnormal valves
- Occur after dental surgeries

MC cause in I/V drug abusers

- Staph aureus (especially with acute presentation)

Acute endocarditis

- Caused by staph aureus (organism of high virulence)
- Onset is rapid
- Valves are normal
- Large vegetations
- Splinter hemorrhages on nail beds are seen
- **Management:**
  - o Multiple blood cultures
  - o Prolonged antibiotic therapy

Terms related to bacterial endocarditis

- **Osler's nodes:** Painful, pea-sized nodules in pulp of fingers/finger or toe pads (SABE)
- **Janeway's lesions:** Non-tender, small erythematous lesions in soles/palm (ABE)
- **Spots in retina:** Roth's spot (round white spots on retina surrounded by hemorrhage)

Conditions and sites of vegetations

- **Libman Sacks:** Both side of valve leaflets

- **NBTE/Marantic endocarditis:** Along the line of closure
- **RHD/Rheumatic fever:** Along the line of closure
- **IE/Infective endocarditis:** On valve cusps, that extends onto valve cords

Modified Duke Criteria for Infective Endocarditis	
MNEMONIC: BE TIMER	
Major Criteria	**Minor Criteria**
Mnemonic-BE	**Mnemonic-TIMER**
• **B**lood culture Positive > 2 times 12 hours apart • **E**chocardiographic evidence of Endocardial Involvement 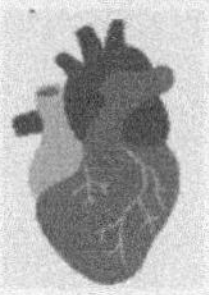	• **T**emperature > 38°C (Fever) • **I**mmunological phenomena (Osler's nodes, Roth sports) • **M**icrobiological Evidence (Positive blood culture not meeting a major criterion) • **E**mbolic Phenomenon (Arterial emboli, septic emboli, conjunctival hemorrhage and painless skin lesions) • **R**isk Factors (Congenital heart condition or IV drug use)
• **Definitive Diagnosis:** Two major criteria OR One major and Three minor criteria OR Five minor criteria. • **Possible Diagnosis:** One major and One minor criteria OR Three minor criteria.	

ANGINA

Stable angina

- Chest pain associated with physical exertion/stress
- In stable angina, enzyme levels are Normal
- Relieved by rest/sublingual nitroglycerine

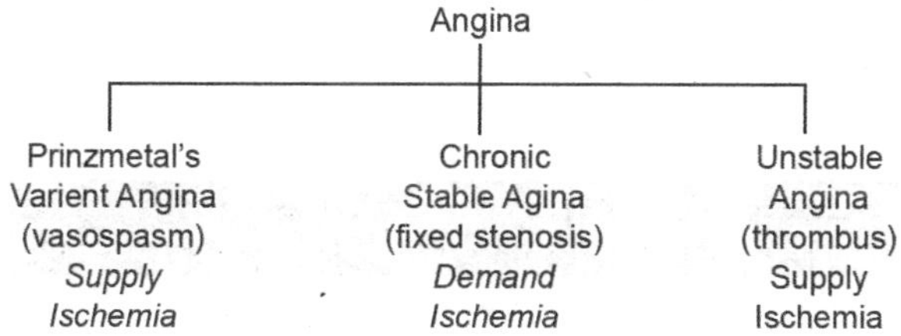

Unstable angina

- Angina pectoris with occurring at rest/minimal exertion
- Severe and new in onset
- Crescendo pattern (worsens with subsequent attacks)
- May turn to MI

Variant/Prinzmetal's angina

- Ischemic pain at rest but **not** usually with exertion
- Focal spasm of an epicardial coronary artery
- Wakes up the patient at night
- Nitrates and calcium channel blockers are used

MYOCARDIAL INFARCTION

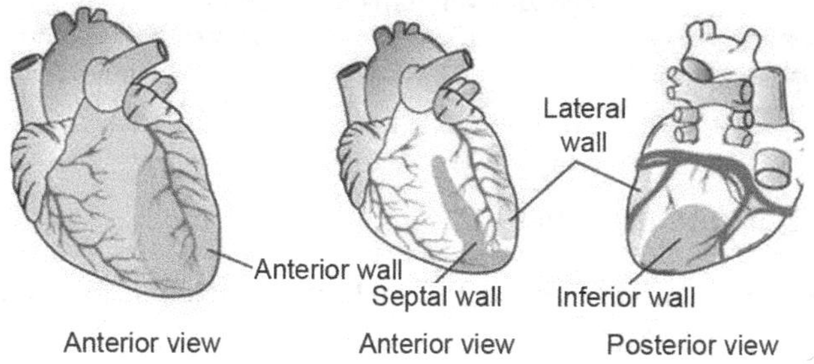

Location of MI by ECG Leads			
I Lateral	aVR	V_1 septal	V_4 anterior
II Inferior	aVL lateral	V_2 septal	V_5 lateral
III Inferior	aVF inferior	V_3 anterior	V_6 lateral

Clinical features

- Chest pain (tightness)
- Sweating
- Silent MI in diabetics
- S4 heart sound

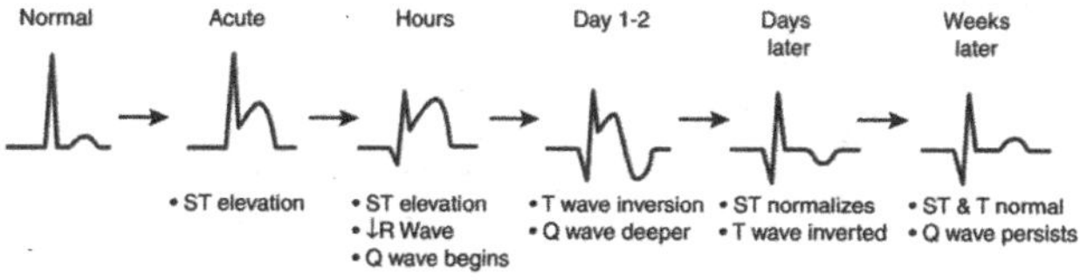

ECG evolution during acute ST elevation myocardial infarction (also termed "acute Q wave myocardial infarction"). However, as described in Chapter 7, if successful early reperfusion of the coronary occlusion is achieved, the elevated ST segments return to baseline without subsequent T wave inversion or Q wave development.

ECG

- **Within few hours:**
  - o ST segment begin to rise
  - o T wave abnormally tall
- **<24 hours:**
  - o ST segment elevation begins to resolve

- o T wave inverts
- **Within few days:** Pathological Q waves

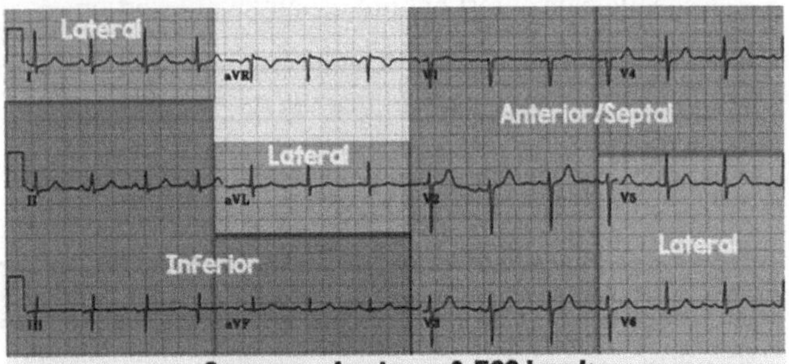

Coronary Anatomy & ECG Leads

Lateral Leads	I, aVL, V5 - V6	LCx or Diagonal of LAD
Inferior Leads	II, III, aVF	RCA and/or LCx
Anterior/Septal Leads	V1 - V4	LAD

Cardiac markers

- **Enzyme to raise at the earliest:** Myoglobin; followed by CK-MB
- **Sensitive marker for MI:** Troponin T

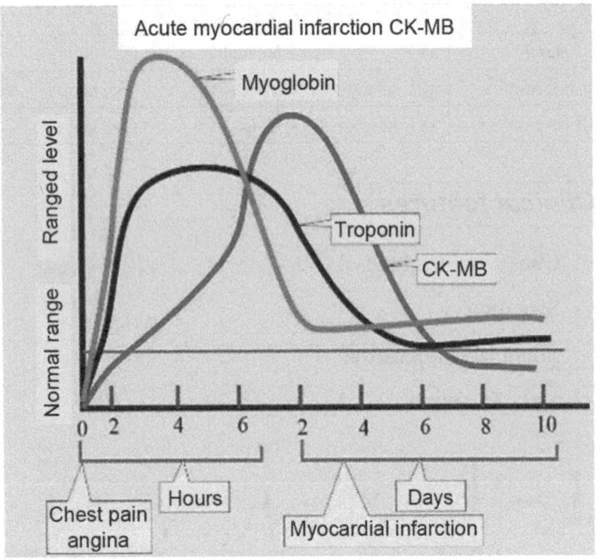

CK-MB

- **Rises at:** 4-8 hours
- **Peaks at:** 16-24 hours
- **Returns to normal at:** 3-4 days

Troponin I

- **Begins to rise at:** 4-6 hours
- **Peaks at:** 12-24 hours (Troponin T at 18-36 hours)
- **Returns to normal at:** 7-10 days (Troponin T at 5-14 days)

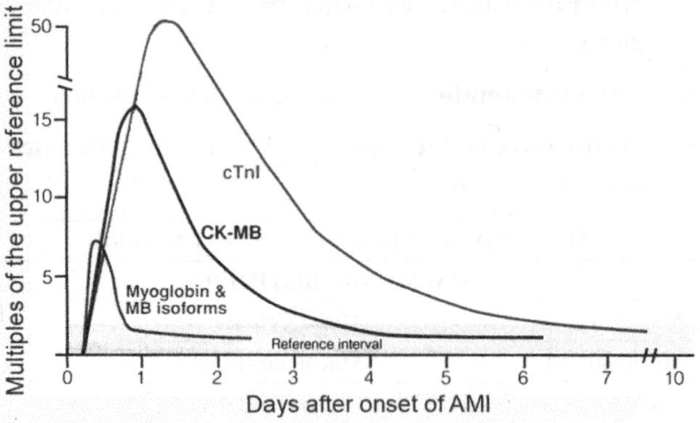

Management (Mnemonic: MONA)

- **M**orphine
- **O**xygen
- **N**itroglycerine
- **A**spirin

Early complications

- Arrhythmia (VT/VF)
- LVF and pulmonary edema
- Cardiogenic shock
- Rupture of ventricular wall (anterior MI)
- Acute MR (inferoposterior MI)
- RVF (inferoposterior MI)

Late complications

- Mural thrombosis and systemic emboli
- Left ventricular aneurysm
- Dressler syndrome
- DVT

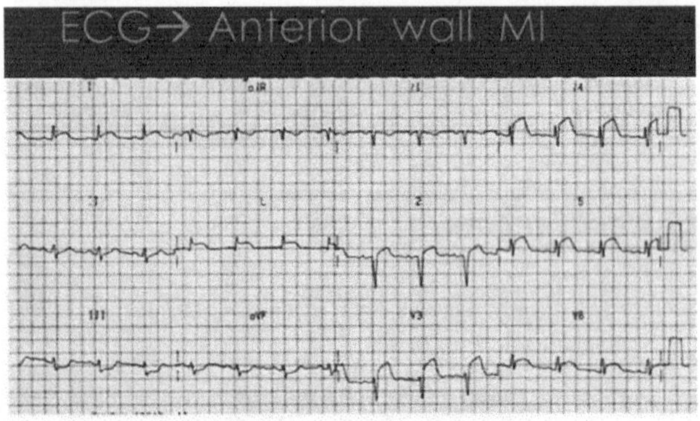

ST elevation in V2-6, I and aVL
Reciprocal ST depression in III and AVF

SECTION 1
MEDICINE

Chapter 11

Respiratory System

Characteristics of Breath Sounds

	Duration of sounds	Intensity of expiratory sound	Pitch of expiratory sound	Locations where heard normally
Vesicular 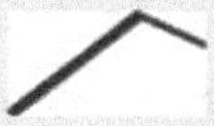	Inspiratory sounds last longer than expiratory sounds	Soft	Relatively low	Over most of both lungs
Broncho-vesicular 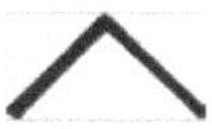	Inspiratory and expiratory sounds are about equal	Intermediate	Intermediate	Often in the 1st and 2nd interspaces anteriorly and between the scapulae
Bronchial 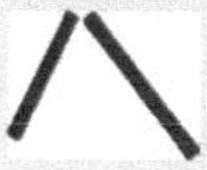	Expiratory sounds last longer than inspiratory ones	Loud	Relatively high	Over the manubrium (larger proximal airways)
Tracheal 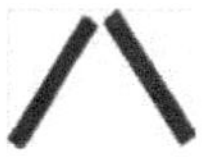	Inspiratory and expiratory sounds are about equal	Very loud	Relatively high	Over the trachea in the neck

Breath sounds

- Vesicular
- Bronchovesicular (vesicular breath sounds with prolonged expiration)
- Bronchial

Paradoxical breathing

- Unilateral Diaphragmatic palsy
- Flail chest

BRONCHIAL BREATHING

Type of breathing	Quality/ Character	Can be immitated by	Suggestive of
Cavernous	Low pitched with hollow character	Auscultating at occipital region of skull	Underlying cavity in the lung Open pneumothorax Pulled trachea syndrome
Tubular	High pitched with tubular or aspirate quality		Pneumonia Pulm infarction Atelectasis or collapse of lung
Amphoric	High pitched with metallic or ECHO like quality	Blowing intensely across the mouth of the bottle	Large cavity in the lungs with smooth walls Pneumothorax communicating with the bronchus

Amphoric breathing

- Open Pneumothorax
- Smooth walled cavities

Cavernous breathing

- Irregular cavity

Tubular breathing

- Consolidation
- Above the level of pleural effusion

SPIROMETRY IN LUNG DISEASES

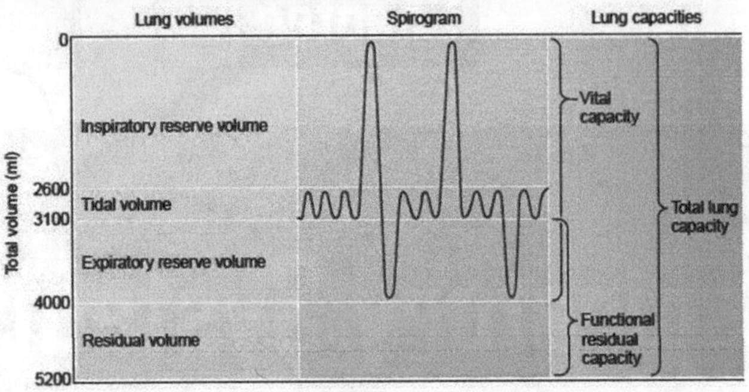

Obstructive lung disease

- **TLC, FVC, RV:** Increased
- **FRC, FEV1, FEV1/FVC:** Decreased

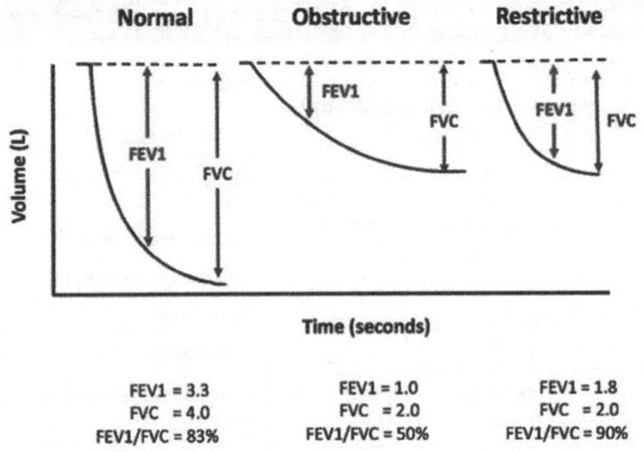

Restrictive lung disease

- All decreased except FEV1/FVC (Normal/increased)

RESPIRATORY FAILURE

Type I respiratory failure

- Hypoxia
- Normocapnia/hypocapnia
- **Acute:** Asthma, pulmonary edema, pulmonary embolism, pneumonia, pneumothorax, ARDS
- **Chronic:** Emphysema, Right to left shunts, lung fibrosis

Type II respiratory failure

- Hypoxia with hypercapnia
- **Acute:** Acute severe asthma, Acute exacerbation of COPD, flail chest
- **Chronic:** COPD, kyphoscoliosis, ankylosing spondylitis, myopathies, kyphoscoliosis

Type III

- Perioperative lung atelectasis

Type IV

- Hypoperfusion of respiratory muscles in patients with shock

ASTHMA

Definition

- Inflammatory disease of the small airways, characterized by episodic, reversible bronchial obstruction due to hyperresponsiveness of tracheobronchial tree

Types

- **Intrinsic/Late onset:** Triggered by aspirin, cold, exercise
- **Extrinsic/Early onset/Atopic:** Type I hypersensitivity

Factors precipitating asthma

- Cold air, dust, emotional stress, exercise, drugs (NSAIDs especially aspirin, beta blockers), allergens (inhaled like dust, ingested like fish)

Pathology

- Bronchial smooth muscle hypertrophy and hyperplasia
- Hypertrophy of submucosal mucus glands
- Bronchial wall edema
- Infiltration with increased number of eosinophils
- Increased leukotriene levels

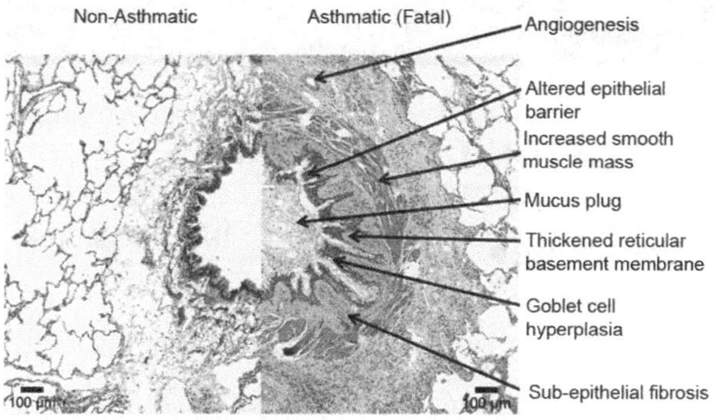

Microscopically

- Curschmann's spirals seen (Whorled mucus plugs),
- Charcot-Leyden crystals (Crystalloid debris of eosinophil membrane)

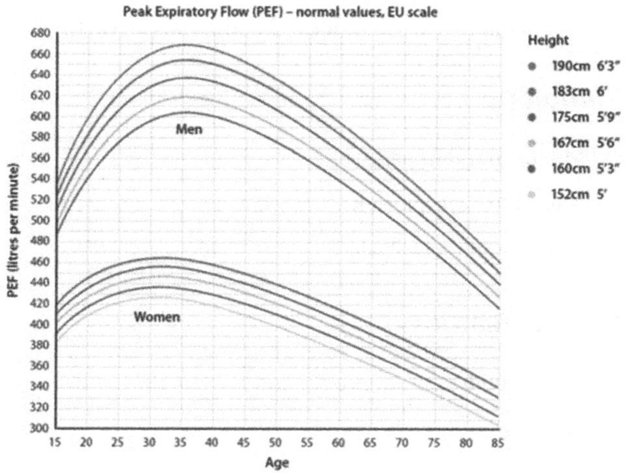

Peak expiratory flow rate

- Diurnal variation of >15-20% is a defining feature of asthma (morning dip)

Nocturnal asthma

- Overnight fall of more than 20% in the FEV1 or PEFR

Management of bronchial asthma

- **Drugs used for prevention of asthma:**
  - o Cromolyn sodium
  - o Ketotifen
  - o Nedocromil sodium
- **Drugs used to reverse bronchospasm:**
  - o Beta-adrenergic (LABA)
  - o Anticholinergics
  - o Methylxanthines
  - o Anti-inflammatory
  - o Leukotrienes antagonist
  - o 5-lipoxygenase inhibitor
  - o Anti-IgE (Omalizumab)
- **Treatment of infection:** Avoidance of allergens and other precipitating factors

EMPHYSEMA

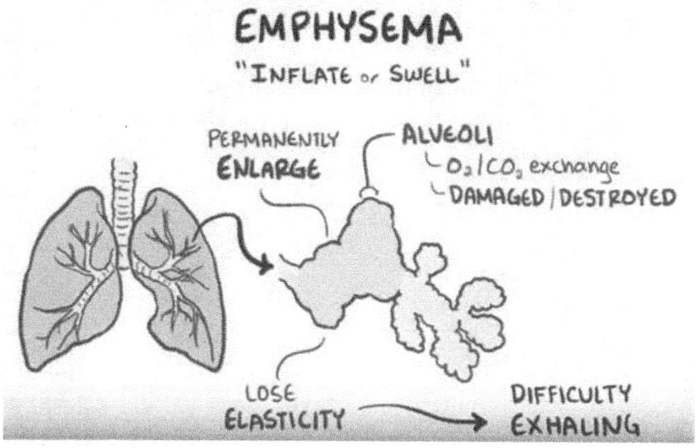

Definition

- Abnormal and permanent dilatation of air spaces distal to terminal bronchioles

3 types

- **Paraseptal:**
  - o Spares proximal
  - o Involves distal acinus
  - o Found near pleura
  - o Result in bullae and blebs which may result in spontaneous pneumothorax
- **Panacinar:**
  - o Associated with Alpha-1-antitrypsin deficiency
  - o Uniform destruction and dilatation of acinus
  - o Predominant in lower basal zones
- **Centriacinar:**
  - o Seen in smokers
  - o Enlargement of central/proximal part of respiratory unit – the acinus
  - o Predominant in upper lobe and apices

Clinical features

- Dyspnea
- Barrel shaped chest
- Respiratory acidosis
- Pulmonary hypertension
- Cor pulmonale

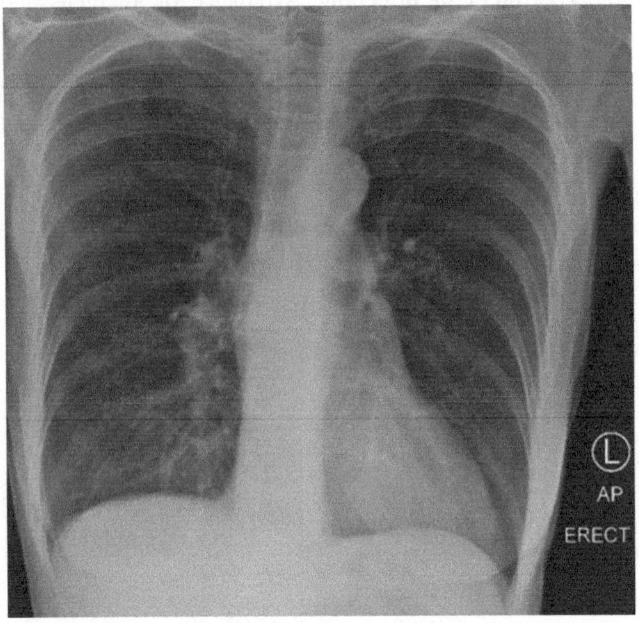

Chest X-ray findings (emphysema)

- Hypertranslucency
- Widened intercostal spaces
- Tubular heart

Pulmonary function test

- FEV1 and VC show an obstructive defect
- Reduced FEV1/VC
- Increase in TLC and RV

Treatment

- Stop smoking
- Long-term O_2 therapy
- Administer influenza and pneumococcal vaccine
- Alpha-1-AT, when it is deficient

CHRONIC BRONCHITIS

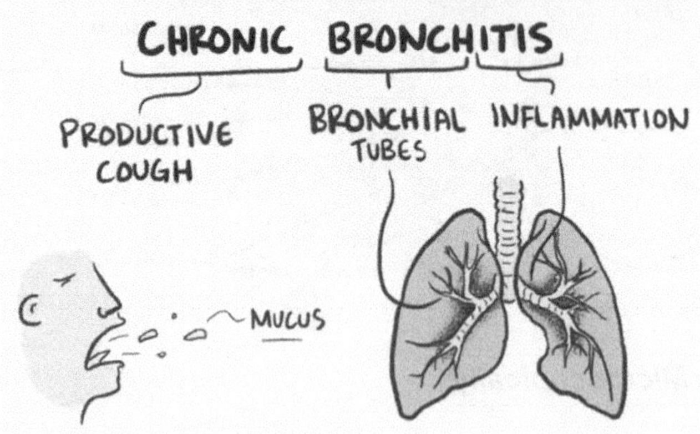

Definition

- Persistent cough with production of sputum for at **least** 3 months in a year for at **least** 2 consecutive years

Pathology

- Mucus gland hypertrophy
- Mucus hypersecretion
- Goblet cell metaplasia

Clinical features

- Cough with sputum production
- Wheezing
- Cyanosis
- Cor pulmonale

Reid's index value

- 0.52 +/- 0.08

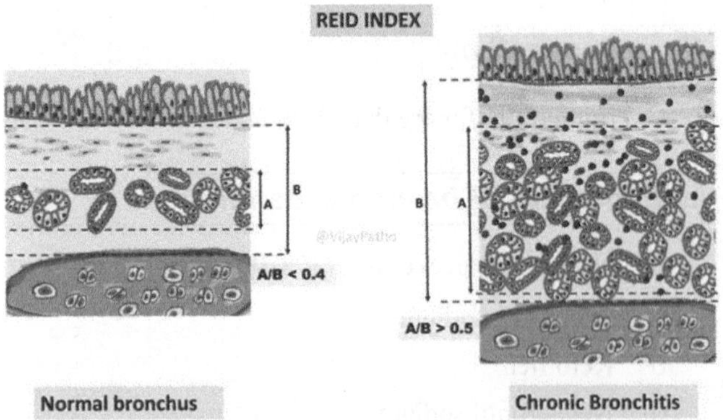

BRONCHIECTASIS

Definition

- Permanently dilated bronchi (by more than 2 mm), purulent sputum, recurrent infections
- Kartagener's syndrome

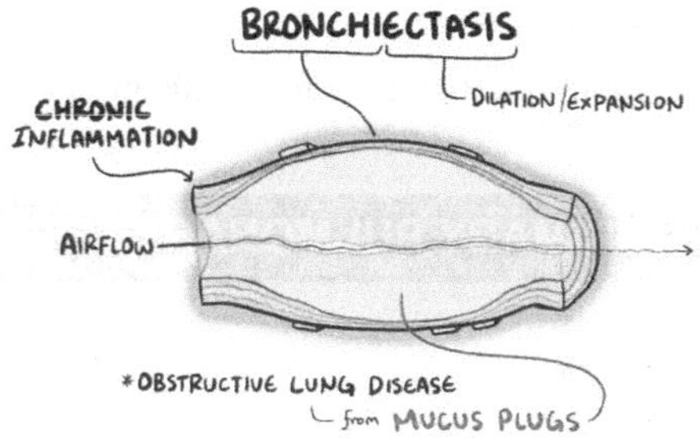

Causes

- Bronchial distension because of chronic obstruction and recurrent infection

MC site

- Lower lobe
- Left lower lobe because the lower lobe bronchus is longer and narrower
- Involvement of upper lobe is uncommon

Clinical features

- Persistent, recurrent cough and large quantity of purulent sputum
- Hemoptysis
- Clubbing

Sputum examination

- Identifying the organism
- 3 layered sputum is seen

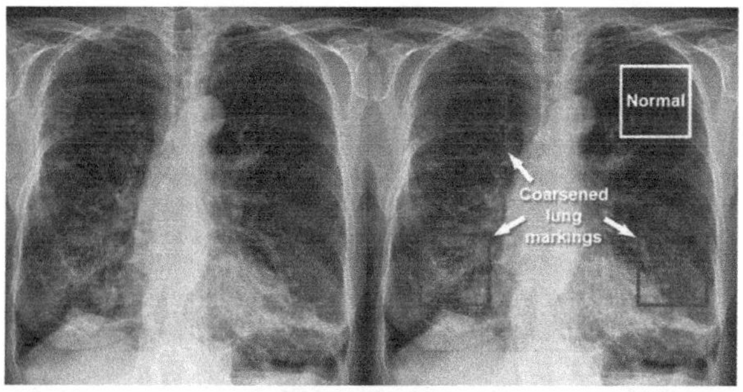

Chest X-ray findings

- Ring shadows
- Tram track sign
- Gloved finger appearance

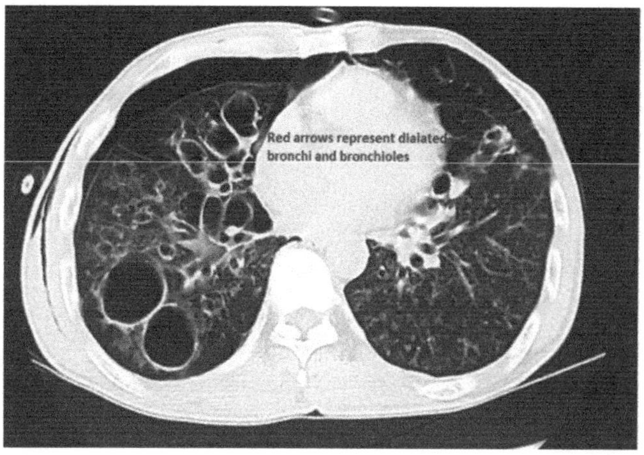

Non-invasive diagnostic test

- CT scan

Confirmation of diagnosis is by

- Bronchography

Treatment

- Control of infections
- Improved clearance of tracheobronchial secretions
- Bronchodilators

PLEURAL EFFUSION

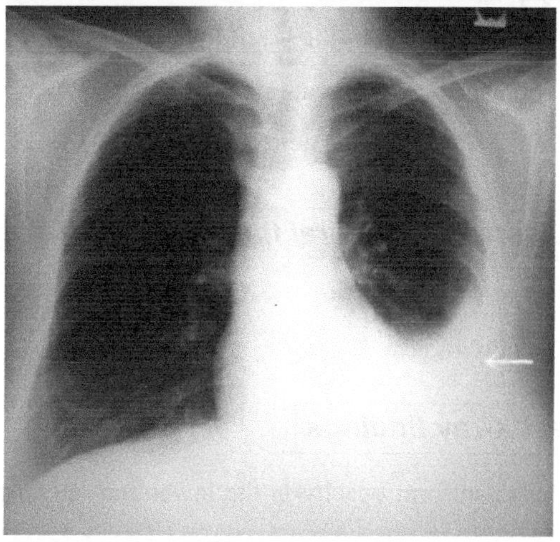

Mechanism of pleural effusion

- Elevation of venous pressure
- Decrease in plasma oncotic pressure
- Increase in pleural space oncotic pressure
- Increased capillary permeability
- Obstruction of lymphatics

2 types

- **Transudate:**
  - o CCF
  - o Cirrhosis liver
  - o Nephrotic syndrome
- **Exudate:**
  - o Infectious conditions
  - o Collagen vascular disease
  - o Meigs' syndrome

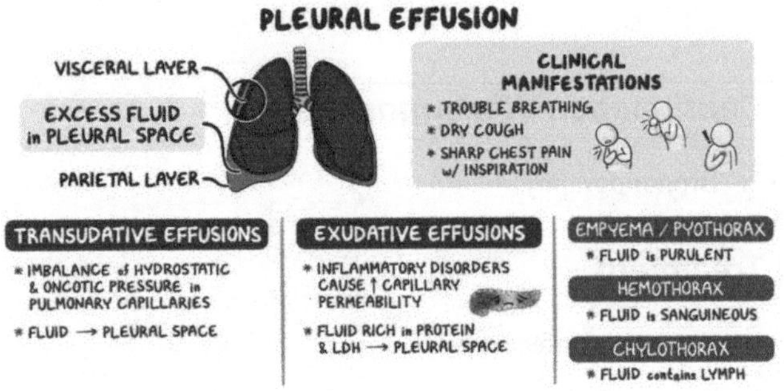

Clinical features

- Pleuritic chest pain
- Dyspnea
- Tracheal and mediastinal shift to opposite side
- Diminished/absent breath sounds
- Stony dull percussion note

Cholesterol in pleural fluid (long standing)

- TB
- Hypothyroidism

Chest X-ray findings

- Dense uniform opacity in the lower and lateral part of the hemithorax shading off above and medially into translucent lung (Ellis 'S' shaped curve)
- Mediastinal and tracheal shift to opposite side
- Obliteration of costophrenic and costodiaphragmatic angles

Treatment

- Treat underlying cause
- Pleural aspiration (not more than 1000 mL in one sitting)

PRIMARY PULMONARY TB

Ghon's focus

- Subpleural focus usually at the lower border of upper lobe or upper border of lower lobe

Ghon's complex

- Ghon's focus + draining lymph nodes

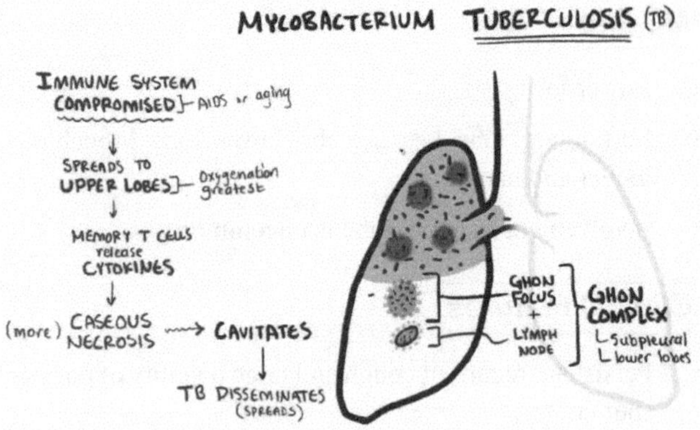

Remnants of healed initial infection

- Ghon's lesions (calcified parenchymal nodules)
- Ranke's complex (calcified hilar nodes)

Clinical features

- Fever
- Loss of appetite
- Cough
- Erythema nodosum
- Phlyctenular conjunctivitis may be associated with primary infection

Miliary TB

- Produced by acute dissemination of TB bacilli via blood stream resulting in the appearance of discrete nodule shadows about the size of millet seeds (2 mm)

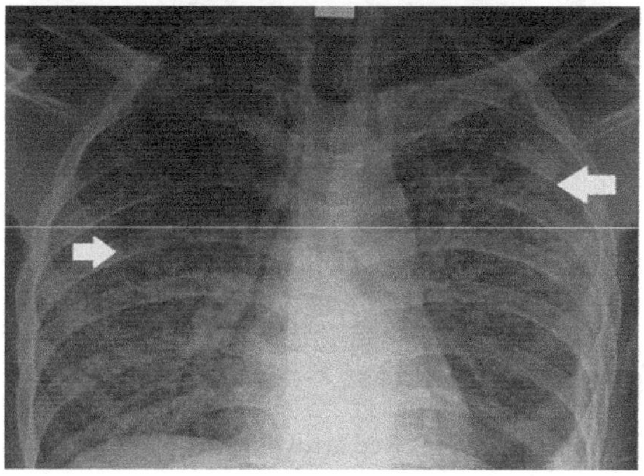

Sputum examination

- At **least** thrice
- For AFB by Ziehl-Neelsen technique (if bacilli are numerous) or Auramine-phenol fluorescent test (if bacilli are small in number)
- >50,000 bacilli/mL of sputum is sputum positivity

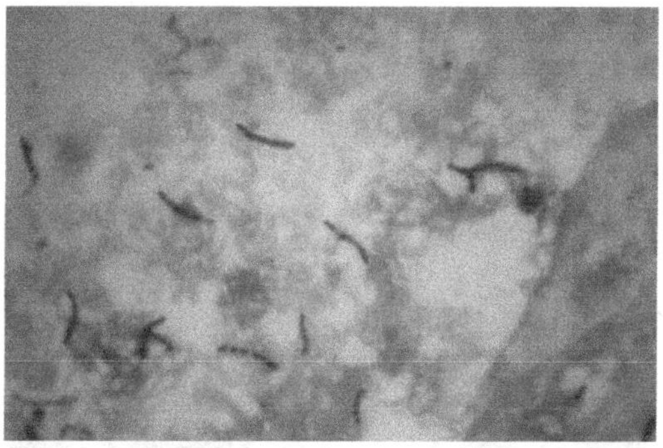

Other methods

- Culture and drug sensitivity tests using BACTEC radiometric method
- PCR technology
- ELISA testing for IgG antibodies

Management

- **First line drugs:**
  - o Rifampicin
  - o INH
  - o Pyrazinamide
  - o Streptomycin
  - o Ethambutol
- **Second line drugs:**
  - o Thiacetazone
  - o Capreomycin
  - o PAS
  - o Ethionamide
  - o Kanamycin
  - o Ciprofloxacin
  - o Cycloserine

PRIMARY PULMONARY TB

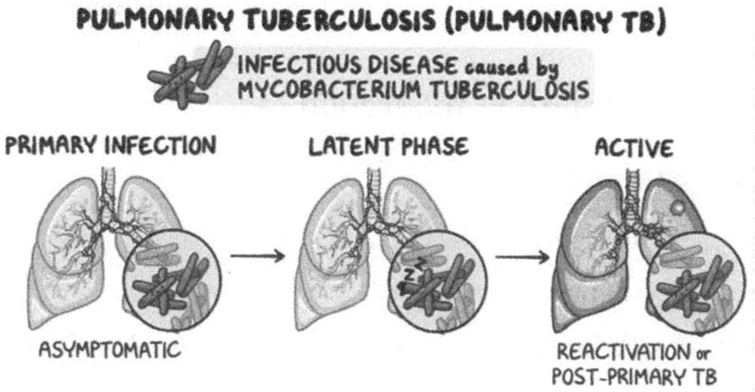

Location of post-primary pulmonary TB

- Usually situated in the posterior segment of apical lobes or apical segment of lower lobe (because of high ventilation perfusion ratios)

Simon focus

- Present in apical or posterior segment of upper lobe.
- Seedling of bacilli in this area is favored by high pO_2 of the region

TUBERCULIN TEST

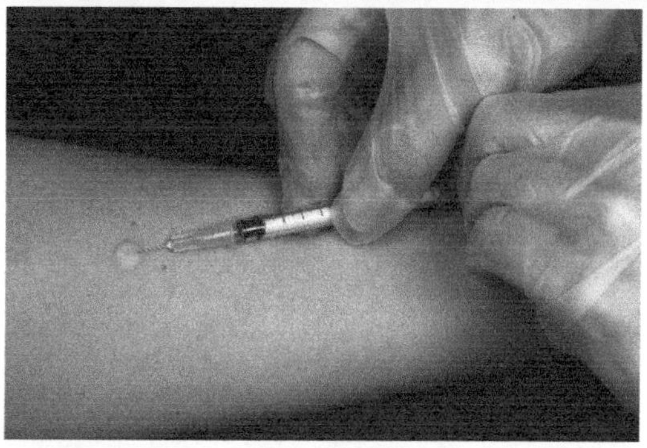

Procedure

- 5U of PPD is injected intradermally on flexor aspect of forearm
- Extent of induration is measured after 48-72 hours

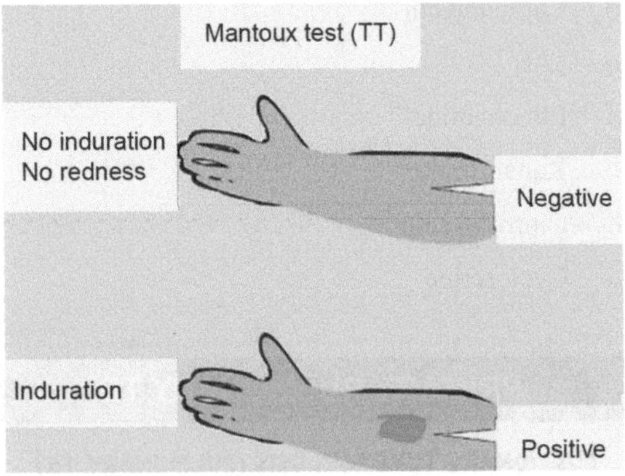

Interpretation of tuberculin test

- **0-4 mm:** Negative
- **5-9 mm:** Doubtful
- **10 mm or more:** Positive
- In HIV infected patients, 5 mm is considered positive

PULMONARY EMBOLISM

Features

- **MC and earliest manifestation:** Dyspnea
- **MC** sign is tachypnea

ECG findings

- S1Q3T3

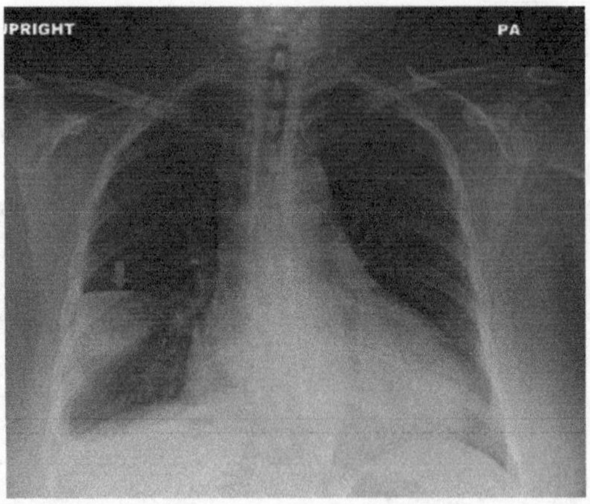

Signs seen on Chest X-ray

- Hampton's hump (Red arrow in X-ray)
- Westermark's sign

Plasma D-dimer ELISA level

- Elevated (> 90%)

Most specific test

- CT scan

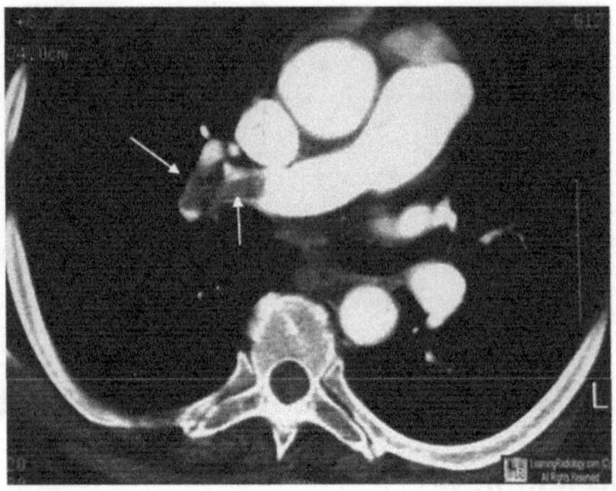

SECTION 2
SURGERY

Chapter 1

ARTERIAL & VENOUS DISORDERS

HEMANGIOMAS

Types

- Capillary (arises from capillaries)
- Cavernous (arises from veins)
- Plexiform (arises from arteries)

Capillary hemangioma

- Salmon patch
- Portwine stain
- Strawberry angioma

Strawberry angioma

- **Strawberry mark/hemangioma: Resolve** spontaneously (by intravascular thrombosis) by 7-8 years

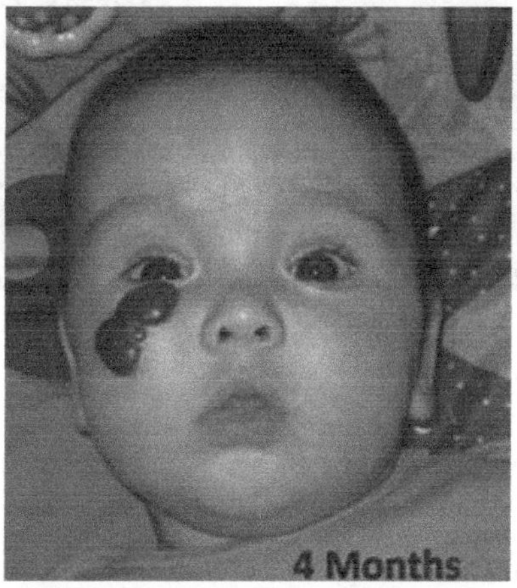

- MC hemangioma
- **NOT** present at birth
- Appears by 1-3 weeks
- It begins to disappear and completely in 7-8 years (70% in 7 years)

Portwine stain

- **Portwine stain/Naevus flammeus:** Persists
- Present at **birth**
- **Persists** throughout life without any change
- **No** spontaneous regression
- Commonly in head & neck
- May be associated with Sturge-Weber syndrome

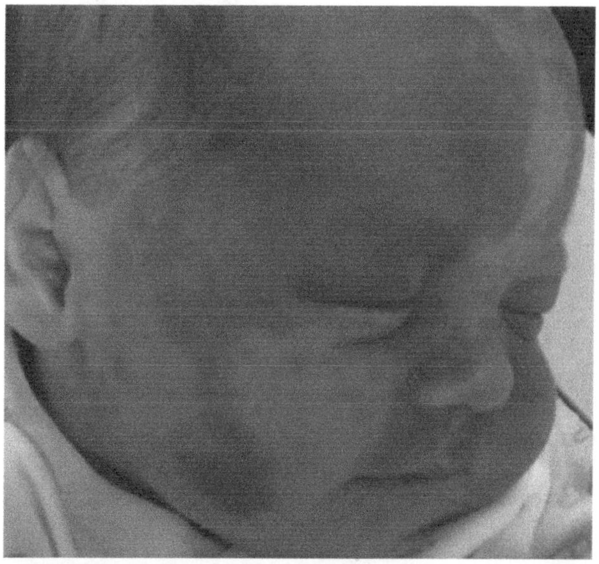

Sturge-Weber syndrome

- **Sturge-Weber syndrome/Encephalotrigeminal syndrome:** Associated with epilepsy, hemiplegia & mental retardation
- Capillary/cavernous hemangioma over face & ipsilateral cerebral hemisphere
- **First symptom:** Focal seizure (on opposite side of skin lesion)
- **Skull X-ray: Tram** track calcification/rail road track
- Hemangiomas + hemiplegia and Jacksonian epilepsy (calcified vascular cerebral and meningeal deposits) + glaucoma

ARTERIAL ANEURYSM

Types

- **True:** All the 3 layers of arterial wall in the wall of aneurysm
- **False:** Single layer of fibrous tissue as a wall of the sac and usually seen after trauma

Types of true aneurysm

- **Fusiform:** Most common, dilatation of entire circumference
- **Saccular:** Dilatation of a part of circumference
- **Dissecting:** Bleeding within the tunica media

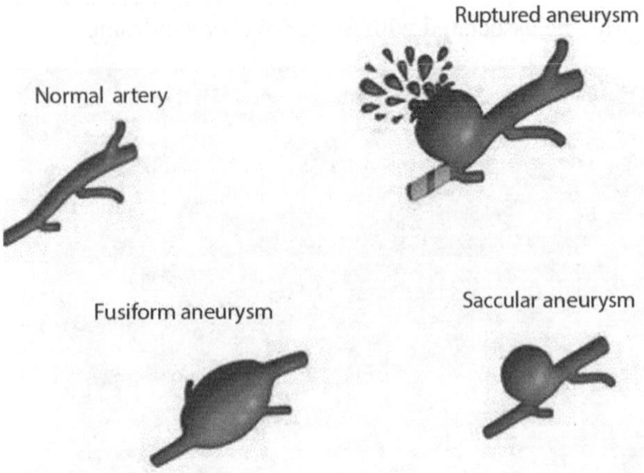

Causes

- Degenerative (atherosclerosis is MC cause)
- Traumatic
- Infective (syphilis, mycotic)
- Collagen diseases (Marfan's syndrome, PAN)

Clinical features

- Pulsatile swelling
- Smooth, soft, warm, compressible
- Thrill & bruit on auscultation
- Swelling reduces in size when pressed proximally

Sites

- **MC (most common) site of aneurysm:** Infrarenal part of abdominal aorta
- **Peripheral** aneurysm is MC in popliteal artery
- Rupture of intracranial saccular aneurysm is the **MC** cause of subarachnoid hemorrhage

Investigations for abdominal aneurysm

- Doppler USG (most widely used non-invasive test; effective screening tool)
- CT scan is more **precise** (investigation of choice as it gives more information regarding extent on sides/neck, size, dimensions, size and site of thrombus, calcification)

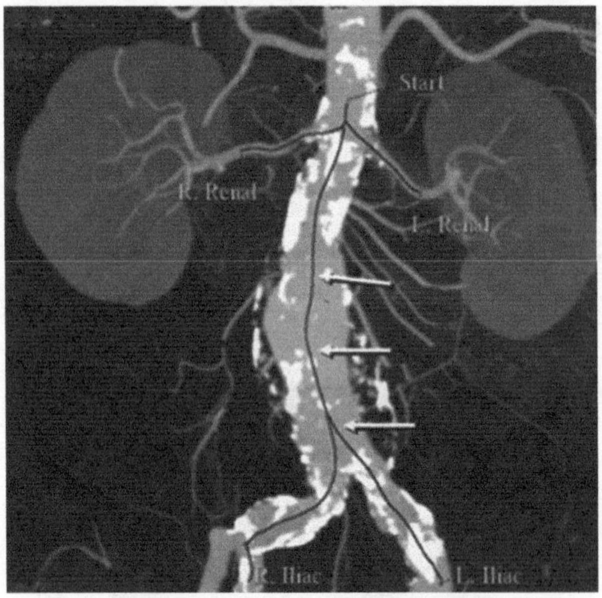

Complication

- **Abdominal aneurysm:** Rupture (commonly in retroperitoneal space)
- **Peripheral aneurysm:** Thrombosis

Treatment

- Aneurysmorrhaphy (excision of the aneurysm & its repair)

Cirsoid aneurysm

- **Cirsoid aneurysm commonly involves:** Superficial **temporal** artery
- Abnormal communication of arteries directly with distended veins (pulsatile swelling)
- Pulsating bag of worms
- Underlying bone thins out because of pressure
- Fall of hair over swelling
- Ligation of feeding artery & excision of the lesion is required

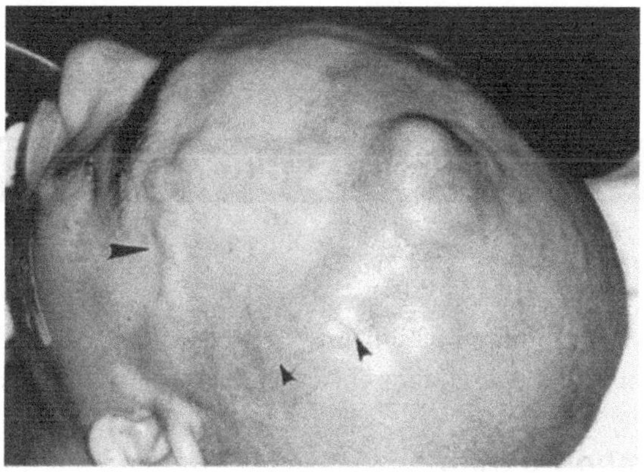

Mycotic aneurysm

- Most commonly caused by **Staphylococcus**
- The arterial wall is weakened

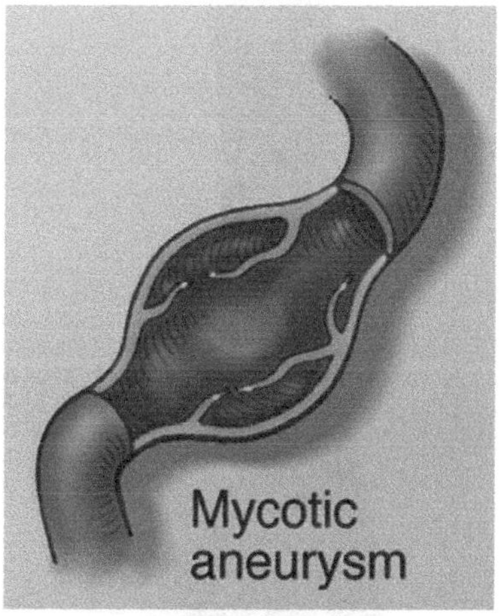

Pseudoaneurysm

- Follows **trauma**
- Actually, a hematoma

THROMBOANGIITIS OBLITERANS/ BUERGER'S DISEASE

Buerger's disease

- It is a vaso-occlusive disease of the small and medium size arteries and veins commonly affecting the lower limb of young male smoker
- **Smoking** is a strong contributory factor
- Medium & small size vessels (arteries & veins) are affected
- Segmental involvement of vessels

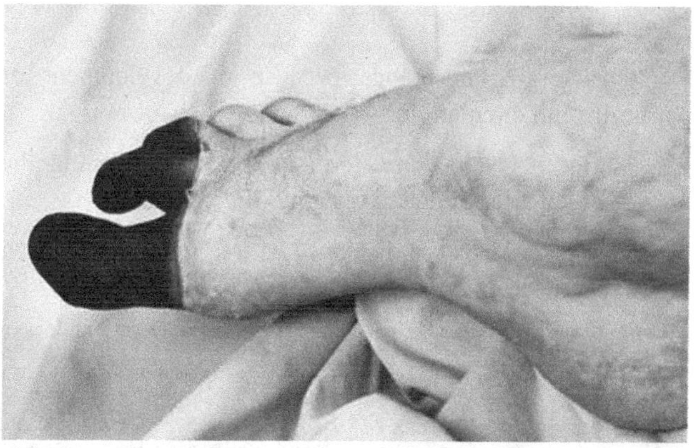

Clinical features

- Male smoker 20-30 years of **age**
- MC in lower limbs
- Migrating thrombophlebitis
- **First symptom:** Numbness and coldness in feet/toes

Other features of arterial occlusion

- Intermittent claudication
- Rest pain
- Colour changes
- Ulceration
- Gangrene

Investigations

- Doppler USG
- Low ankle pressure index is low (ankle Systolic Blood Pressure/arm SBP; normally >1)

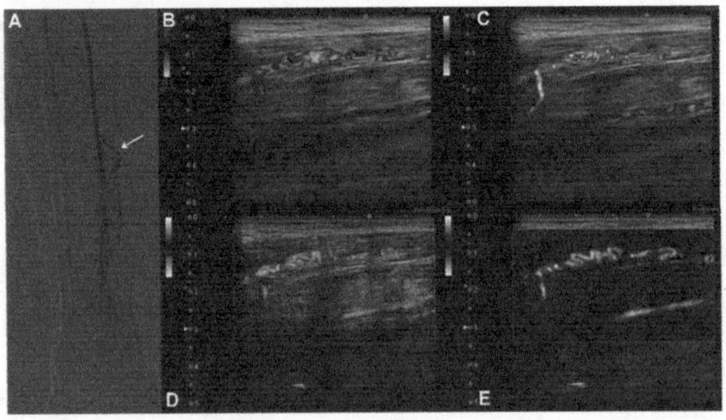

Arteriography

- Multiple occluded segments in small & medium sized arteries
- **Corkscrew** appearance because of development of collateral circulation
- Martorell's sign (fine, tortuous vessels, replacing the diseased arteries due to opening of collaterals)
- Fine **collaterals** are displayed as tree root or spider leg appearance on arteriography

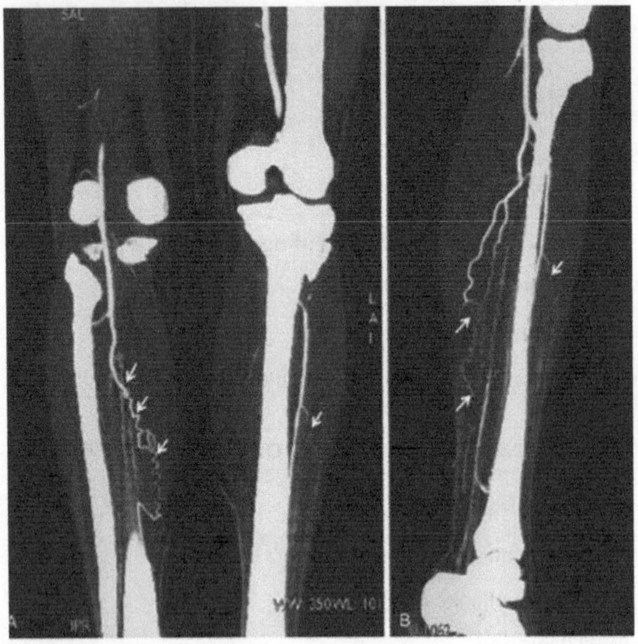

Management

- Stop smoking
- **Relief of pain:** Vasodilators (phentolamine/phenoxybenzamine), pentoxyfylline, xanthinol nicotinate, analgesic, paravertebral or common peroneal nerve block

Lumbar sympathectomy done if

- Rest pain
- Ischemic ulceration not responding to conservative treatment
- Preserve **L1** (otherwise dry ejaculation may occur)

Amputation

- If the lumbar sympathectomy fail to heal the ulcers and gangrenous lesions of the limb
- Omentopexy
- Arteriovenous/AV fistula (between popliteal artery & popliteal vein)

DEEP VENOUS THROMBOSIS

DVT

- Venous thrombi are mainly composed of RBC & fibrin whereas arterial thrombi are mainly formed of platelets

Virchow's triad

- Stasis of blood
- Trousseau's sign (hypercoagulability of blood)
- Changes in endothelial lining of vessel wall

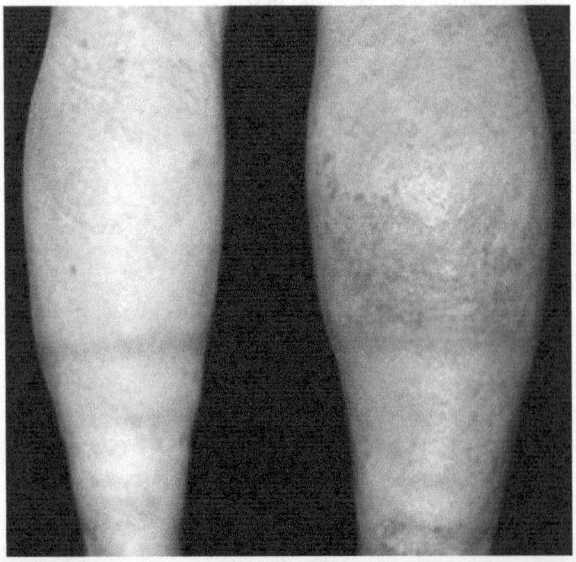

Phlegmasia

- **Phlegmasia alba dolens/white leg:** Deep femoral vein thrombosis associated with lymphangitis
- **Phlegmasia caerulea dolens/blue leg:** Extensive DVT of iliac & pelvic veins

Features

- **MC site:** Calf veins
- **Earliest sign of DVT:** Rise in temperature
- **Clinical presentation:**
  - o Unilateral leg swelling
  - o Local warmth
  - o Erythema
  - o Pain
- **Homans sign in DVT:** Forced dorsiflexion of foot causes calf pain

Investigations

- Contrast phlebography (gold standard)
- Fibrinogen uptake test
- **Duplex USG (image below):**
  - o Investigation of **choice**
  - o Allows accurate visualization of deep vein
  - o Make a positive diagnosis of DVT

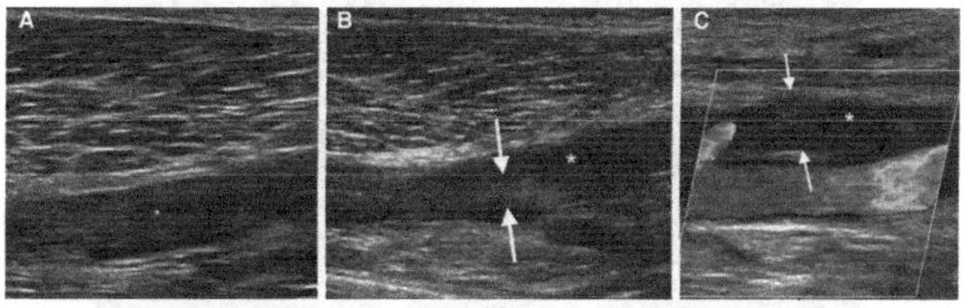

Management

- Bed rest
- Anticoagulation (Heparin/warfarin)
  - o **LMW Heparin:** Decreased dosing schedule & less risk of heparin induced thrombocytopenia
- Aspirin
- Calf length pneumatic compression devices
- Thrombolytic therapy (streptokinase/urokinase)
- Operative thrombectomy

VARICOSE VEINS

2 types

- **Primary varicose veins:** Incompetent valve in superficial system alone; may be inherited
- **Secondary varicose veins:** Incompetent communicating and deep veins of the leg

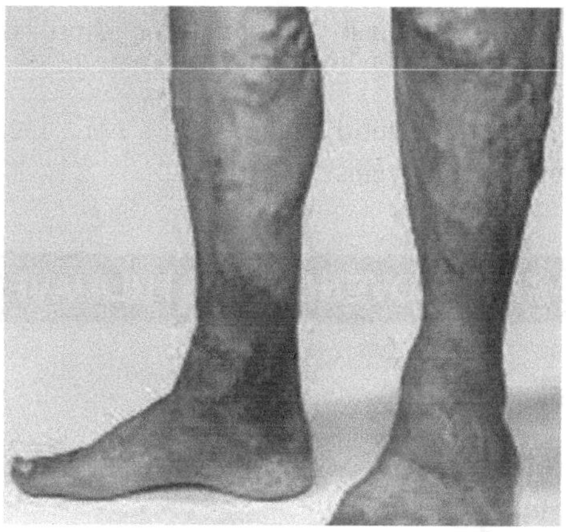

Features

- Varicose veins are dilated, tortuous superficial veins
- MC site is leg
- **Test to demonstrate saphenofemoral incompetence:**
  - o Brodie-Trendelenburg I test
  - o Trendelenberg II for perforator incompetence

Gold standard investigation

- Duplex imaging

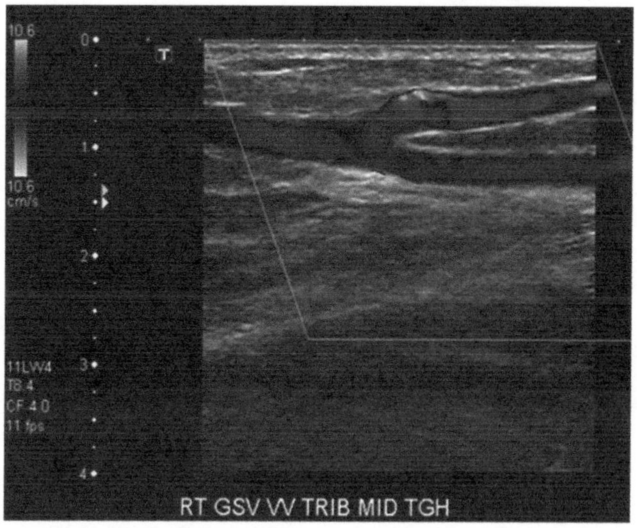

Management

- **Palliative:** Elastic stockings/bandage
- **Sclerosant injection:** 5% Ethanolamine oleate (injection given to promote thrombosis and sclerosis of veins)
- **Surgery:**
  - o **Saphenofemoral flush ligation:** For long saphenous varicosity
  - o **Popliteal flush ligation:** For short saphenous varicosity
- **Cockett & Dodd operation:** For incompetent communicating veins

ARTERIOVENOUS FISTULA/AVF

Types

- **Acquired:** Usually progressive; because of penetrating injuries
- **Congenital:** Stationary

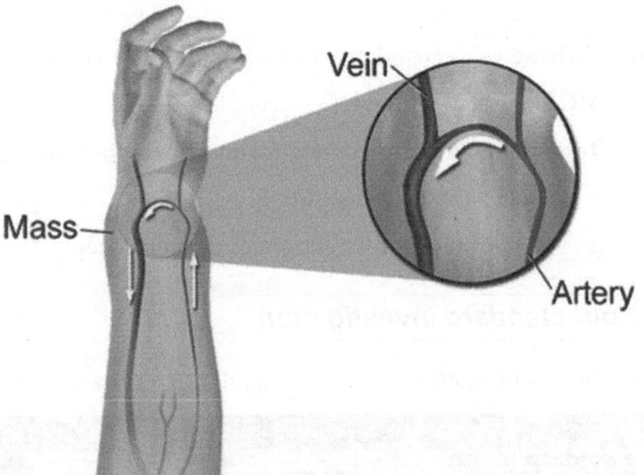

Arteriovenous Fistula

Features

- Communication between an artery and a vein
- Veins become arterialized (dilated, tortuous & thick) because of excessive blood flow through them
- AV fistula **increases** pulse rate, cardiac output leading to high output cardiac failure
- Pulsatile swelling
- **Palpation:** Thrill
- **Auscultation:** Continuous bruit
- **Physiological effects of AVF:**
  - o Enhanced venous return & increased cardiac output
  - o May cause overgrowth of limb later (if in young) etc.
- **Nicoladoni/Branham sign:**
  - o Pressure on the artery proximal to fistula causes
  - o Swelling to reduce in size, a thrill/bruit to cease
  - o Fall in pulse rate & pulse pressure returns to normal

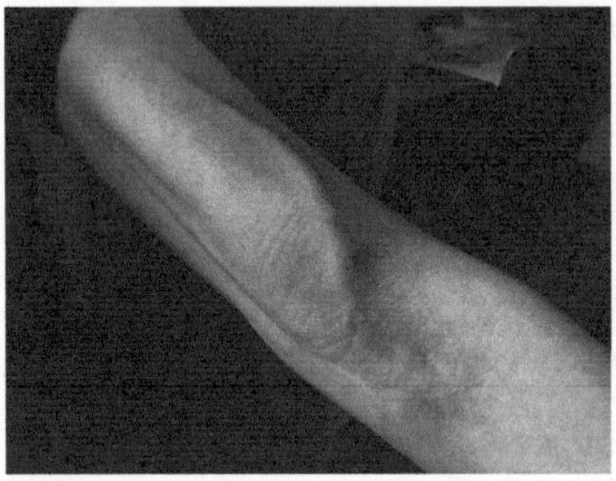

Investigation

- Arteriography confirms the lesion

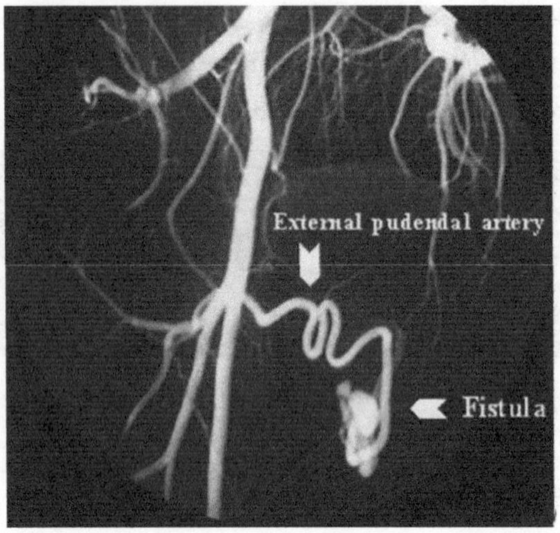

Management

- Acquired lesion is progressive so need operation
- Vessels separated & repaired
- **Quadruple ligation:** Ligating the involved artery & vein above and below the lesion

Chapter 2

WOUND HEALING & TISSUE REPAIR

WOUNDS

Surgical classification of wounds

- **Clean wound:**
  - o Infection rate less than 2%
  - o **Examples:**
    - ♦ Herniorrhaphy
    - ♦ Excisions
    - ♦ Surgeries of the brain, joints, heart transplant
- **Clean contaminated wound:**
  - o Infective rate is around 10%
  - o **Examples:**
    - ♦ Appendicectomy
    - ♦ Bowel surgeries
    - ♦ Gallbladder, biliary & pancreatic surgeries
- **Contaminated wound:**
  - o Infective rate is 15 – 30%
  - o **Examples:**
    - ♦ Open fresh accidental wounds
    - ♦ Acute abdominal conditions
- **Dirty infected wound:**
  - o Infective rate is 40 – 70%
  - o **Examples:**
    - ♦ Abscess drainage
    - ♦ Pyocele
    - ♦ Empyema gallbladder
    - ♦ Faecal peritonitis

WOUND HEALING

Healing by primary/1st intention

- Closed wounds
- Edges approximated
- **Example:** Clean skin incision closed with sutures
- Clean cut wound with edges approximated, no infection

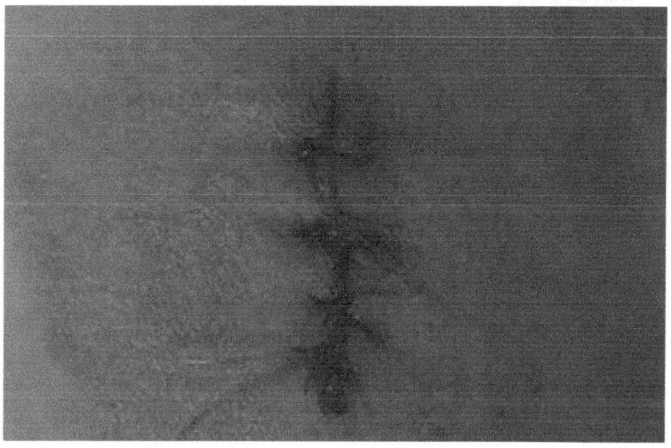

Healing by secondary intention

- Wound is infected, edges not approximated properly and significant tissue loss is present

- Slow healing
- More scar formation

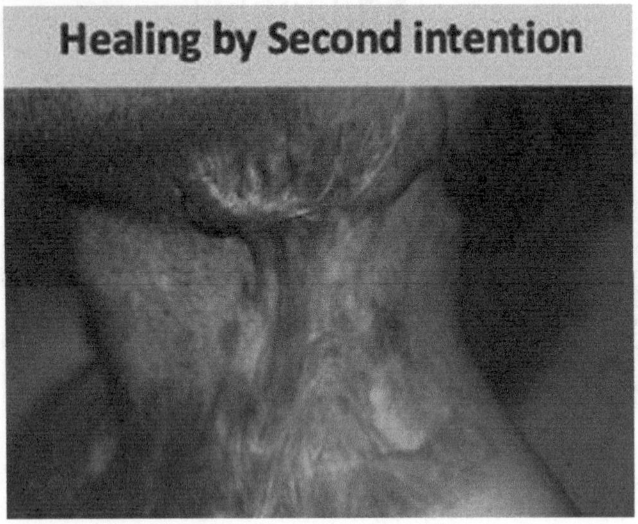

Factors delaying wound healing

- Vitamin C deficiency
- Deficiency of trace metals (zinc, copper etc.)
- Absence of oxygen (reduced perfusion)
- Presence of vitamin E (inhibitory role)
- Anemia
- Infection etc.

KELOID

Features

- MC site is sternum
- May spread into normal tissue not affected by injury
- True keloid continues to get worse even after a year
- May be familial
- Rarely subsides
- Recurrence is common
- May turn malignant
- **Appears after:** Appears after few days of surgery
- Recurrence is common after excision and resuture
- **Treatment:**
    - o Treatment is difficult
    - o Shaving away the excess tissue, avoiding incision into normal skin & thin skin graft
    - o Intralesional steroid

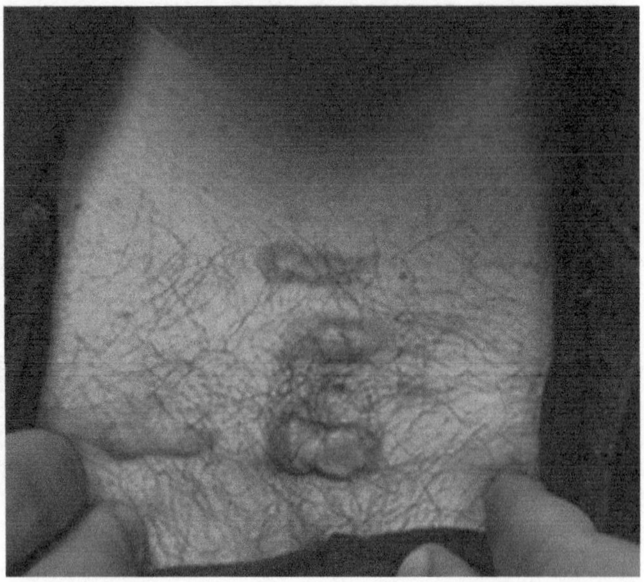

SUTURES

Types

- **Absorbable sutures:**
    - o Catgut
    - o Dexon (polyglycolic acid)
- **Non absorbable sutures:**
    - o Prolene
    - o Silk

SKIN GRAFTS

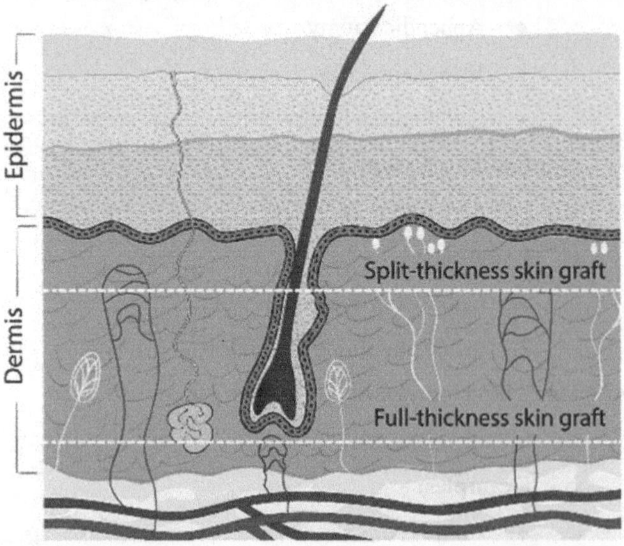

Partial thickness (Thiersch) graft

- Contains epidermis + upper capillary dermis
- Vascularized by ingrowth of capillaries from underlying tissue

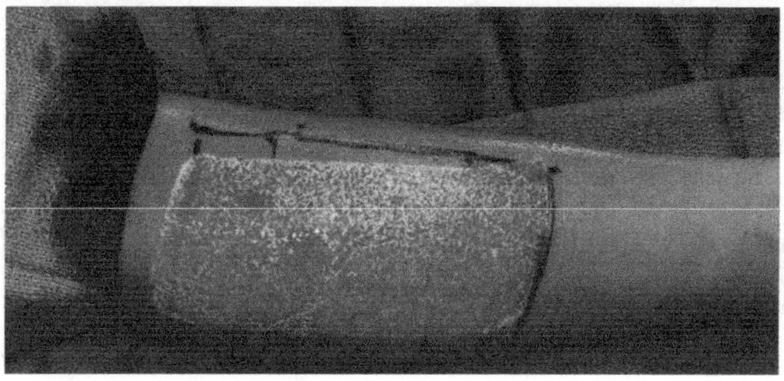

Full thickness (Wolfe) graft

- Contains epidermis + whole of dermis
- Has normal skin texture and reduced tendency of contracture
- 'Take' is also reduced
- Can be taken from areas of thin skin (ear, upper eyelid or scalp)

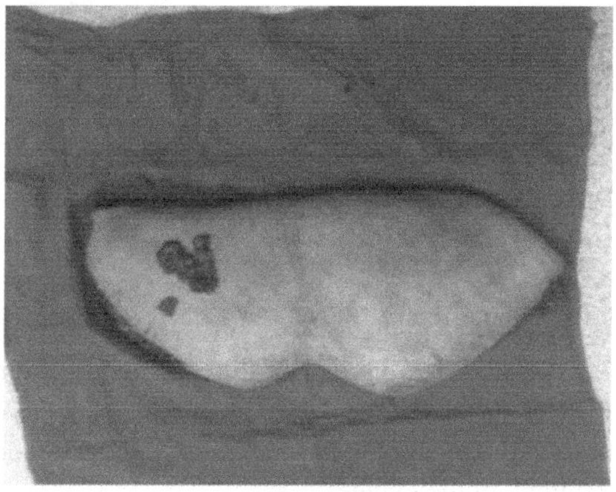

Figure: Full thickness from the back

Fasciocutaneous flap

- Inclusion of deep fascia into a cutaneous flap allows greater extension and mobility of the graft

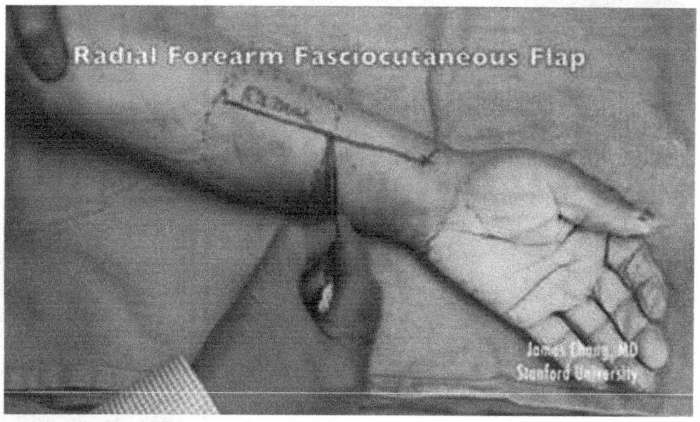

Myocutaneous flap

- Muscle with overlying skin is of special value in covering bare bone (latissimus dorsi myocutaneous flap)

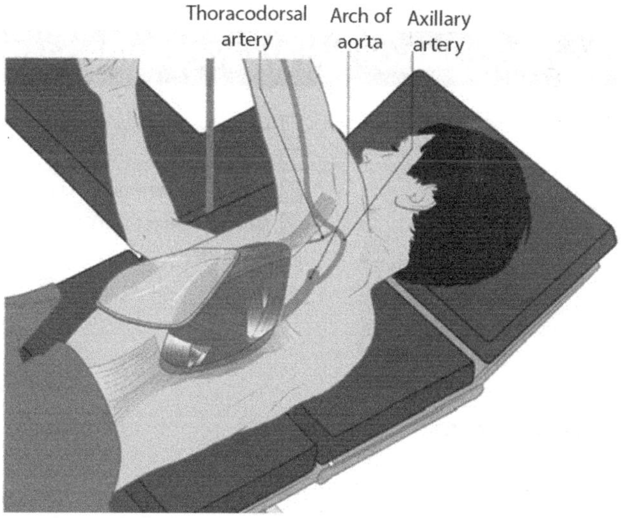

Microvascular free flap

- Free skin flap based on a neurovascular bundle is re-anastomosed by microvascular surgery to a donor pedicle in another area of body

Composite grafts

- Consist of skin & some underlying tissue (fat, cartilage etc.)

SECTION 2

SURGERY

Chapter 3

SALIVARY GLANDS

ANATOMY OF SALIVARY GLANDS

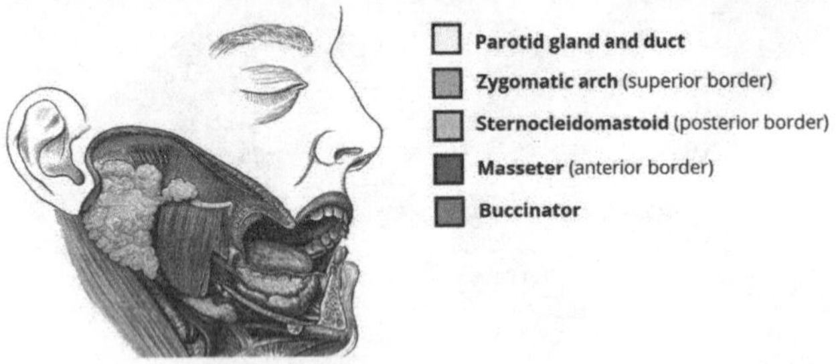

Parotid gland

- **Largest** of all salivary glands
- Para means around & Otis means ear
- It is situated between the ramus of mandible and sternocleidomastoid muscle
- **Parts:**
  - o Superficial part (80%)
  - o Deep part (20%)
- **Parotid duct: Stensen's** duct emerges from the anterior surface of the gland, runs over the surface of masseter, passes through buccinator muscle and opens into the oral mucosa opposite to the crown of upper second molar tooth
- **Nerve supply:**
  - o Parasympathetic is secretomotor from **auriculo-temporal** nerve
  - o Sympathetic is vasomotor from plexus around the external carotid artery

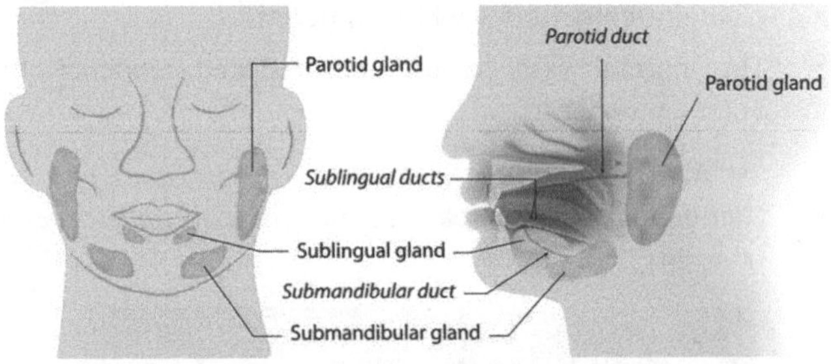

Submandibular gland

- J shaped salivary gland
- Situated in the anterior part of digastric triangle
- **Parts:** Superficial & deep
- Submandibular (**Wharton's**) duct emerges from the anterior surface of the deep part of the gland, enters the floor of the mouth, on the summit of papilla besides the frenulum of the tongue

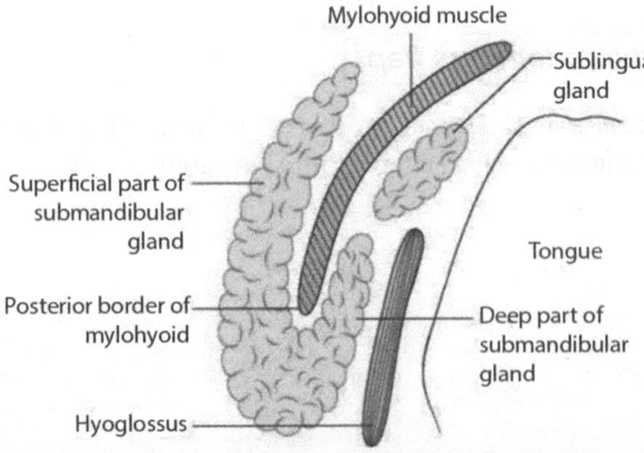

Minor salivary glands

- 450 minor salivary glands which are distributed in lips, cheeks, palate and floor of the mouth
- They may also be present in oropharynx, larynx, trachea and paranasal sinuses

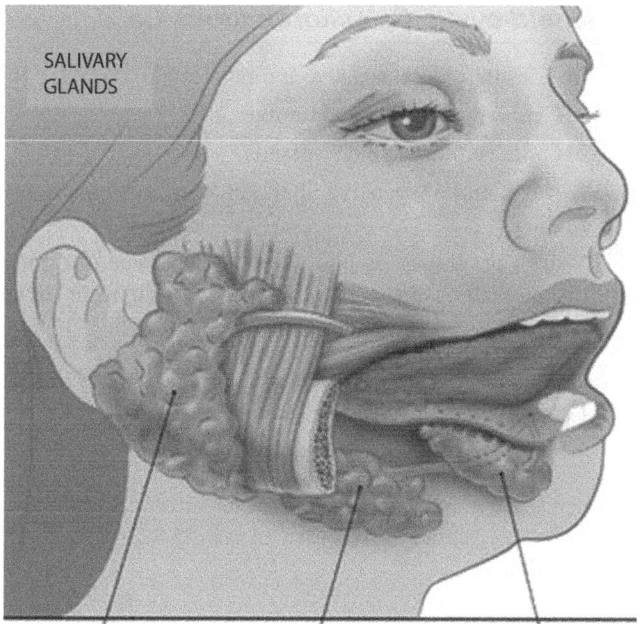

- **Sublingual glands:**
  - o One on each side
  - o Located in the anterior aspect of the floor of mouth
  - o Gland opens directly into mucosa or through a duct which drains into submandibular duct
  - o This duct is called **Bartholin** duct
- Minor salivary glands are not present in gingivae and anterior portion of hard palate

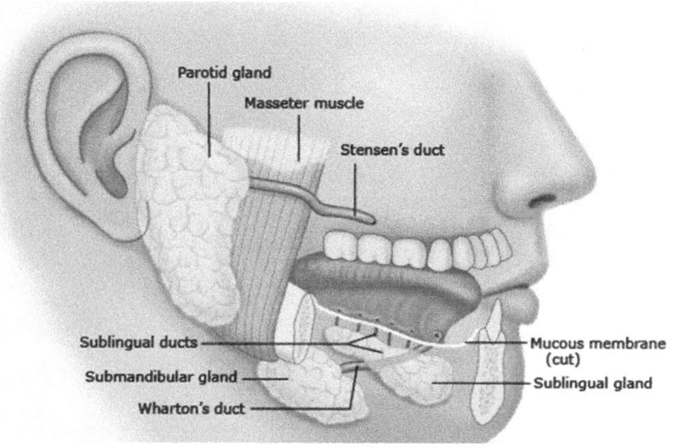

TUMOURS OF SALIVARY GLAND

Pleomorphic adenoma/Mixed salivary tumour

- **Most common** of the salivary gland tumours in adult (80%)
- **MC** (most common) tumor of parotid (80%)
- Mixed parotid tumor (Cartilage + epithelial cells)
- **MC** in females
- Usually present as solitary mass
- Firm, lobulated, painless swelling over parotid region
- Free from skin & deeper tissues (masseter)
- **No** involvement of facial nerve
- Superficial lobe is usually involved
- **MC** malignancy developing in pleomorphic adenoma is adenocarcinoma (otherwise in a normal parotid, it is mucoepidemroid Ca)
- **Malignant transformation (seen in 2-10%) is suggested if:**
  - o Feels stony hard
  - o Facial nerve is involved
  - o Fixed to skin or deeper tissue
  - o Swelling grows rapidly
  - o Becomes painful
  - o Involvement of cervical lymph nodes
- Diagnosis is made by needle **biopsy** (per oral route)

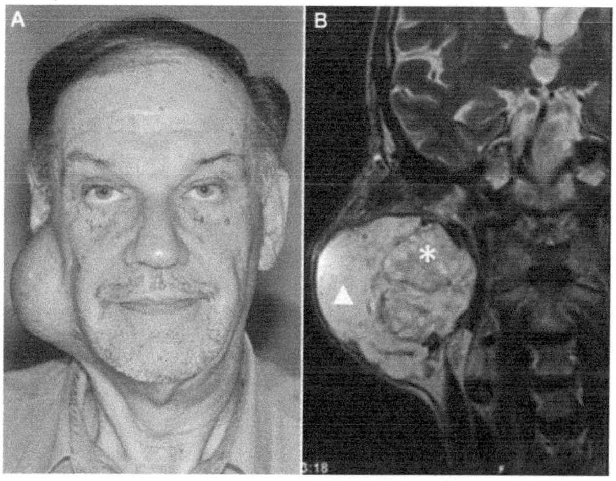

- **MC benign parotid gland tumour:** Pleomorphic adenoma (MC benign tumour of major & minor salivary glands)

- **Treatment of pleomorphic adenoma:** Superficial parotidectomy (**Patey's** operation)
- Surgical procedure done is superficial/partial parotidectomy with conservation of facial nerve

Warthin's tumour (adenolymphoma/papillary cystadenolymphomatosum)

- **It consists of:** Epithelial & lymphoid elements (adenolymphoma)
- **Exclusively** located in parotid
- **Only** tumour to produce hot spot with Tc^{99}
- Benign neoplasm of parotid
- 10% cases are bilateral
- Produces a hot spot in Tc-99 pertechnetate scan, so a **clean-cut** diagnosis can be made preoperatively without need of biopsy
- Partial parotidectomy with conservation of facial nerve
- **Treatment of Warthin's tumour: Superficial** parotidectomy

Adenoid cystic Ca/cylidromatous Ca

- Invades Perineural space & lymphatics
- **MC** minor salivary gland tumour
- **MC** site is minor salivary glands
- Always more extensive than on clinical signs/X-ray findings
- **Worst** prognosis as the tumour infiltrates for long distance along the perineural spaces of adjacent nerve and may invade medullary bone

SECTION 2
SURGERY

Chapter 4

BREAST

BREAST

Anatomy

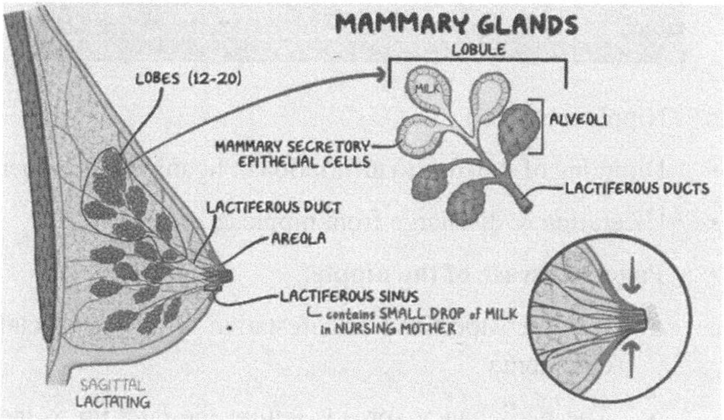

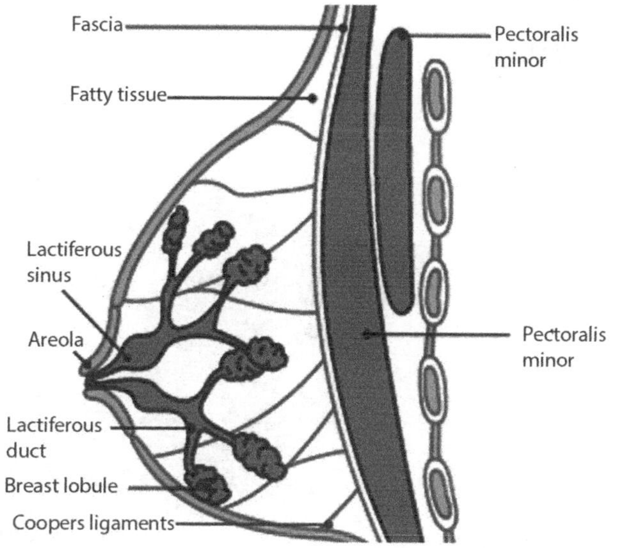

- Modified sweat gland
- Derived from ectoderm
- Extends from 2nd to 6th rib in the midclavicular line & lies over pectoralis major, serratus anterior and external oblique muscle
- Horizontally it extends from side of sternum to the mid-axillary line
- **Axillary tail of Spence:** Prolongation from the outer part of the gland which passes up to the level of the 3rd rib in the axilla through a defect in deep fascia, where it is in direct contact with the main lymph node of the breasts (anterior axillary lymph node)
- **Ligament of Cooper:** Breast is anchored to the underlying skin and to the underlying pectoral fascia by bands of connective tissue called ligament of Cooper
- **Lymphatic drainage:**
  - **Axillary LN (lymph nodes): 75%**
    - **Anterior group (Pectoral, external mammary) lies along lateral thoracic vessels:** Main
    - **Central group:** Next common node. Easily palpable during clinical examination
    - **Posterior (subscapular):** Rare to be involved in tumour
    - **Lateral group:** Lies along axillary vein; rarely involved in tumour
    - Apical
  - Later they drain into supraclvicular lymph nodes
  - 25% drains mainly from the medial half of the breast into 2nd to 4th intercostal space internal mammary LN

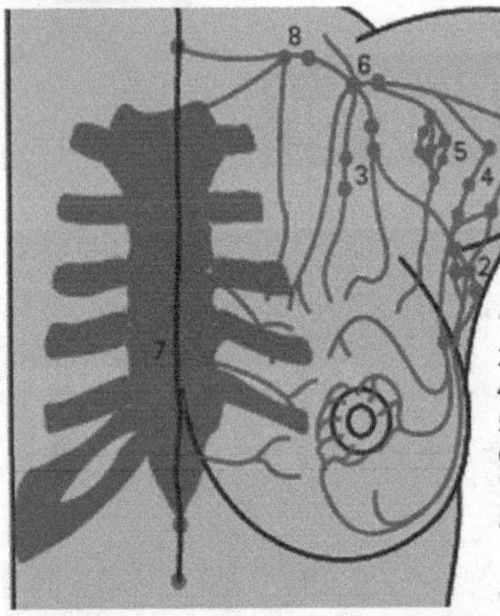

CARCINOMA BREAST

Aetiology

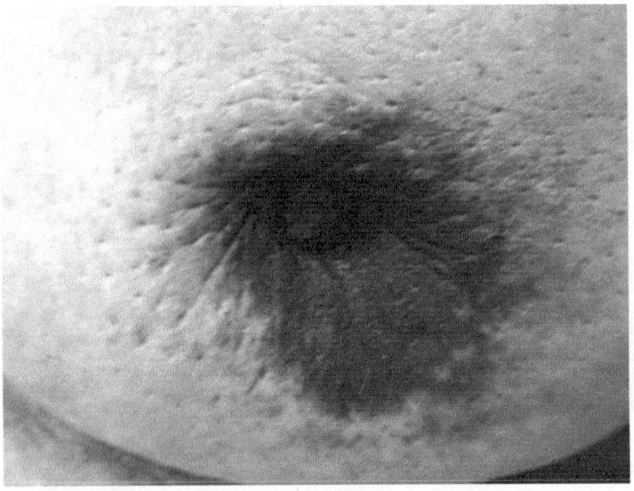

- More common in developed Western world
- **Risk factors for breast Ca:**
  - o Positive family history
  - o Nullipara
  - o Attaining early menarche and late menopause have high-risk
  - o Early child-bearing & breastfeeding reduces the risk
  - o Obese
  - o Benign breast disease with atypia, hyperplasia and epitheliosis has got higher risk
  - o MC in individuals who are on oral contraceptive pills & hormone replacement therapy for more than 5 years
- **BRCA:**
  - o **BRCA 1:** 17q (long arm of chromosome 17)
  - o **BRCA 2:** 13q (long arm of chromosome 13)

Features

- **MC site:** Upper outer quadrant
- **Peau'd orange:**
  - o Due to obstruction of dermal lymphatics, opening of the sebaceous glands & hair follicles get buried in the oedema giving rise to orange peel appearance

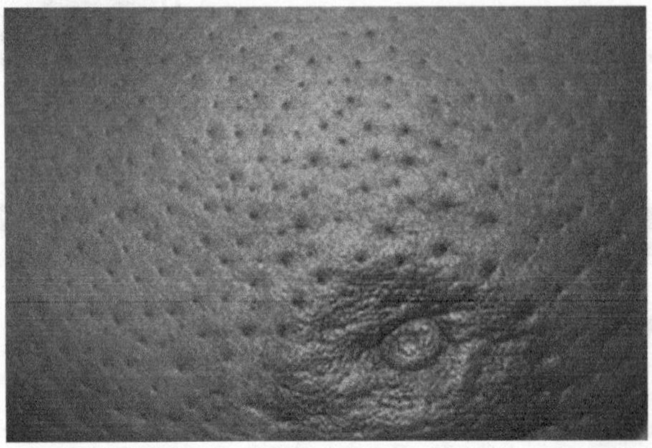

- Nipple retraction
- Dimpling of skin due to infiltration of ligament of Cooper
- Ulceration & discharge from nipple & areola
- **Paget's disease of the nipple:**
  - o It is the superficial manifestation of an intraductal carcinoma
  - o The malignancy spreads within the duct up to the skin of the nipple and down into the substance of the breast
  - o It **mimics** eczema of nipple and areola

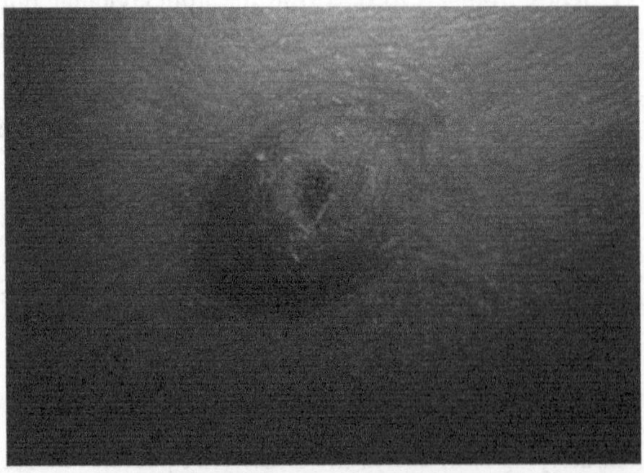

Early Paget's disease

Investigations

- Breast Imaging Reporting & Data System for mammographic findings (**BIRADS** grading)
- **Triple examination (PCR):**
  - o **P**athological examination
  - o **C**linical examination
  - o **R**adiological examination
- **MRI:**
  - o Screening of breast carcinoma in high-risk cases
- **Mammography**:
  - o Used for screening in old age
  - o Carries risk of radiation so not used in reproductive age group

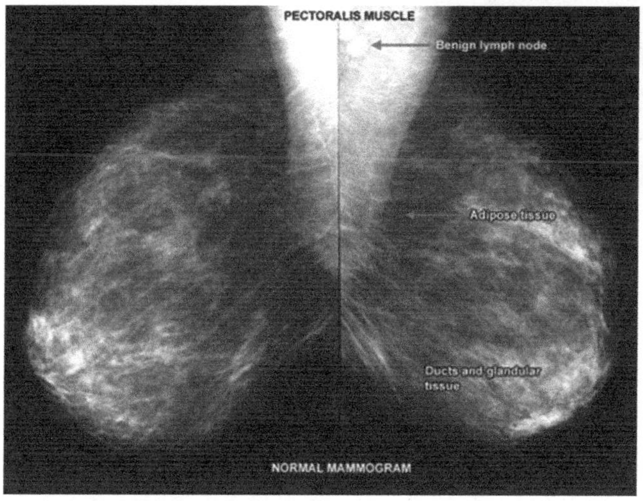

- Best prognostic factor is status of Lymph nodes
- **Sentinel lymph node biopsy/SLNB:**
  - o The first axillary LN draining the breast (by direct drainage) is designated as the SLN
  - o SLN is the first node involved by tumours cells and presence or absence of its histological involvement, when assessed will give a predictive idea about the further spread of tumour into other nodes
  - o It is **done** in all cases of early breast cancers, T1 and T2 without clinically palpable nodes
  - o It is **not** done in clinically palpable axillary nodes as there is already distortion of lymphatic flow due to tumour
  - o The incidence of involvement of other nodes without SLN is less than 3% and so if SLNB is negative, nodal dissection can be avoided but needs regular follow-up

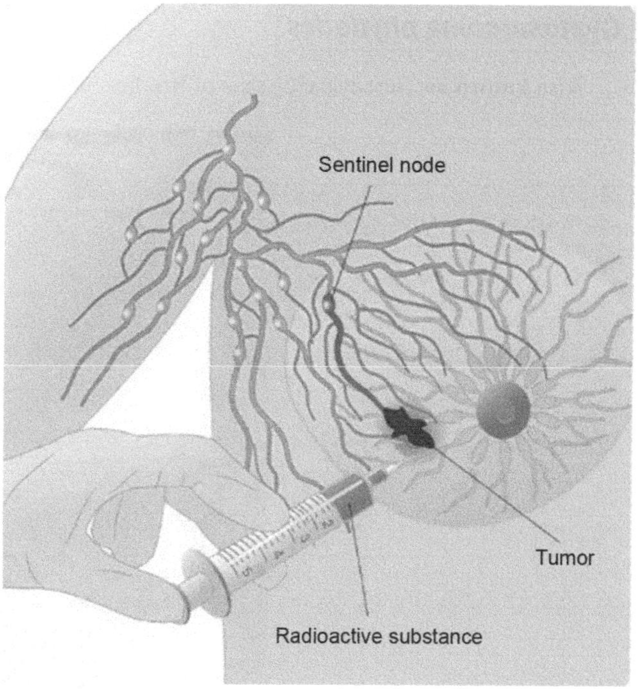

Management

- **Treatment of Estrogen receptor positive (ER+) in a pre-menopausal woman:** Tamoxifen (Tamoxifen increases risk of uterine Ca)
- **Management of stage I & II of breast Ca:** Lumpectomy/ breast conservative therapy + axillary clearance + radiotherapy

OTHER CONDITIONS OF BREAST

Mondor's disease

- Spontaneous thrombophlebitis of the superficial veins of the breast and anterior chest wall

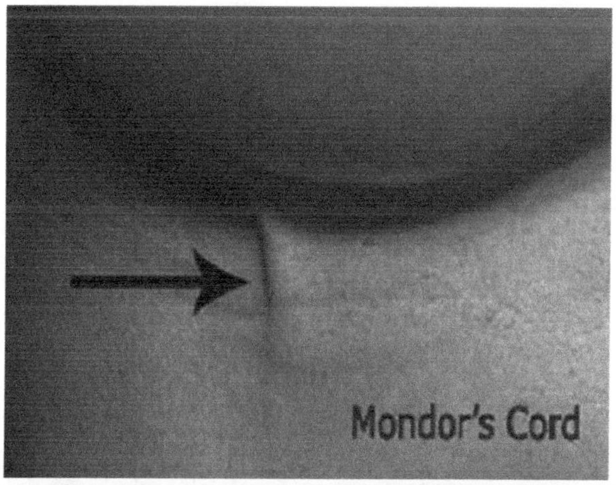

Cystosarcoma phyllodes

- **Also known as:** Serocystic disease of Brodie
- They show a wide spectrum of activity, varying from almost a benign condition (85%) to a locally aggressive and sometimes metastatic tumour (15%)

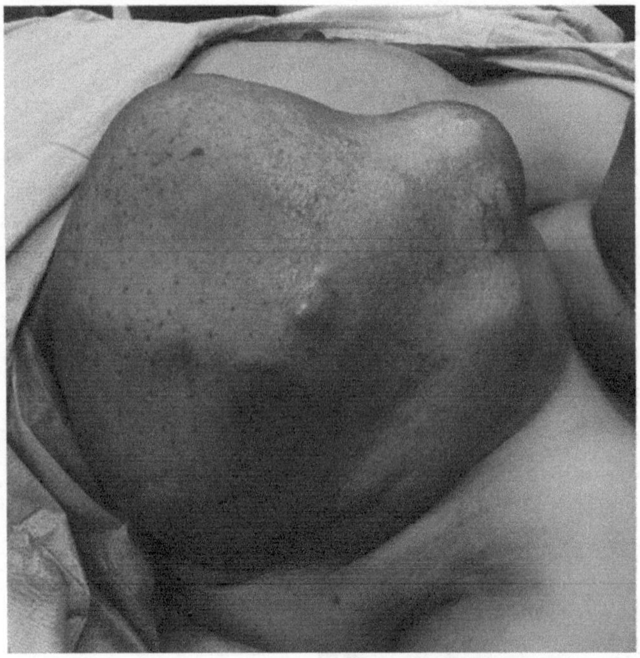

SECTION 2

SURGERY

Chapter 5

NECK

CERVICAL RIB

Pathology

- It is an extension of costal element (anterior part) of transverse process of **C7** vertebrae more than 2.5 cm (normal)
- The resultant **syndrome** is called as cervical rib syndrome, thoracic inlet syndrome, thoracic outlet syndrome, scalene syndrome
- More **common** in females, usually on the right side
- **Cervical rib can cause:**
  - Constriction of the subclavian **artery** (ischemia in the hand & forearm)
  - Compression of **C8 & T1** causes tingling & numbness along its distribution, i.e., in the little finger, medial side of hand & forearm

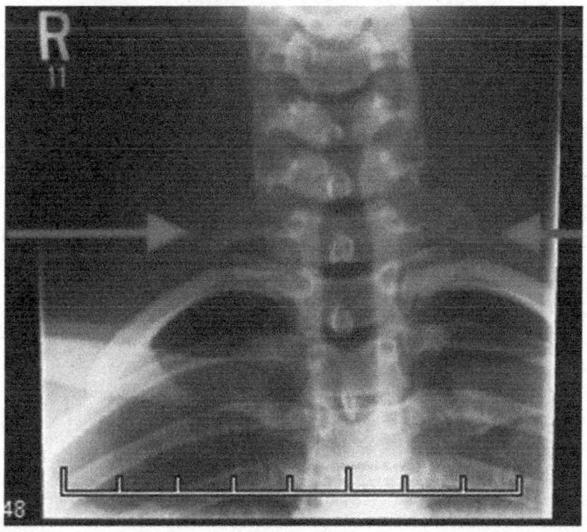

Features

- **Majority** of the patients are asymptomatic (80%)
- **Vascular manifestations:**
  - Pain (due to ischemia of muscle)
  - Upper limb claudication
  - Positive Adson's test
  - Allen's test
- **Neurological features:**
  - Pain on the medial side, weakness of the medial side of hand
  - Positive Card test for weakness of interossei muscles
  - Positive Froment's sign to detect weakness of adductor pollicis muscle

CYSTIC HYGROMA

Origin

- It is a cystic swelling due to sequestration of a portion of jugular lymph sac from lymphatic system, during the development period in utero
- Fluid filled lesions of lymphatic origin (**lymphangioma**)
- In posterior triangle of neck

Associated with

- Turner's syndrome
- Trisomies

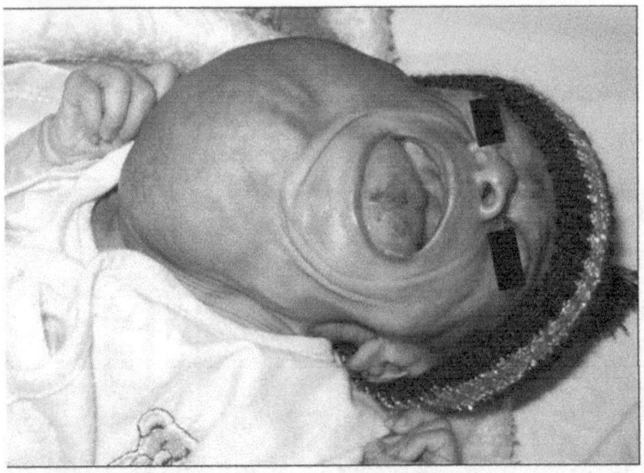

Clinical findings

- Brilliantly **translucent**
- Cough impulse is **positive** (during crying the swelling size increases)

Management

- Excision is the treatment of **choice**

BRANCHIAL CYST

Features

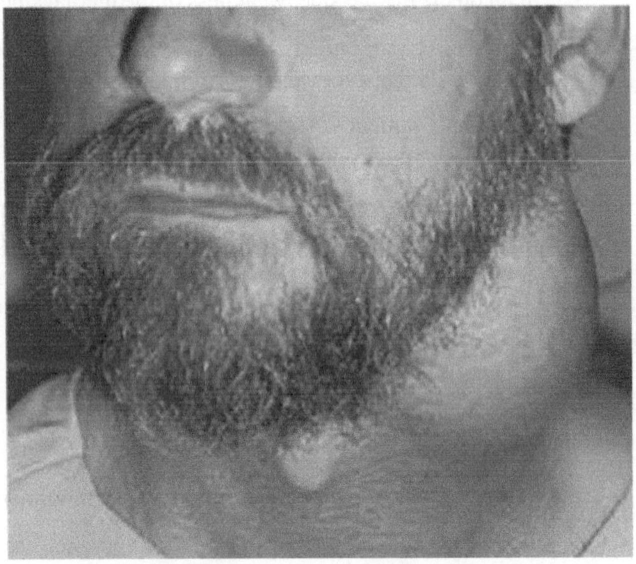

- It arises from the remnants of **second** branchial cleft
- Normally 2nd to 4th clefts disappear to form a smooth neck
- Persistent 2nd cleft is called cervical **sinus** of His which eventually gets sequestrated to form a branchial cyst
- It is located in **upper** part of neck, beneath the anterior border of the upper third of sternocleidomastoid muscle
- Cyst wall is made up of lymphoid tissue
- Histologically it is lined by squamous epithelium

THYROGLOSSAL CYST

Features

- It is a swelling occurring in the neck in any part along the **line** of thyroglossal tract
- Beneath the hyoid **commonly** (subhyoid)
- Occupies the **midline**, towards the left
- Swelling moves upwards on **protrusion** of the tongue
- Also moves on **swallowing**
- Patient is asked to open the mouth and keep the lower jaw still
- Examiner holds the cyst between the thumb and forefinger. When the patient is asked to protrude the tongue, a '**tugging** sensation' can be felt
- Papillary Ca of thyroid may develop in thyroglossal cyst (1%)
- Sistrunk's operation is done
- Infection of thyroglossal cyst which burst opens or after inadequate removal of the cyst leads to the formation of thyroglossal **fistula**

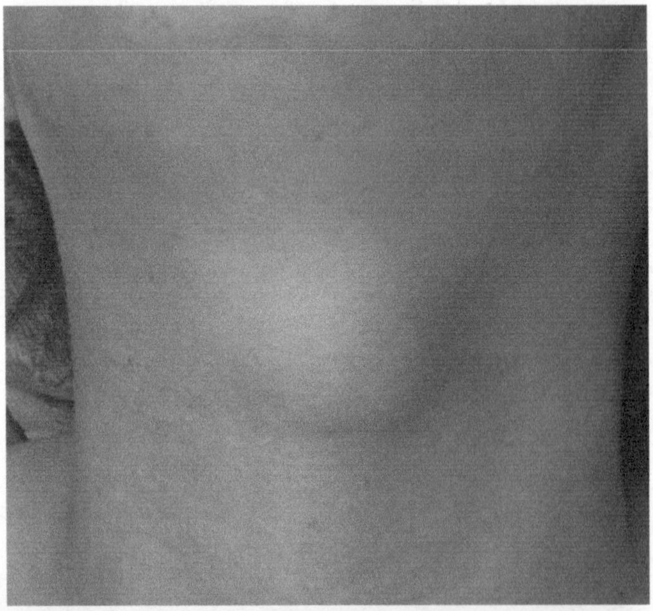

SECTION 2

SURGERY

Chapter 6

THYROID

RELEVANT ANATOMY AND PHYSIOLOGY

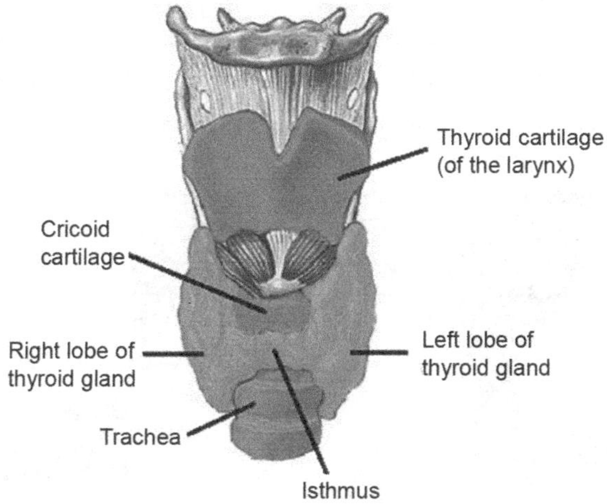

Anatomy

- **Weight:** 20 grams
- **Extent:** C5 to T1 vertebrae
- Located in anterior triangle of neck
- **Parts:**
  - o Right & left lateral lobes
  - o Isthmus connects the two lateral lobes in midline extending from 2nd to 4th tracheal rings
- **Blood supply:**
  - o Superior thyroid artery (branch of external carotid artery)

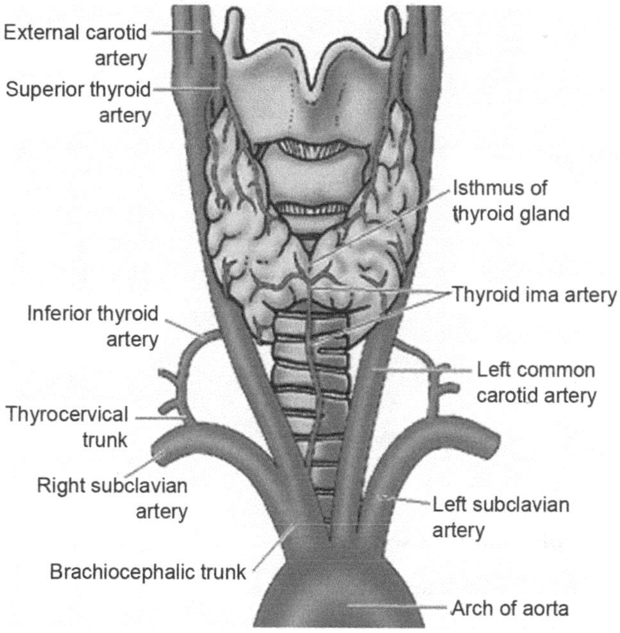

  - o Inferior thyroid artery (branch of thyrocervical trunk)
  - o Thyroidea **ima** artery (branch of aorta or brachiocephalic artery)
- **Venous drainage:**
  - o Superior thyroid vein
  - o Middle thyroid vein drains into internal jugular vein
  - o Inferior thyroid vein
  - o **Kocher's** vein

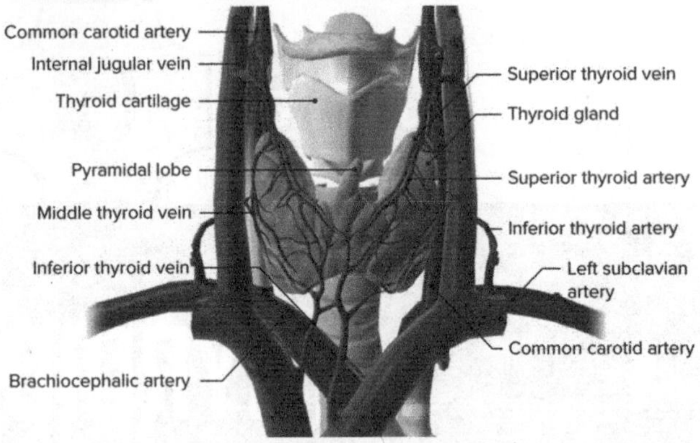

Hormones secreted by thyroid

- Thyroid gland has **two** secretory cells

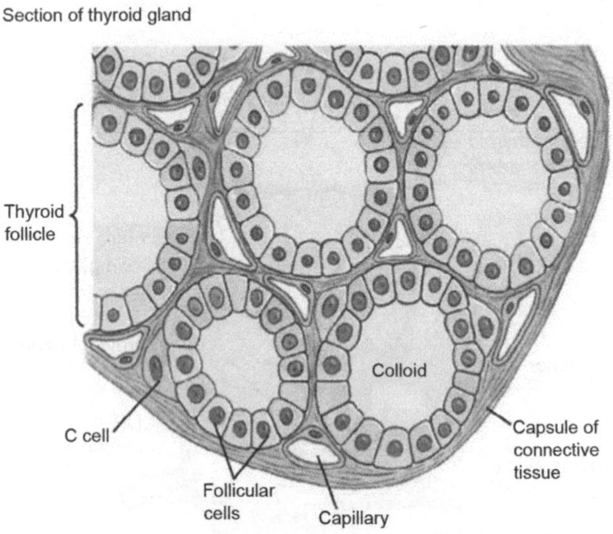

- **Follicular cells secrete:**
  - o T_3 (Tri-iodo-thyronine)
  - o T_4 (Thyroxine)
- Parafollicular/C cells secretes calcitonin

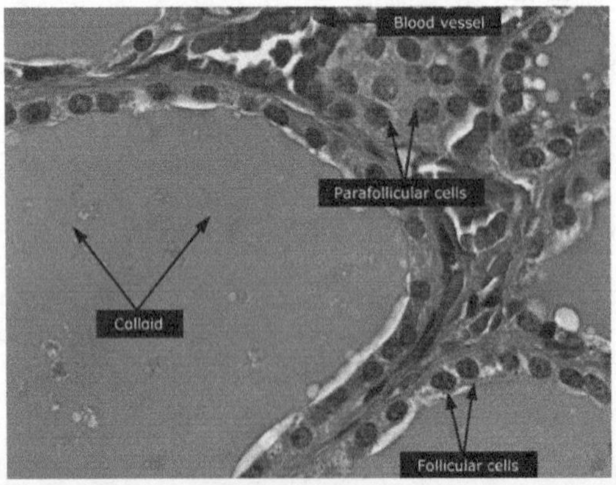

SOLITARY THYROID NODULE

Solitary thyroid nodule

- Single palpable nodule in thyroid on clinical examination, in an otherwise normal gland. Rest of the gland is impalpable
- **Causes:**
  - o Thyroid adenoma (20%)
  - o Papillary Ca thyroid (20%)
- **Most common in:** Female
- **Types (as per RAIU):**
  - o **Hot:** Nodule is overactive
  - o **Warm:** Normally functioning nodule
  - o **Cold:** Non-functioning nodule
- **Initial investigation of choice is:** FNAC
- **Surgical procedure:**
  - o Hemithyroidectomy if it is a nontoxic nodule due to any cause
  - o If it is papillary Ca of thyroid, then near total thyroidectomy is done

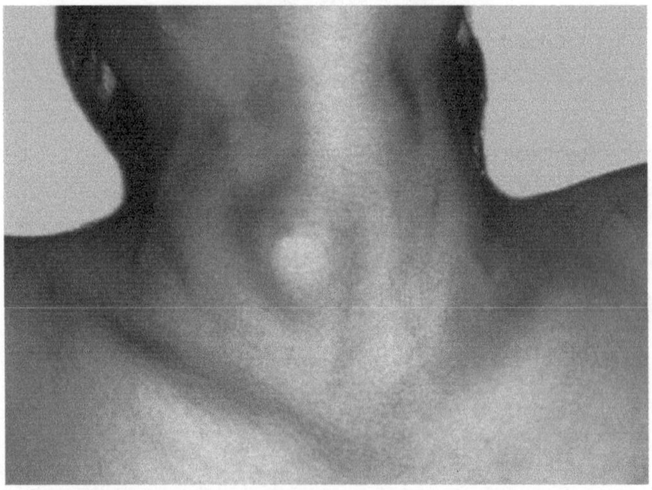

THYROID TUMOURS

Medullary Ca

- Uncommon type of thyroid Ca (5%)
- **Arises** from parafollicular/C cells of thyroid
- Contains characteristic **amyloid** stroma wherein malignant cells are dispersed

Medullary Thyroid Carcinoma

Microscopic Features

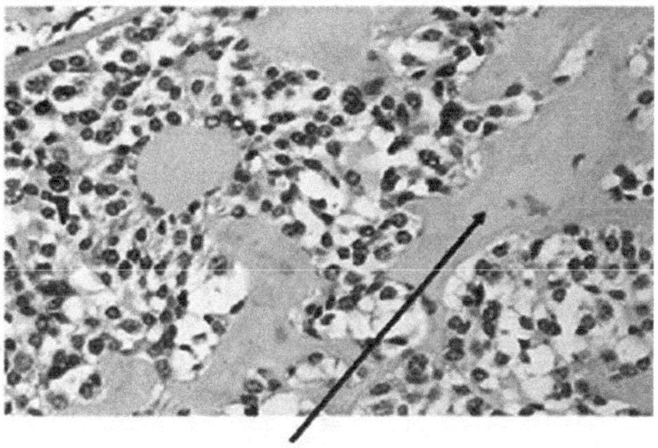

Amyloid stroma

- In these patients, blood levels of **calcitonin** is high, a very useful tumour marker
- Associated with **MEN**-IIa or MEN-IIb and pheochromocytoma with hypertension
- **Management: Total** thyroidectomy is the treatment of choice with central node dissection

Papillary Ca

- **Most common** thyroid tumour (60%)
- Common in females
- May develop after radiation exposure (either external or radioactive iodine therapy)
- **Microscopy:**
    - o Psammoma bodies are seen
    - o **Orphan** Annie eye nuclei

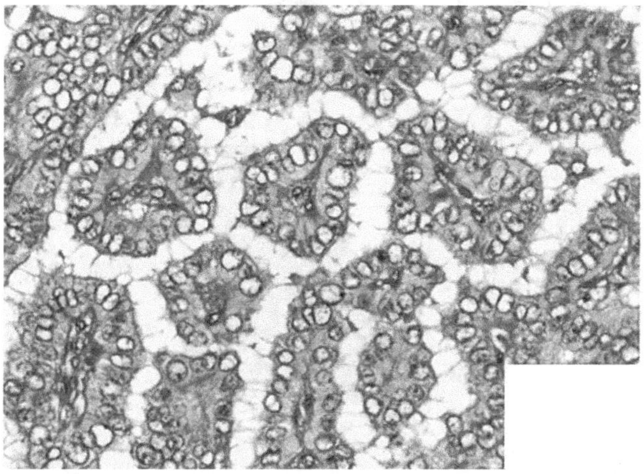

- Compression features are uncommon
- **Lymphatic spread:** Often discrete lymph nodes are palpable
- Least malignant
- **Treatment: Total** or near-total thyroidectomy, with central node compartment dissection (level VI)

Follicular Ca

Follicular thyroid cancer with angioinvasion

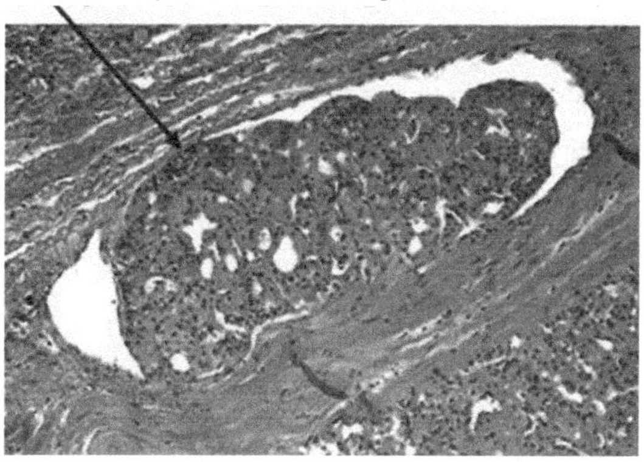

- 17% common
- Seen in females
- Can occur de novo or in a pre-existing **multinodular** goiter
- More aggressive tumour
- Recurrent laryngeal nerve compression causes hoarseness of voice (positive **Berry's** sign), indicating advanced malignancy
- FNAC is **inconclusive**, because capsular and angioinvasion, which are the main features in follicular Ca, are not detected by FNAC

Thyroidectomy

- **Neck swelling immediately following thyroid surgery is due to:** Tension **hematoma** (so open immediately)

MEN SYNDROME

MEN-I/Wermer syndrome

- Parathyroid neoplasm
- Pancreas neoplasm
- Pituitary (anterior) adenoma

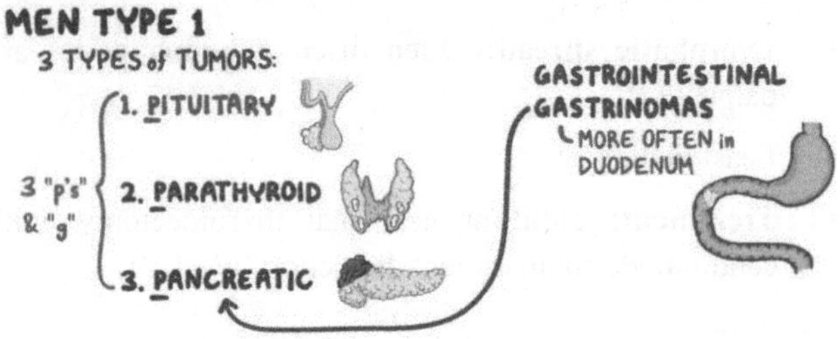

MEN-IIA/Sipple syndrome

- Medullary Ca thyroid
- Phaeochromocytomas
- Parathyroid hyperplasia

MEN-IIB

- Medullary Ca (thyroid)
- Phaeochromocytomas
- Mucosal neuromas (with distinctive marfanoid habitus)
- Parathyroid (rare)

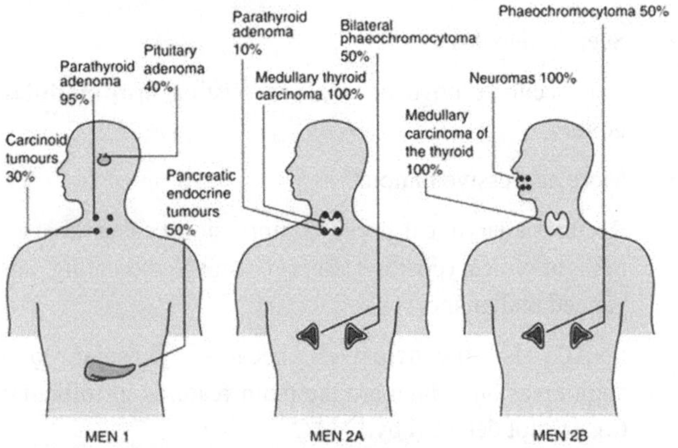

THYROID DYSFUNCTION

Hypothyroidism

- **Children:** Cretinism
- **Adults:** Myxedema
- Due to iodine deficiency
- Dry inelastic skin
- Loss of hair in lateral eyebrow
- Hoarseness of voice
- Menorrhagia
- **Cold** intolerance
- Delayed ankle jerk
- Increased sleepiness
- Gain in weight/**obese**

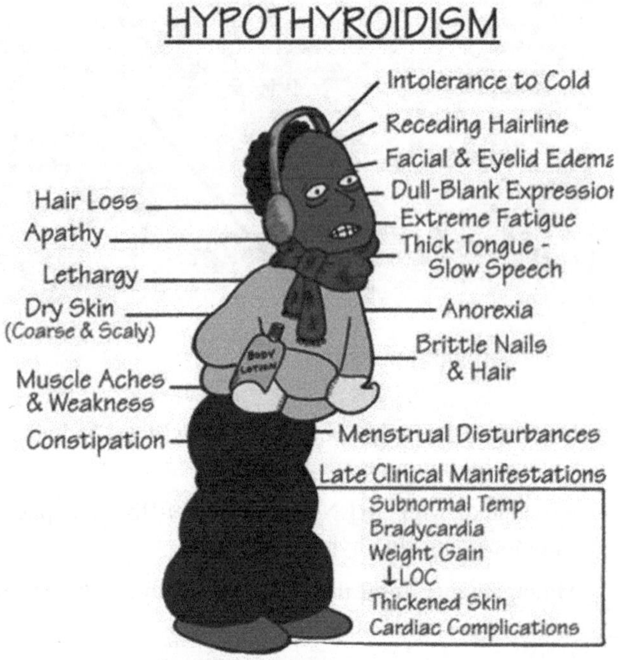

Hyperthyroidism

- **Diffuse toxic goitre:** Graves' disease

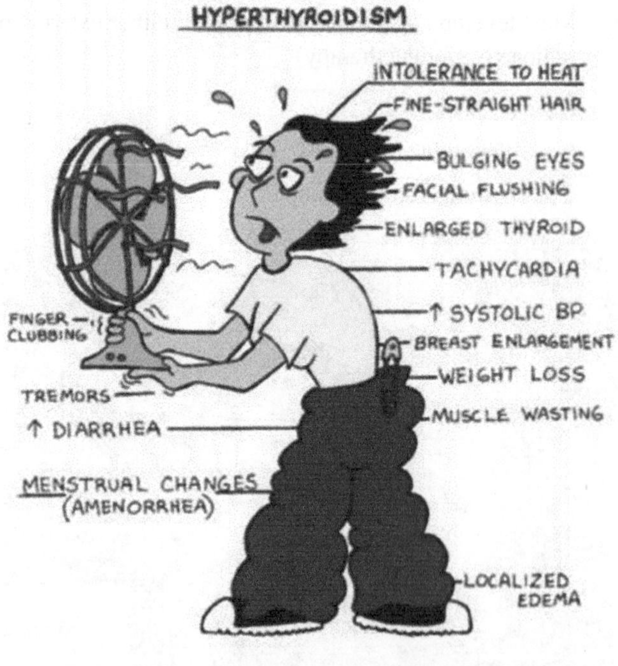

- Tremor

- Insomnia
- **Heat** intolerance
- Sweating
- Palpitations
- Weight **loss**
- Oligomenorrhea
- **Graves' disease (primary thyrotoxicosis):**
  - o Most **common** cause of hyperthyroidism
  - o Seen most commonly in females
  - o **Eye** signs and central nervous system (CNS) signs are common manifestations
  - o Pretibial myxedema
  - o T_3 and T_4 are increased; TSH is low
  - o **Radioisotope study: Elevated** RAIU (RadioActive Iodine Uptake)
  - o In **90%** cases, TSH-R and TSAB (Thyroid Stimulating AntiBody) are increased
  - o Anti-TPO antibodies are elevated in 75% of cases

THYROIDITIS

Acute thyroiditis

- Follows upper respiratory infection (Streptococcal infection usually)
- Seen commonly in children
- No HLA association
- **Normal** thyroid profile

Subacute (De Quervain's) thyroiditis

- Occurs after a few weeks of viral infection
- Seen in young women
- HLA-B35
- Patient is initially **hyperthyroid**

Hashimoto's thyroiditis

- Also known as lymphocytic thyroiditis
- Most common type of thyroiditis leading to **hypothyroidism**
- Presents as painless neck mass (anterior), which is granular and nodular
- In 90% of cases, anti-Thyroid PerOxidase **(anti-TPO)** antibodies are seen
- Hurthle cells are seen on FNAC

Reidel's thyroiditis

- Associated with autoimmune disease
- Painless mass in neck
- May present with pressure symptoms
- It presents as woody non-tender thyroid
- FNAC **cannot** be done
- Open biopsy is done

SECTION 2
SURGERY

Chapter 7

ESOPHAGUS

ANATOMY

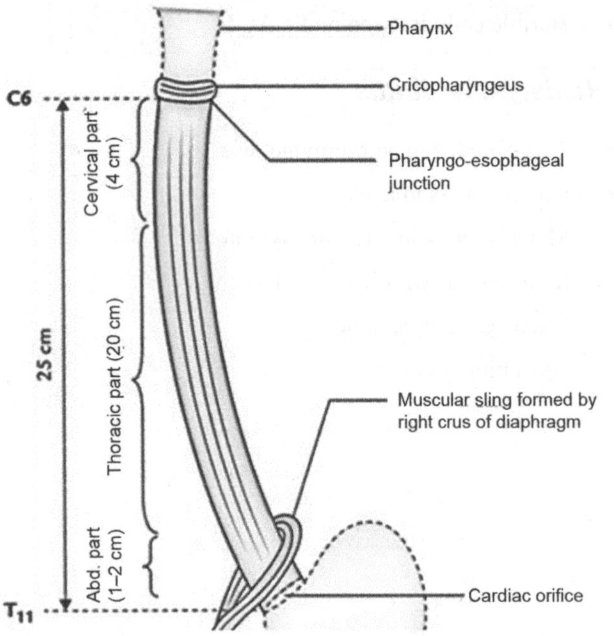

Anatomy

- **Esophagus pierces diaphragm at a distance of:** 15 inches (from incisor)
- **Length of esophagus:** 25 cm
- **Esophagus commences at:** Lower end of cricoid
- **Extent:** C6 – T11
- **Epithelium of esophagus:** Stratified squamous non-keratinized

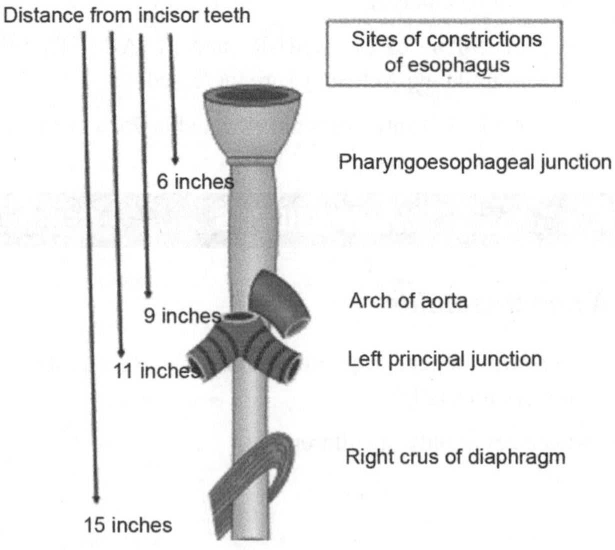

Constrictions of esophagus (distance from central incisor)

- 15 cm (Cricopharynx)
- 25 cm (Aortic arch)
- 27 cm (Left bronchus)
- 40 cm (Diaphragmatic entry)

Esophagus shown three indentations on radiographic study; from above downwards they are

- Aortic arch
- Left bronchus
- Left atrium

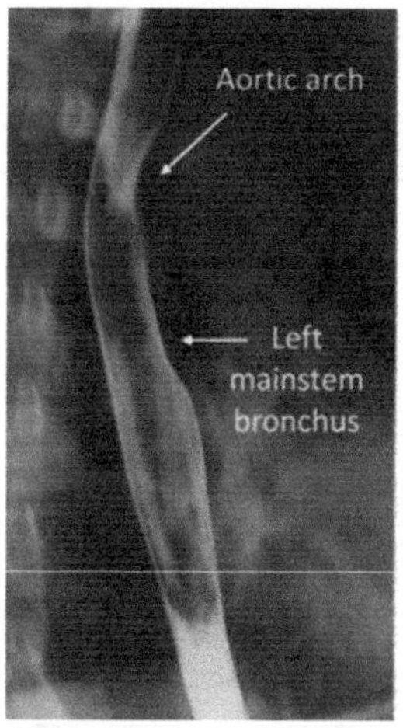

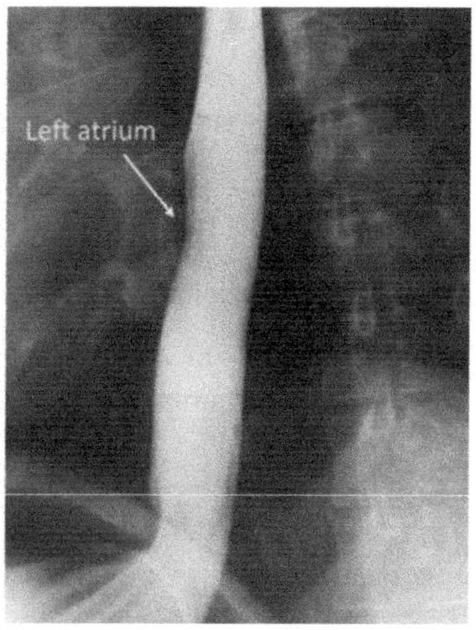

Blood supply of esophagus

- **Upper third:** Inferior thyroid artery
- **Middle third:** Branches from descending thoracic aorta;
- **Lower third:** Left gastric artery

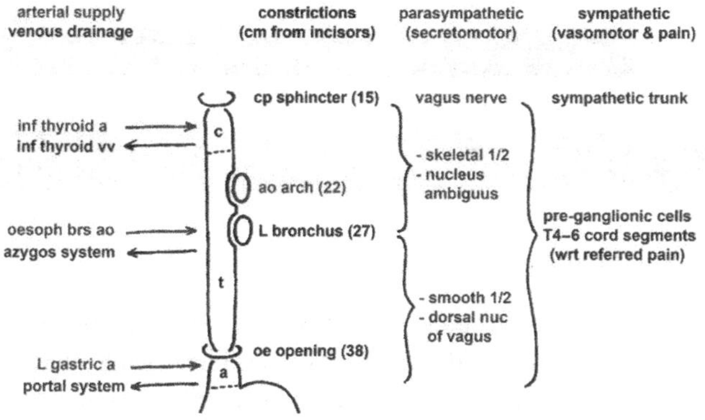

GASTROESOPHAGEAL REFLUX DISEASE

Features

- It is a pathological reflux of acid from the stomach into the lower esophagus
- There is **reduced** LES (lower esophageal sphincter) pressure
- **Clinical presentation:**
  - o Chest pain & heart burn (pyrosis)
  - o Appearance of symptoms within seconds of ingestion of food is **typical** presentation
  - o Regurgitation
- **Complications:**
  - o Barrett's esophagus
  - o Adenocarcinoma of esophagus
  - o Stricture of lower end of esophagus
- **Investigations:**
  - o 24 hours esophageal pH monitoring is **gold** standard
  - o De-Meester scoring system
- **Treatment:**
  - o Proton pump inhibitors
  - o **Anti-reflux surgery (Fundoplication): Nissen's** posterior total fundoplication

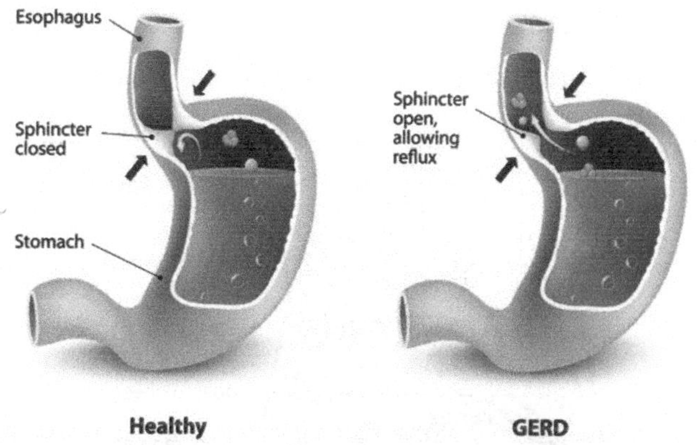

HIATUS HERNIA

Types

- **I: Sliding hiatus hernia (Most common)**
  - o Upward displacement of the gastroesophageal junction into the posterior mediastinum
  - o Stomach remains in its usual longitudinal alignment
- **II: True paraesophageal**
  - o Normally positioned intraabdominal gastroesophageal junction
  - o Upward herniation of the stomach alongside it
- **III:** Mixed paraesophageal (I & II)
- **IV:** Paraesophageal containing other intra-abdominal organs

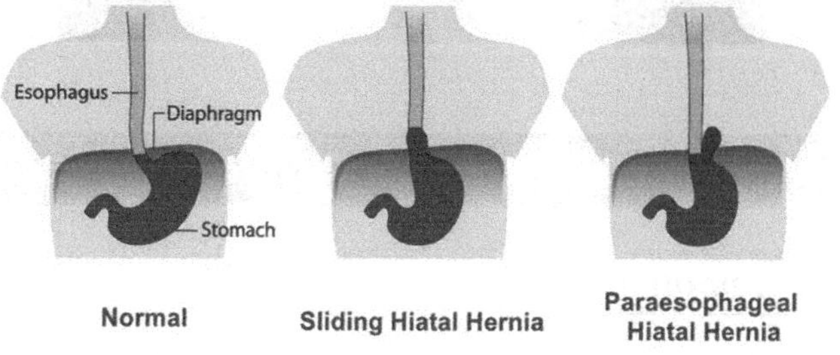

CONGENITAL DIAPHRAGMATIC HERNIA

Features

- It is also known as Bochdalek hernia/posterolateral hernia
- Around **80%** are on right side of diaphragm
- **Classical triad:**
    - o Respiratory distress
    - o Dextrocardia
    - o Scaphoid abdomen

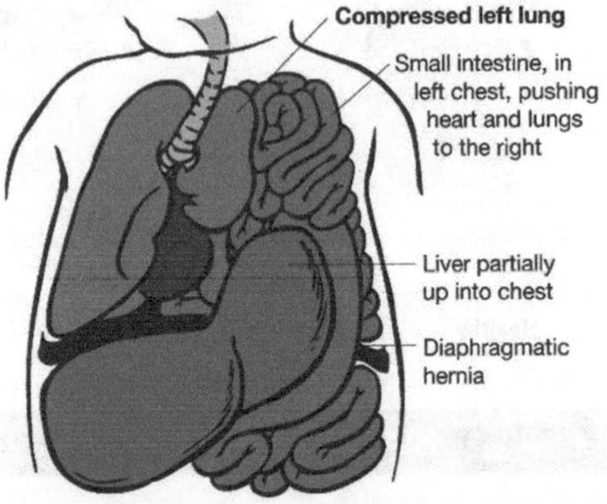

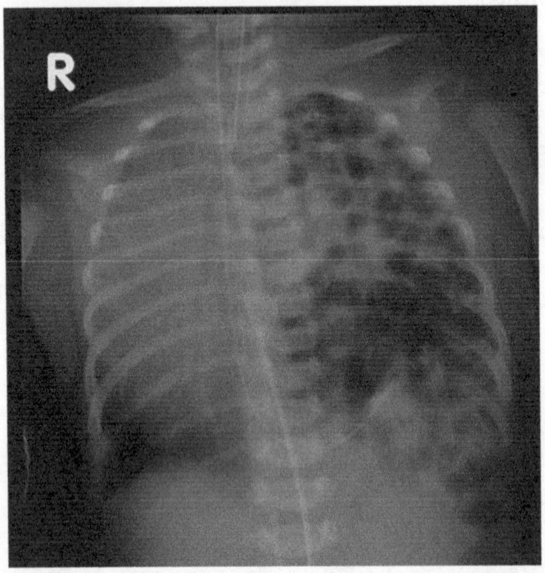

MALLORY-WEISS SYNDROME

Common in

- Alcoholics

MC site

- Cardia of stomach (**NOT** esophagus)

Pathology

- **Partial vertical** tears
- Pylorus closed & closed lower esophageal sphincter/ LES (barotrauma)

Feature

- Hematemesis

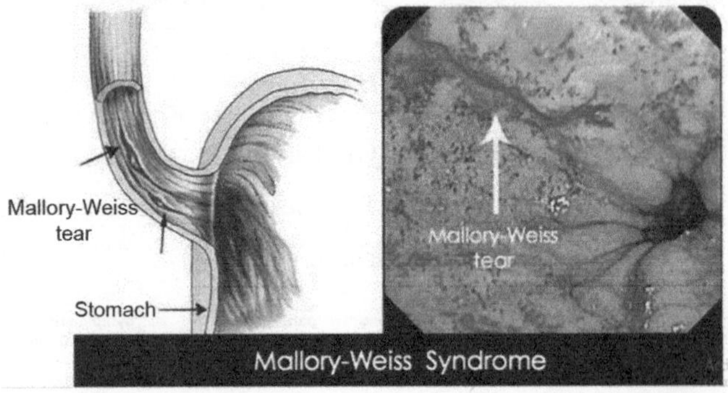

BOERHAAVE'S SYNDROME

Definition

- Spontaneous rupture of esophagus usually involving left posterolateral side of the distal esophagus into the left pleural cavity or just above gastroesophageal junction

Mechanism

- Forceful vomiting (against a closed glottis)
- May produce **perforation** of the esophagus (**transverse**, posterolateral part)
- Cricopharynx & pylorus are closed

Clinical presentation

- **Mackler's triad:**
    - o Acute chest (thoracic) pain
    - o Cervical subcutaneous emphysema
    - o Vomiting

Investigation

- **Chest X-ray:** Hydropneumothorax

- Diagnosis **confirmed** by contrast esophagogram
- Chest CT scan shows mediastinal air & fluid at the site of perforation

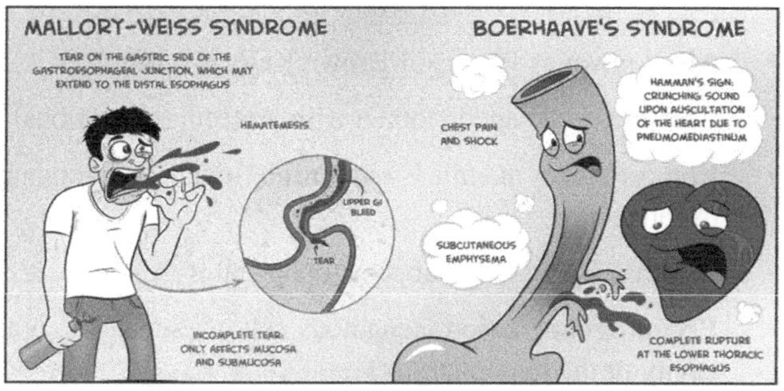

ACHALASIA CARDIA

Definition

- Achalasia means failure to relax

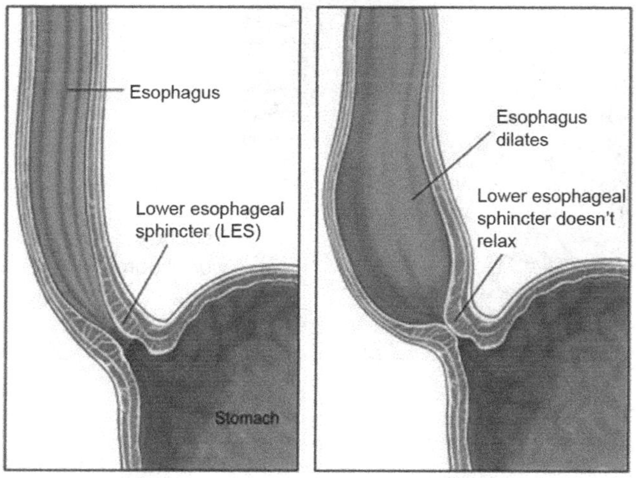

Normal Achalasia

Clinical feature

- Dysphagia is the **presenting** symptom. It is initially for liquids but later on for both liquids & solids
- **Classical triad:**
    - o Dysphagia
    - o Weight loss
    - o Regurgitation
- **Premalignant** condition (leads to squamous cell Ca of esophagus)

Pathology

- **Failure** of relaxation of lower esophageal sphincter/LES
- Destruction of the nerves to LES is primary pathology
- Degeneration of neuromuscular function of the body of esophagus is secondary

Investigation

- **Gold** standard test is manometry (**Findings:** Increased pressure in LES)
- **Barium study shows: Bird beak**/Rat tail/Pencil tip appearance

Treatment

- **Heller's** myotomy

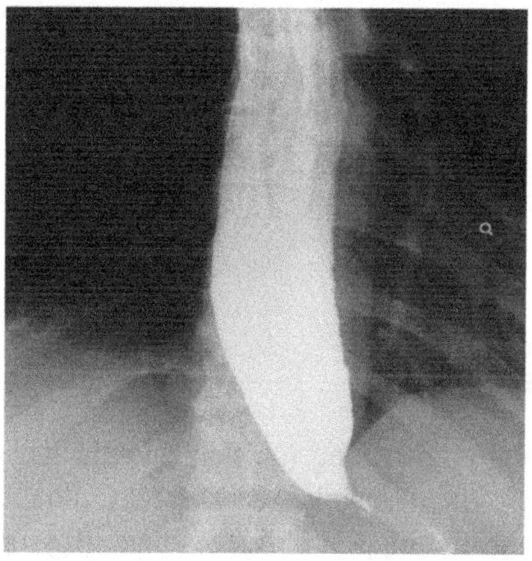

DIFFUSE ESOPHAGEAL SPASM

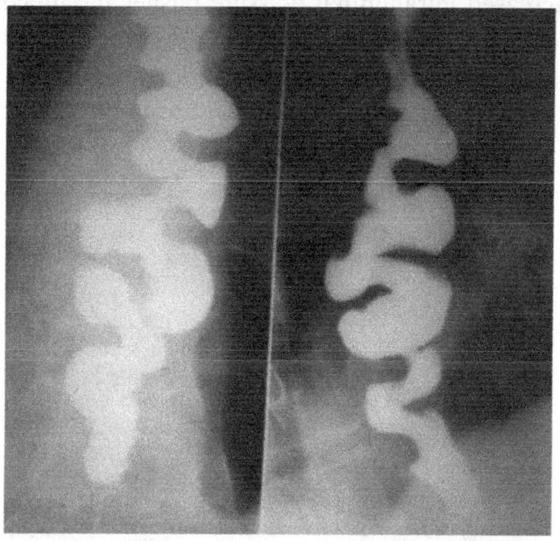

Features

- There are repetitive, simultaneous and high amplitude esophageal contractions
- Barium swallow shows **corkscrew** or rosary-bead esophagus, segmental spasm or pseudodiverticulosis appearance

- Manometry is **gold** standard for diagnosis

ZENKER'S DIVERTICULUM

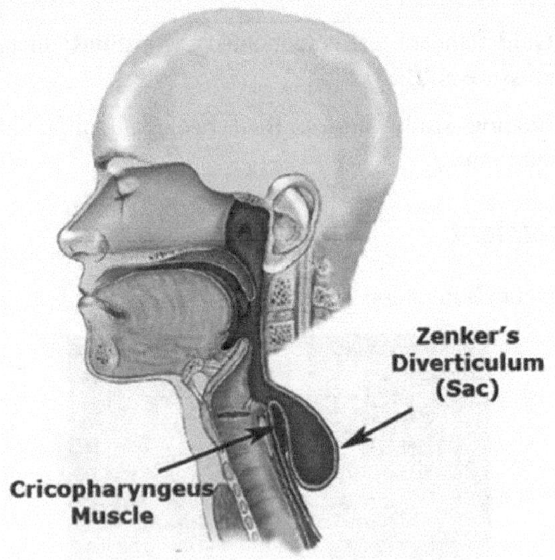

Features

- Mucosal outpouching (pulsion diverticulum) occurring through the triangular bare area (Killian's triangle) between the upper oblique fibers (thyropharyngeus muscle) and lower horizontal fibers (cricopharyngeus muscle) of the inferior constrictor muscle
- Increased intraluminal pressure pushes the mucosa and submucosa through a muscular defect in the wall of the esophagus causing a pulsion diverticulum
- Barium swallow is **diagnostic**

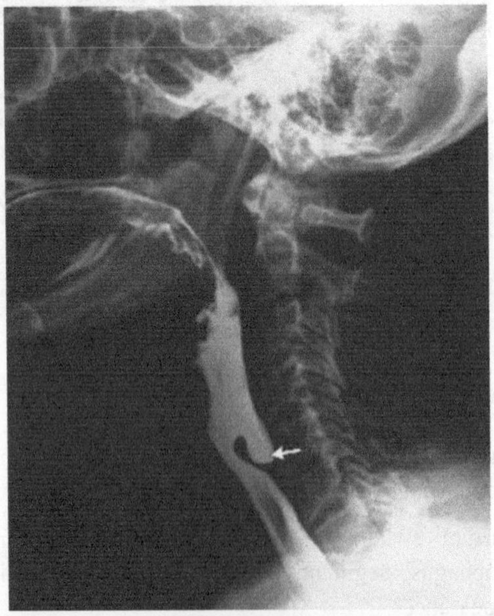

PLUMMER VINSON SYNDROME

Features

- Also known as Patterson-Brown Kelly syndrome
- Seen in middle aged women without teeth (edentulous)
- Iron deficiency anemia is a **common** finding (sideropenic dysphagia)
- Dysphagia due to the upper esophageal web
- **Premalignant** lesion (squamous cell of esophagus, oral cavity or the hypopharynx)
- Koilonychia (brittle, spoon shaped fingernails)

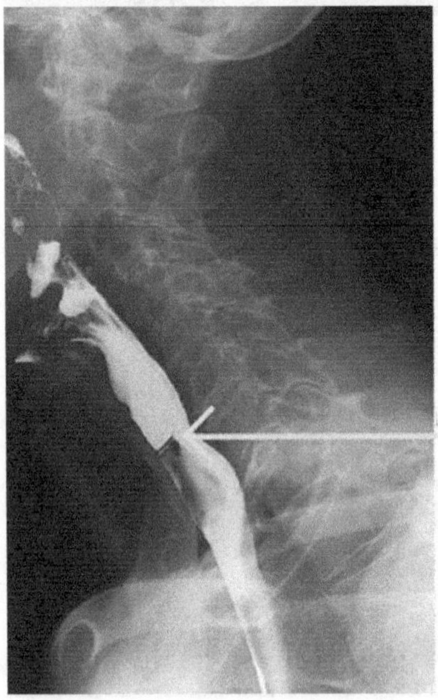

Esophageal web on videofluoroscopy

DYSPHAGIA LUSORIA

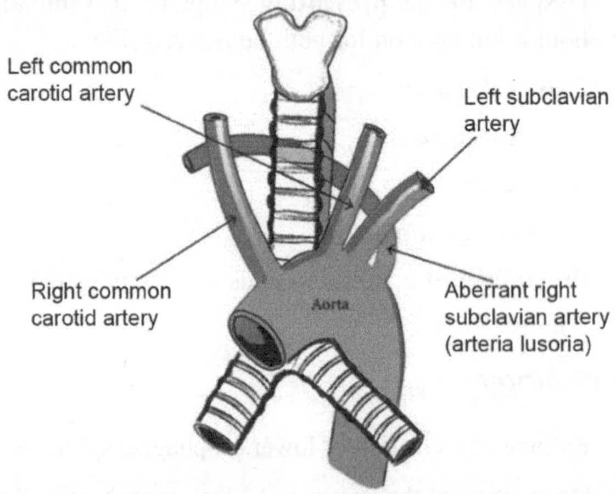

Features

- A disorder of swallowing caused due to vascular anomalies
- Vascular rings and pulmonary slings occur as a result of developmental abnormalities of the great vessels that cause compression of the esophagus
- **Most common** anomaly is **right** subclavian artery arising from descending aorta and moves behind esophagus which might cause significant posterior compression of the esophagus

TRACHEOESOPHAGEAL FISTULA

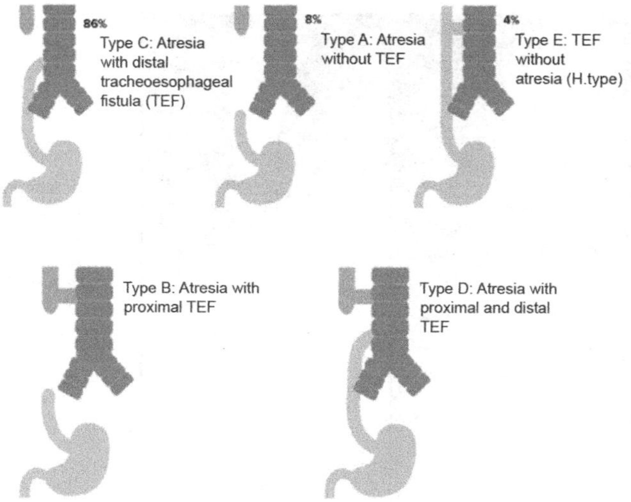

Features

- An abnormal communication (fistula) between the esophagus and trachea
- Diagnosis is **suggested** by an infant presenting with excessive salivation along with coughing or choking during the first oral feeding
- Associated with:
  - o V: Vertebral body segmentation defect
  - o A: Anal atresia
  - o C: CVS disorders (Patent ductus arteriosus, Ventricular septal defect)
  - o T: Tracheoesophageal fistula
  - o R: Renal agenesis (unilateral)
  - o L: Limb anomalies (radial ray hypoplasia)

BARRETT'S ESOPHAGUS

Pathology

- Metaplasia is seen at lower end of esophagus
- **Type of metaplasia:** Squamous to columnar epithelial metaplasia is seen
- Most **common** type is intestinal metaplasia

Predisposing factor

- As a result of prolonged GERD

Complication

- **Premalignant** condition (development of adenocarcinoma)
- Barrett's ulcer (chronic peptic ulceration)
- Stricture (high/mid-esophageal & long)

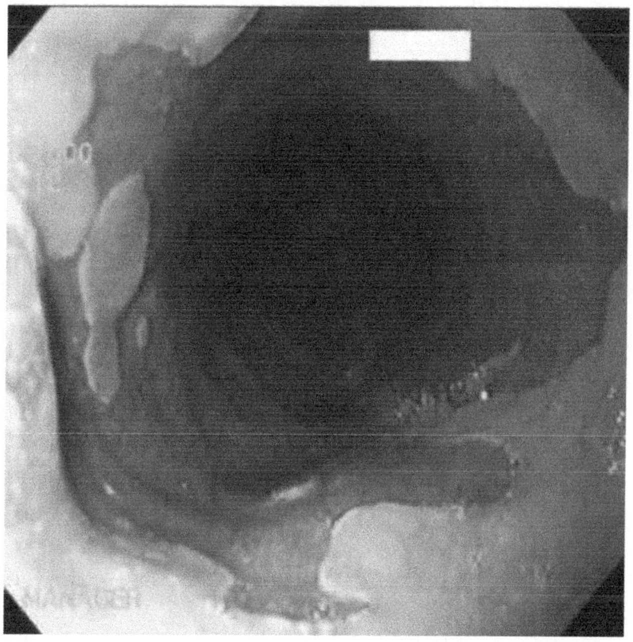

SCHATZKI'S RING

Features

- It consists of concentric symmetric narrowing representing an area of restricted distensibility of lower esophagus
- Lies at squamocolumnar gastroesophageal junction

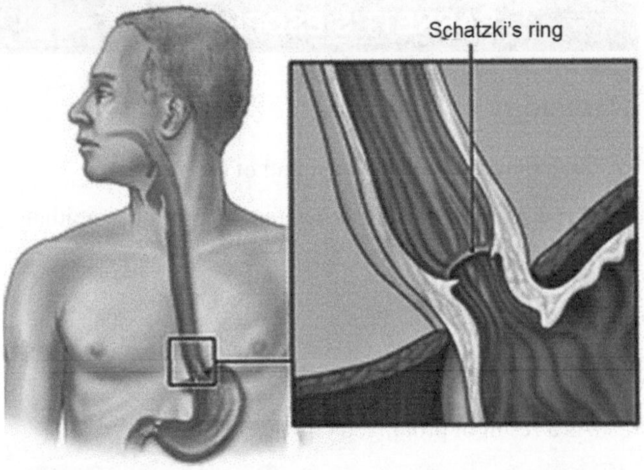

ESOPHAGEAL CA

Predisposing factors

- Smoking
- Chronic achalasia
- Tylosis
- Plummer-Vinson syndrome
- Barrett's esophagus (adenocarcinoma)

MC (Most common) in esophageal Ca

- **MC histological type worldwide:** Squamous cell Ca
- **MC site:** Middle third of esophagus
- **MC esophageal Ca in United States/Western world:** Adenocarcinoma
- **MC site of adeno Ca:** Lower end
- **MC site of squamous cell Ca:** Middle 1/3rd

Other important points

- **First investigation: Barium swallow:**
  - o Shows irregular rat tail filling defect (not to be confused with rat tail appearance of achalasia cardia)
  - o Apple core lesion
- **Investigation of choice:** Endoscopy with biopsy
- **Chemotherapeutic agents used:** Cisplatin, bleomycin and 5-FU

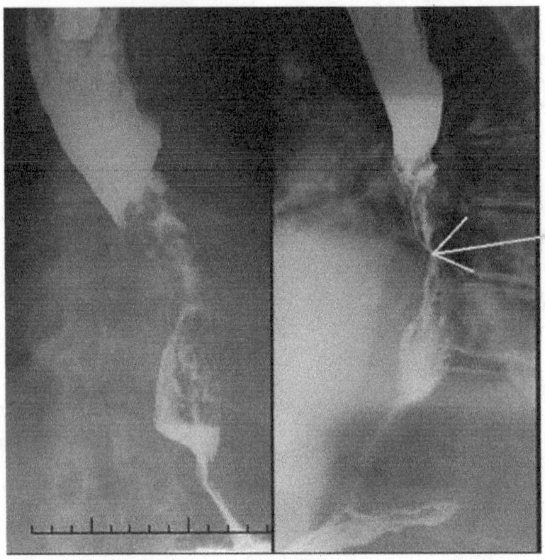

SECTION 2
SURGERY

Chapter 8
STOMACH

STOMACH

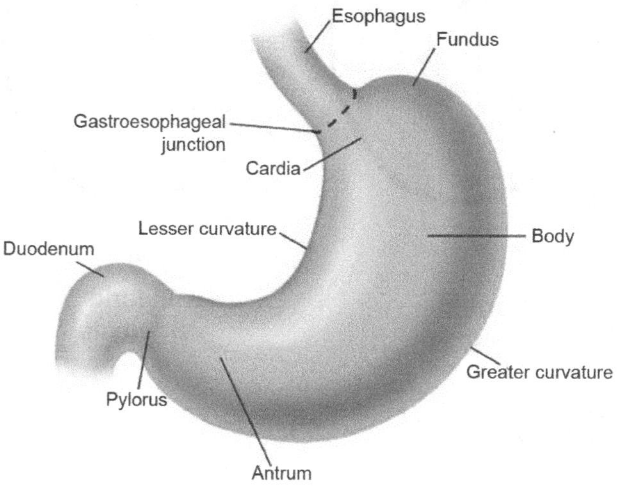

Blood supply of the stomach

- **Right gastric artery (Hepatic artery) supplies:** Lower right part of the stomach
- **Short gastric artery (Splenic artery) supplies:** Fundus
- **Left gastric artery (Celiac artery) supplies:** Lower third of esophagus upper right part of the stomach
- **Left gastroepiploic artery (Splenic artery) supplies:** Upper part of greater curvature
- **Right gastroepiploic artery (Gastroduodenal artery) supplies:** Lower part of greater curvature

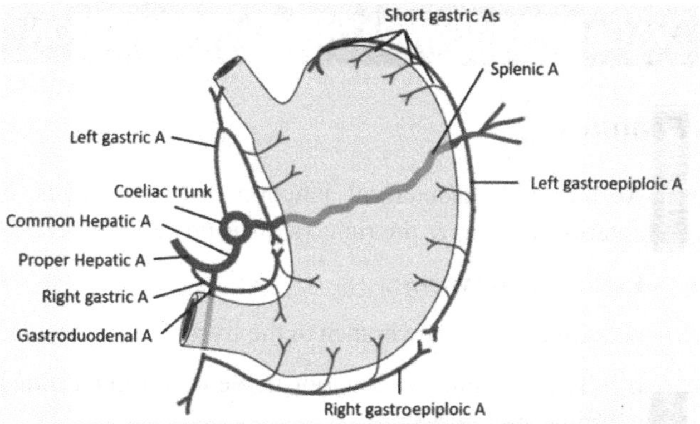

DUODENUM/D

Divided into four parts

- **D1 (superior part):** 5 cm
- **D2 (descending part):** 7.5 cm
- **D3 (horizontal part):** 10 cm
- **D4 (ascending part):** 2.5 cm

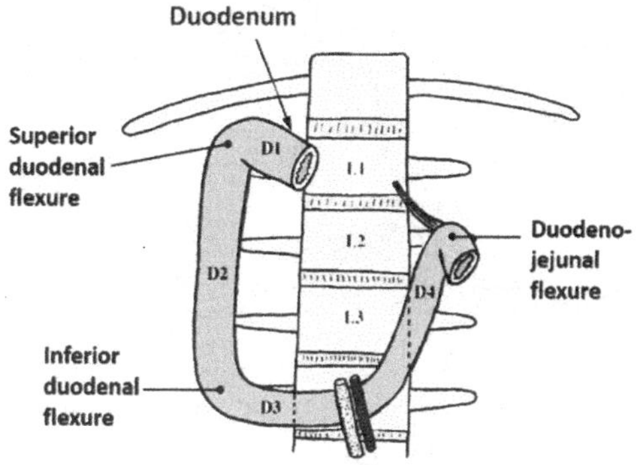

Brunner's gland

- Main function of these glands is to produce mucus rich alkaline secretion which protects duodenum from gastric acid

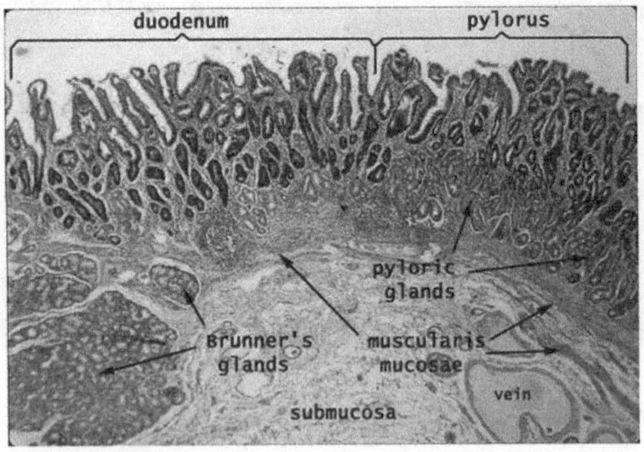

VAGAL/PARASYMPATHETIC INNERVATION

Features

- At the gastroesophageal junction, the left vagus is anterior (Le-An) & the right vagus is posterior
- **Left/Anterior vagus:**
  - o Gives of hepatic branch to the liver
  - o Then continue as anterior nerve of **Latarjet** along the lesser curvature
- **Right/Posterior vagus:**
  - o First branch is criminal nerve of **Grassi** (potential etiology of recurrent ulcers, if it is not divided)
  - o Another branch is given to celiac plexus which continue posteriorly along the lesser curvature

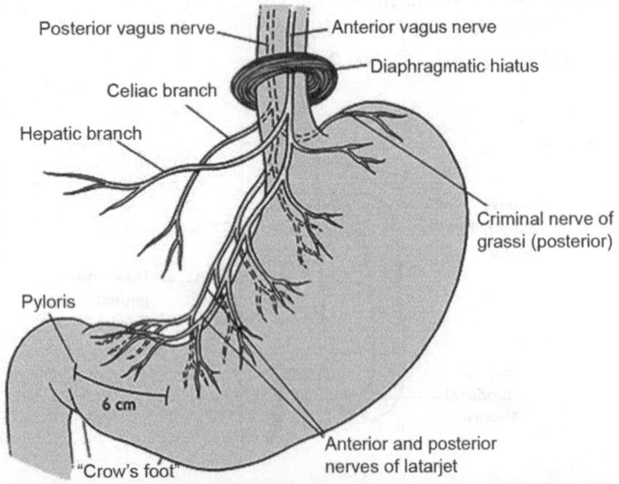

VAGOTOMIES

Vagotomies

- **Truncal vagotomy:**
  - o Vagus nerve is cut above the celiac & hepatic branches of the vagi
- **Selective vagotomy:**
  - o Vagus nerve is cut below the celiac and hepatic branches if vagi

IHPS/IDIOPATHIC HYPERTROPHIC PYLORIC STENOSIS

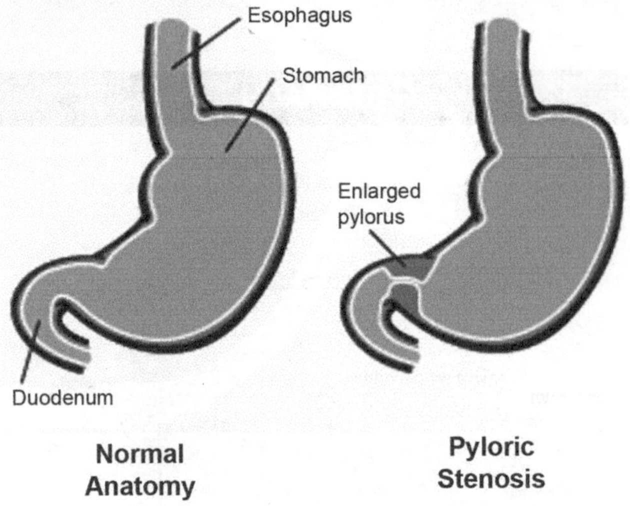

Presents at

- About **4** weeks after birth
- **Never** congenital, therefore terminology has been changed from congenital HPS to idiopathic HPS

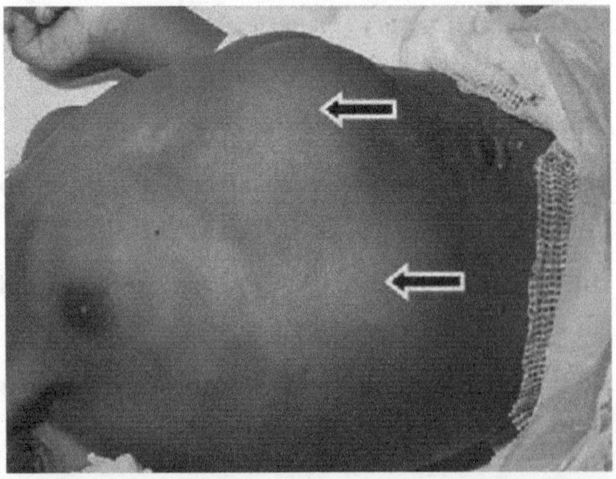

Feature

- Weight loss
- **Projectile** vomiting
- **Non-bilious**
- Hypochloremic hypokalemic metabolic alkalosis

Fluid of choice

- Isotonic Dextrose normal saline

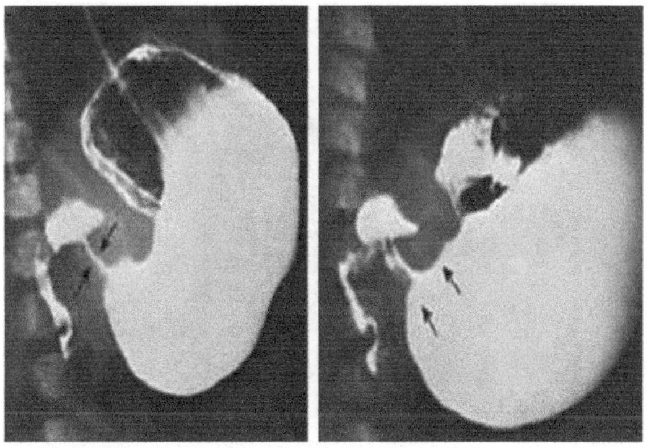

Infantile Hyperthophic Pyloric Stenosis

GASTRIC CA

MC site

- Pylorus & Antrum

Predisposing factors

- **Organism:** H. pylori (causes gastritis, gastric atrophy)
- **Blood group: A** blood group
- Long-term nitrates ingestion (dried, smoked, salted foods)
- Pernicious anemia
- Menetrier's disease
- Atrophic gastritis

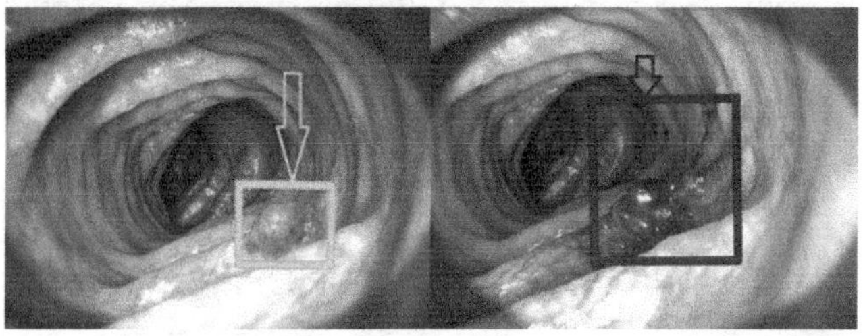

MC features

- Weight loss
- Virchow's nodes/**Troisier's** sign (Left supraclavicular lymph node enlargement)
- Krukenberg's tumour
- **Sister** Mary Joseph node
- Blumer's shelf (Pouch of Douglas)
- Linitis **plastica**

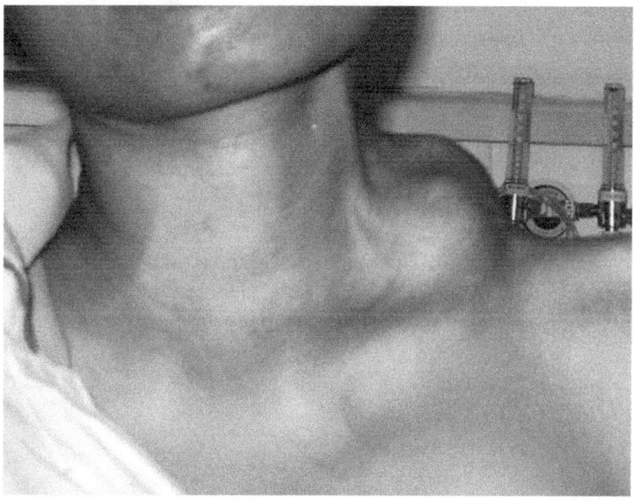

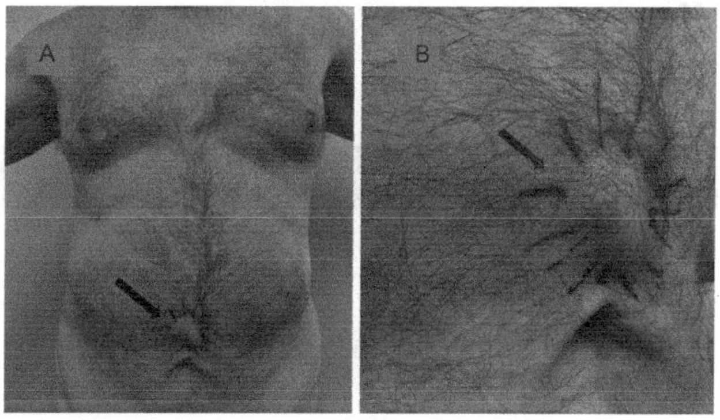

Early gastric Ca

- Primary lesion limited to mucosa & submucosa
- Excellent prognosis

Sister Mary Joseph's nodule

- Metastatic involvement of **paraumbilical** nodes from intrapelvic/intra-abdominal malignancies (stomach)

GIST/GASTROINTESTINAL STROMAL TUMOURS

Pathology

- **MC site:** Stomach
- **Arises from:** Cells of **Cajal**

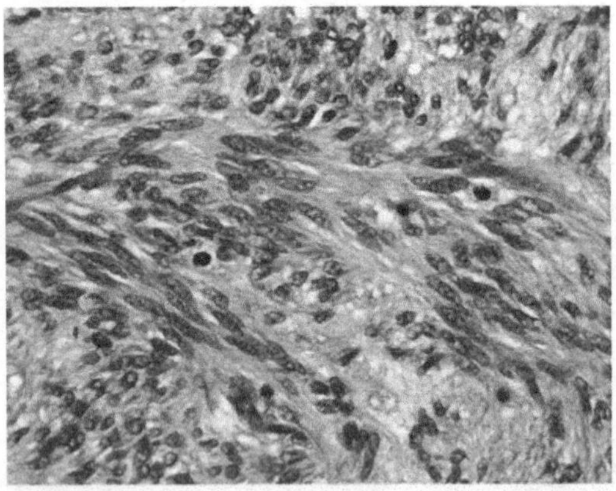

Stomach GIST composed of spindle cells with lightly eosinophilic, wispy cytoplasm and few scattered mitotic figures (high power)

Diagnosis

- PET scan

Management

- Excision → if recurrence → Sunitinib/Imatinib

HELICOBACTER PYLORI

Features

- Spiral shaped, gram-**negative** rod, motile with lophotrichous flagella

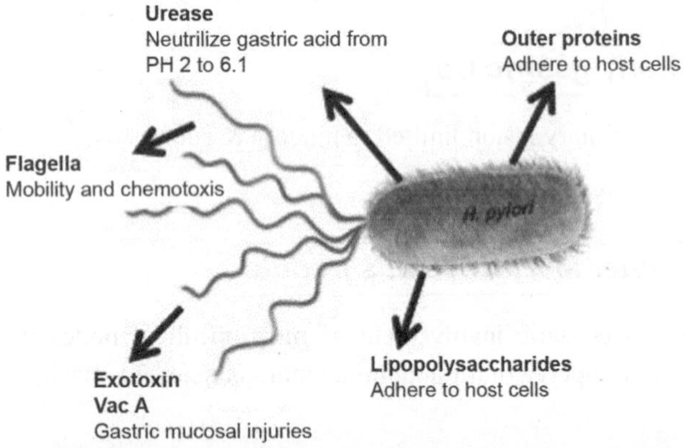

- Grows optimally at a pH of 6-7
- It produces **urease**, which converts urea to ammonia
- This ammonia buffer acid
- 90% of duodenal ulcer & 75% of gastric ulcer are caused by H. pylori
- H. pylori also increases risk of adenocarcinoma of stomach and gastric MALT lymphoma

GASTRIC ULCER

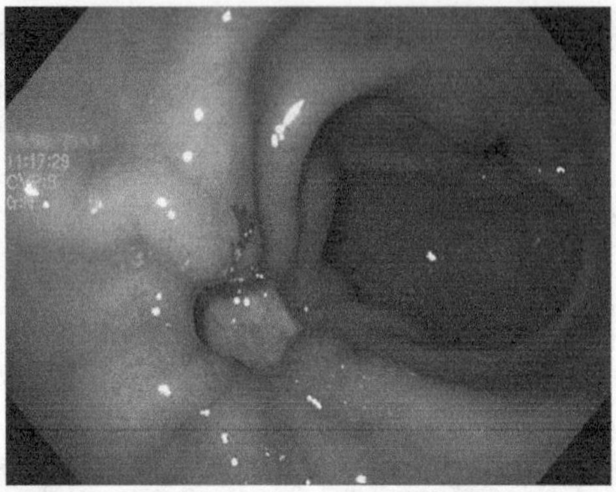

Features

- There is altered mucosal barrier function
- **MC** site along the incisura angularis in lesser curvature
- Pain occurs in the epigastrium after taking food
- So, the patient is hesitant to eat (as it aggravates pain) and there is **loss** of weight
- Hematemesis is common
- **Complications:**
  - o Perforation into lesser sac
  - o Hourglass contracture
  - o Teapot stomach
  - o Malignancy

DUODENAL ULCER

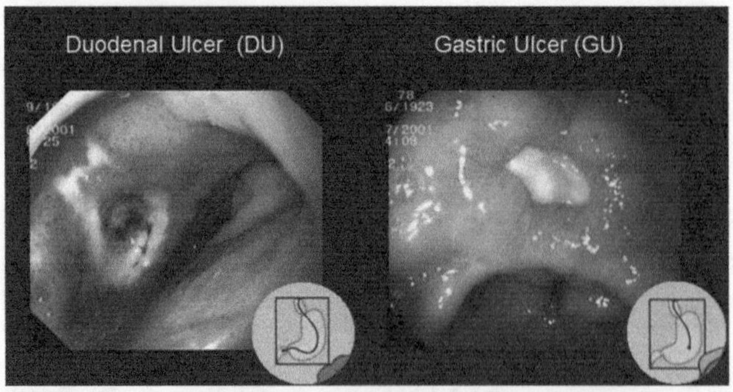

Pathology

- Associated with stress & anxiety (hurry, worry & curry)
- **Blood group: O** positive
- **MC site of duodenal ulcer:** 1st part of duodenum
- First part of duodenum is overall the MC site of peptic ulcers
- Pain is common during night and decreases after taking food (hunger pain)
- Patient eats frequently and there is weight **gain**
- Melena is common
- Bariums meal shows deformed/absent duodenal cap (because of spasm)
- Bleeding is the **MC** complication
- **Source of bleeding in duodenal ulcer:** Gastroduodenal artery
- Perforation is more on anterior wall
- Duodenal ulcers are benign (no conversion to malignancy)

VAGOTOMY

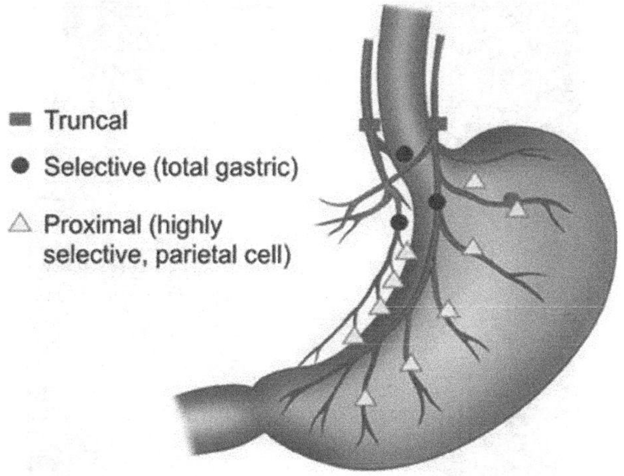

Types of vagotomy

- **Highly selective vagotomy/Proximal gastric vagotomy/parietal cell vagotomy:**
  - Procedure of choice for chronic/intractable duodenal ulcers
  - Nerve of Latarjet supplying the antrum is **preserved** and hence gastric motility
  - Drainage procedure is not required
  - Reduce down chances of dumping syndrome & gastric atony
  - But relatively high recurrence
- **Vagotomy & drainage:**
  - Truncal vagotomy is done
  - **MC** procedure done for duodenal ulcers
- **Vagotomy & antrectomy:**
  - Done to lower down chances of **recurrence**
  - So, procedure of choice for recurrent duodenal ulcers
  - High mortality & morbidity

PERFORATED PEPTIC ULCER

Perforated peptic ulcer

- Perforated peptic ulcer is a surgical emergency (acute abdomen)
- **Diagnosis:**
  - Upright chest X-ray shows **free air** under diaphragm

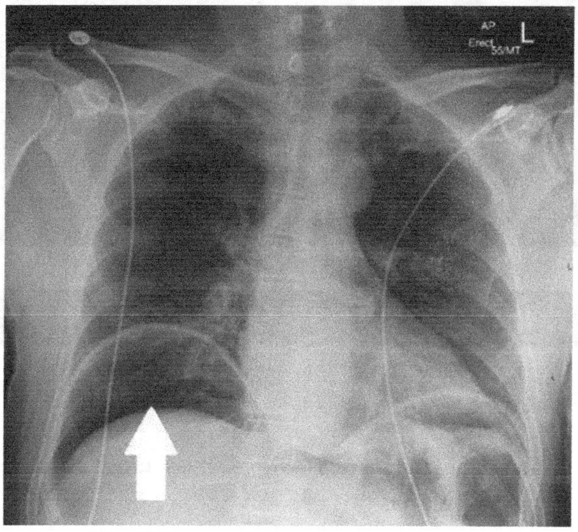

- **Treatment:**
  - Surgery is always indicated
  - Exploratory **laparotomy**
  - Nil by mouth (NBM)
  - Nasogastric suction
  - Acid suppression
  - Antibiotics

MENETRIER'S DISEASE

Features

- Also known as hypoproteinemic hypertrophic gastropathy
- Acquired, premalignant disease characterized by massive gastric folds in the fundus and the corpus of the stomach giving the mucosa a cobblestone or cerebriform appearance
- Associated with protein **loss** from the stomach

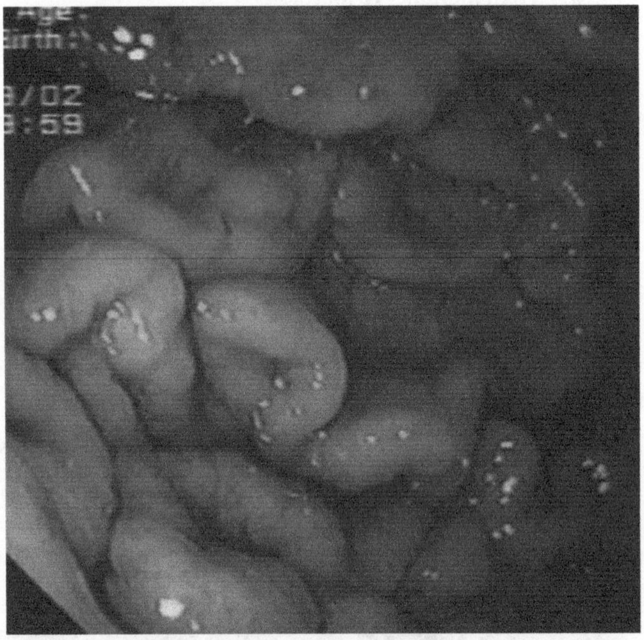

STRESS GASTRITIS

Features

- Also known as stress ulcers/stress erosive gastritis/hemorrhagic gastritis
- **Cushing ulcers:**
    - o Seen in setting of head **trauma**/CNS disease/raised intracranial tension
- **Curling's ulcer:**
    - o Seen in thermal **burn** injury involving more than 30% body surface area
    - o In the body & fundus (NOT in antrum or duodenum)

DUODENAL ATRESIA

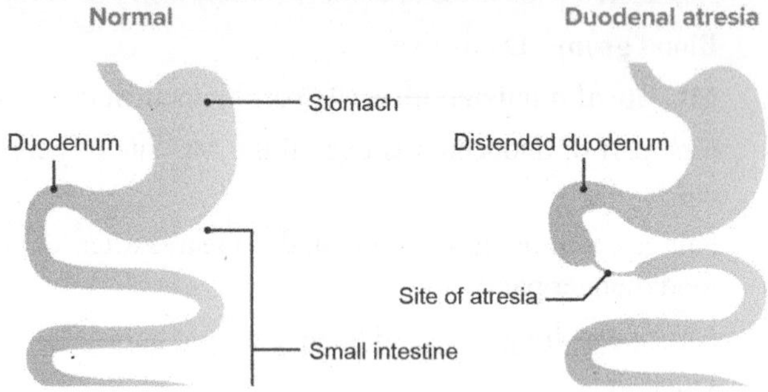

Features

- Due to result of failure of vacuolization of the duodenum from its solid cord stage
- Usually, the atresia is distal to the ampulla of Vater
- Infant presents with bilious vomiting
- **X-ray abdomen: Double** bubble sign (air filled in stomach & duodenal bulb)
- **Treatment:** Diamond shaped **duodenoduodenostomy** is done

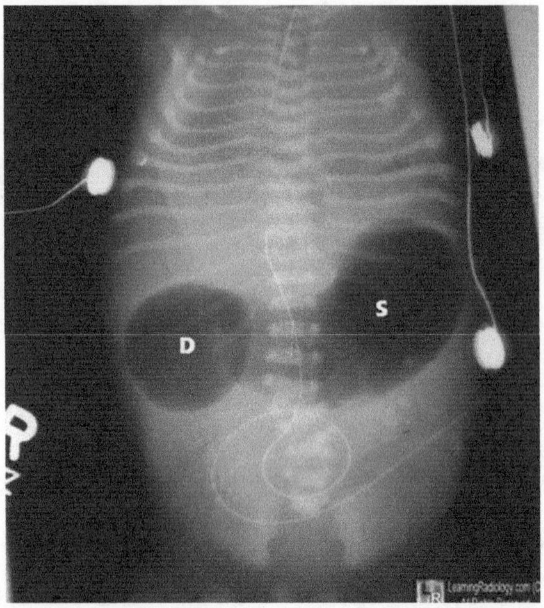

BEZOARS

Features

- Collection of non-digestible material

- **Phytobezoar:**
  - o Seen in patient who had undergone surgery of the stomach or who have impaired gastric emptying
- **Trichobezoar:**
  - o Concretions of hair
  - o Seen in **psychiatric** long-haired girls, who often deny eating their own hair

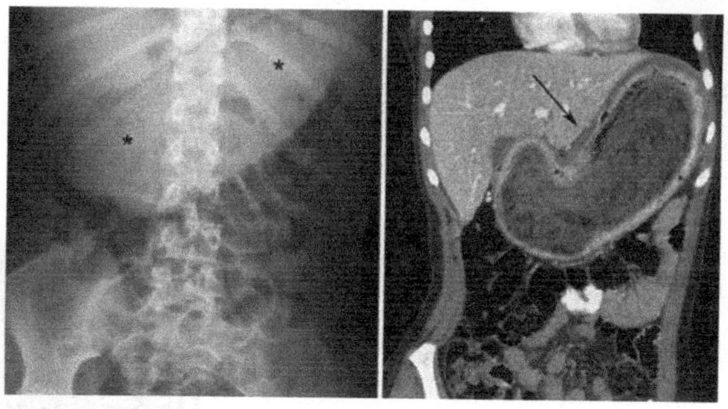

Chapter 9

SMALL AND LARGE INTESTINE

MECKEL'S DIVERTICULUM

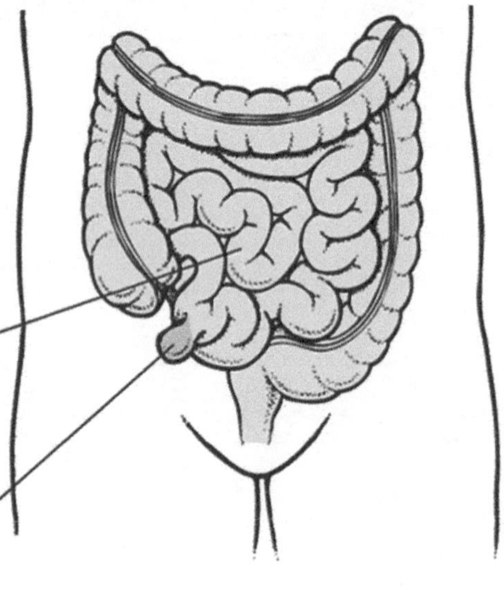

Features

- **True** congenital diverticulum
- Vestigial **remnant** of omphalomesenteric duct/vitelline duct
- **Rule of 2:**
  - o 2 feet from ileocecal valve
  - o 2 types of ectopic tissue are common (Gastric & pancreatic)
  - o Seen in 2% population

Complications

- Torsion may lead to obstruction, ischemia & necrosis
- It can be a leading point of intussusception

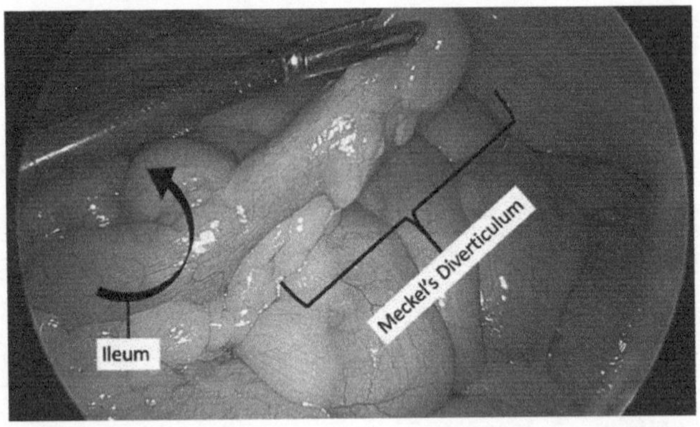

IOC

- **Technetium-99m pertechnetate (99mTc):** Most **accurate** diagnostic test in children

INTUSSUSCEPTION

Features

- **Outer tube is known as:** Intussuscipiens
- **Inner tube is known as:** Intussusceptum
- **Sign de dance:** Emptiness in Iliac fossa
- **MC type:** Ileo-colic
- Red **currant** jelly stools

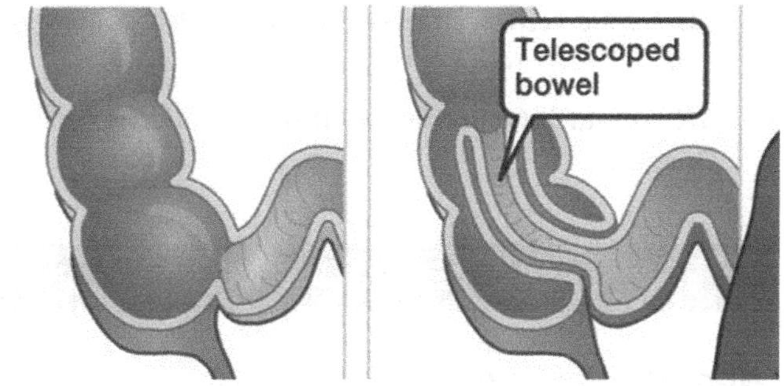

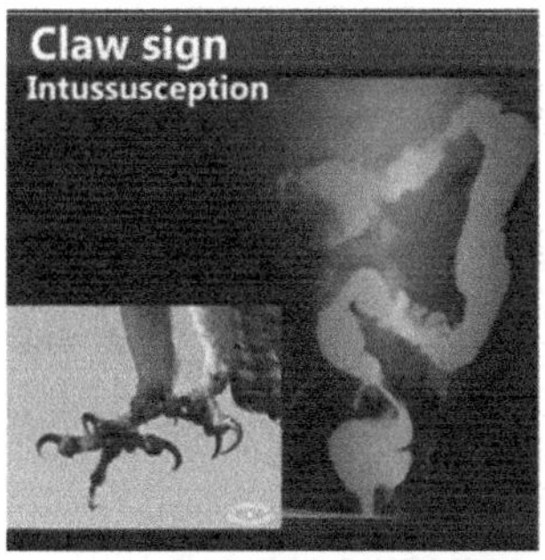

ANATOMY OF APPENDIX

Features

- Length of 2 – 20 cm
- Base of appendix is located at the convergence of taenia coli along the inferior aspect of the cecum
- **MC location:** Retrocecal

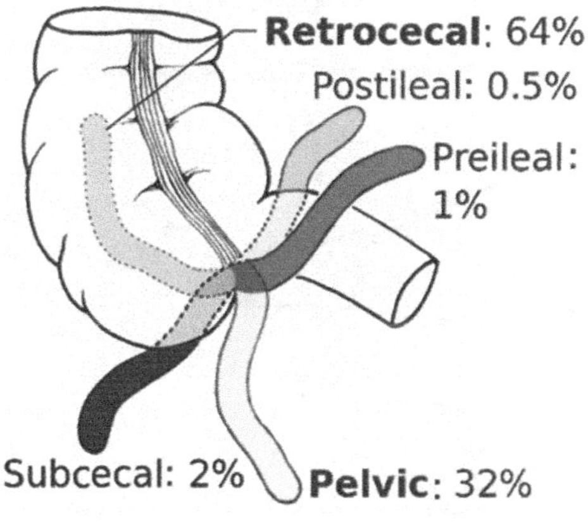

ACUTE APPENDICITIS

Appendicitis

- Most **common** surgical emergency
- Obstruction of the lumen is supposed to be the major cause
- **Clinical signs:**
  - o **Rovsing's sign:** Pain in the right lower quadrant during palpation of the left lower quadrant
  - o **Obturator sign:** Pain on internal rotation of the hip (pelvic appendix)
- **Most tender area: McBurney's** point

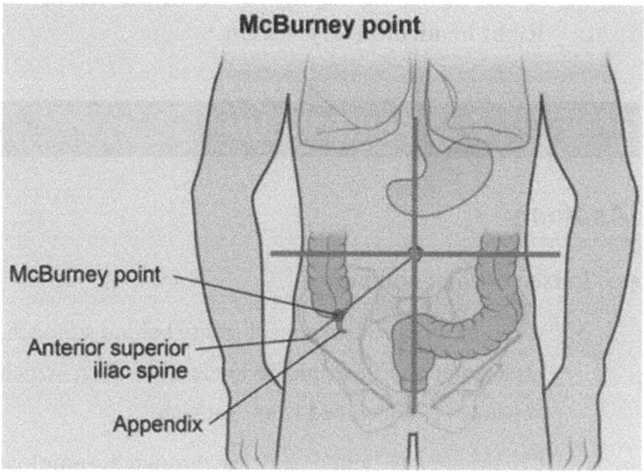

- **Imaging modalities:**
  - o CECT confirmatory (but diagnosis is clinical)
- Managed by appendicectomy
- **Ochsner-Sherren regimen:**
  - o If an appendix mass is present & the condition of the patient is satisfactory, the standard treatment is the conservative Ochsner-Sherren regimen

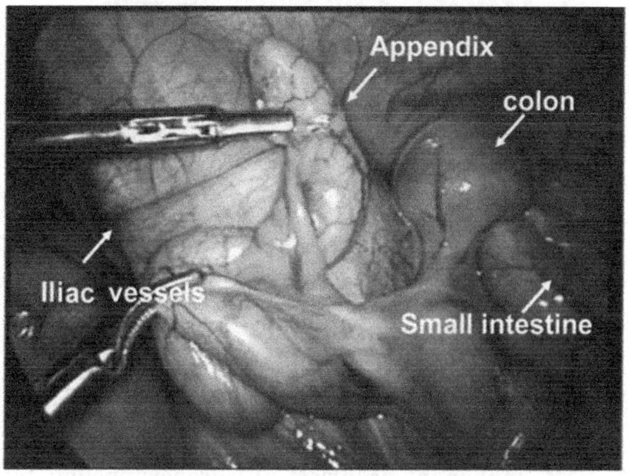

Figure: The appendix and surrounding structures

APPENDICULAR CARCINOID

Features

- **MC** in distal third of appendix (tip)
- **Mean tumour size:** 2.5 cm
- Rarely metastasize
- **Management:**
  - o Appendicectomy (<1 cm)
  - o **Right hemicolectomy:** >2 cm

PERITONEUM

Anatomy

- **Lesser sac/omental bursa:**
  - o A larger recess of peritoneal cavity behind stomach, lesser omentum & caudate nucleus of liver, which separates stomach bed from stomach
  - o Communicates with greater sac through the epiploic foramen/Foramen of Winslow
- **Mesentery:** Fan shaped fold of peritoneum that connects jejunum & ileum to the posterior abdominal wall

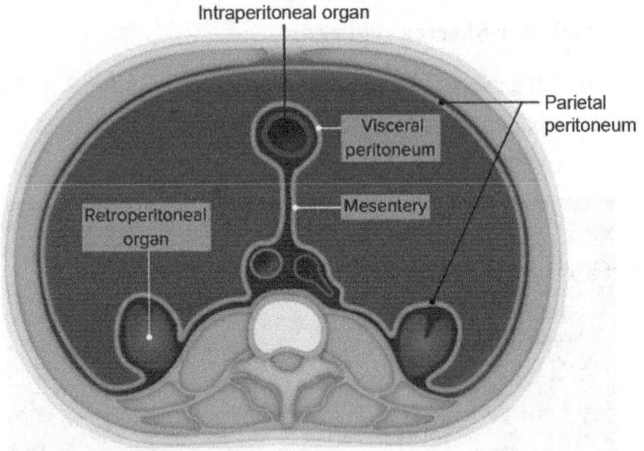

Some important points

- **Peritoneal mesotheliomas are associated with:** Asbestos exposure
- **MC malignant neoplasm of retroperitoneum:** Lymphoma & retroperitoneal sarcoma
- **Idiopathic retroperitoneal fibrosis is also known as:** Ormond's disease
- **MC site of intraperitoneal abscess:** Pelvic (Pouch of Douglas)

COLORECTAL POLYPS

Non-neoplastic polyps

- Hyperplastic polyp
- **Hamartomatous polyp:**
  - o Juvenile polyps
  - o Peutz-Jeghers syndrome
- Inflammatory polyp

Malignant potential

- **Classic FAP (Familial adenomatous polyps):** 100%
- **Villous/tubulovillous adenoma:** 20%
- **Adenomatous:** 5%

RECTUM

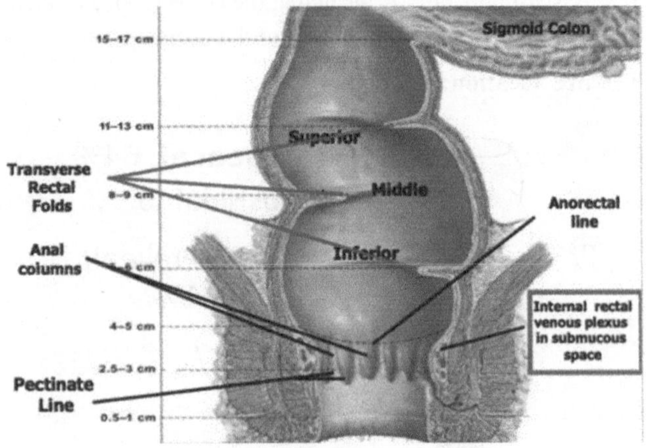

Parts of rectum

- Upper one-third is covered by peritoneum on anterior surface
- Middle third is covered by peritoneum on anterior surface
- Lower third is not covered by peritoneum hence it is the most mobile part

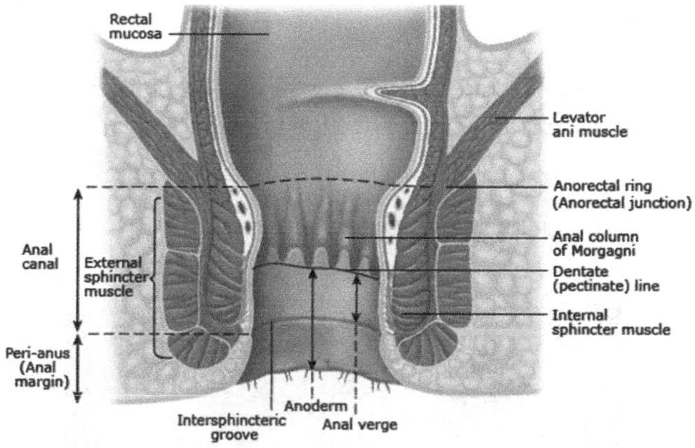

COLORECTAL CA

Pathology

- **MC site:** Rectum (38%)
- **MC site in colon:** Sigmoid colon (21%)
- **MC type (histology):** AdenoCa

Presentation

- **Right sided tumour:**
  - o Fungating/cauliflower type growth
  - o **Anemia** because the lesion ulcerate
  - o Melena
  - o Good prognosis
- **Left sided tumour:**
  - o Annular, constricting or stenosing growth
  - o Obstruction/**pain**
  - o Alteration of bowel habits
  - o Poor prognosis
- **MC site of metastasis:** Liver (33% patient may have metastasis)
- **Barium enema:** Apple core or napkin ring lesion in constricting Ca
- **Gold standard for diagnosis:** Colonoscopy

Risk factors

- Increased dietary fats & oil
- Low fiber diet
- Elevated serum cholesterol
- Ulcerative colitis & Crohn's disease
- Familial adenomatous polyps

Treatment of choice

- Surgery

HIRSCHSPRUNG'S DISEASE

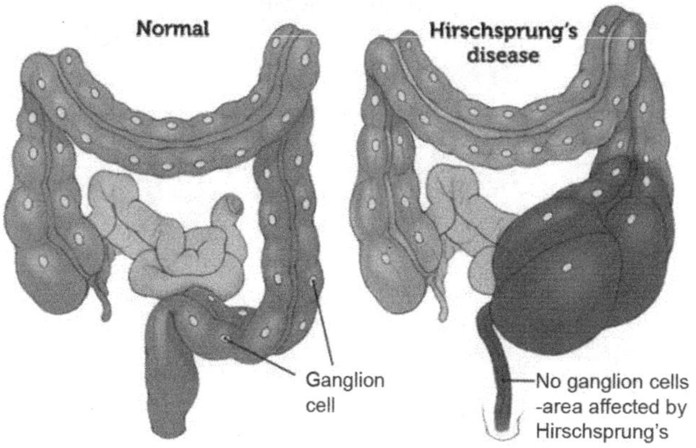

Features

- Pathologically absent ganglion cells in the myenteric (Auerbach's) and submucosal (Meissner's) plexus with hypertrophy of nerve trunks in the plexus
- **MC affected site:** Rectosigmoid (75%)
- Rectal biopsy is **gold** standard for diagnosis

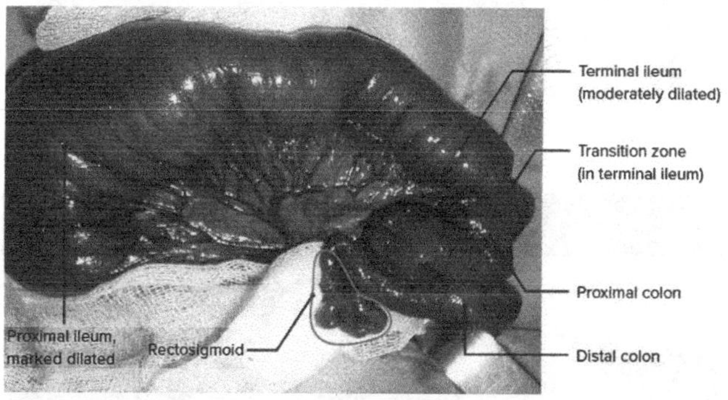

CROHN'S DISEASE

Features

- Chronic transmural inflammatory disease of the GIT
- Can involve any part of the GIT from mouth to anus but usually involves small intestine (terminal ileum) & colon
- Involves entire thickness of bowel

- **Skip areas:** Diseased bowel is separated by areas of grossly appearing normal bowel
- **Cobblestone appearance:** Linear ulcers may coalesce to produce transverse sinuses with islands of normal mucosa in between
- String sign of **Kantor**
- **Serology:** Anti-Saccharomyces cerevisiae/ASCA auto-antibodies

Crohn's Disease

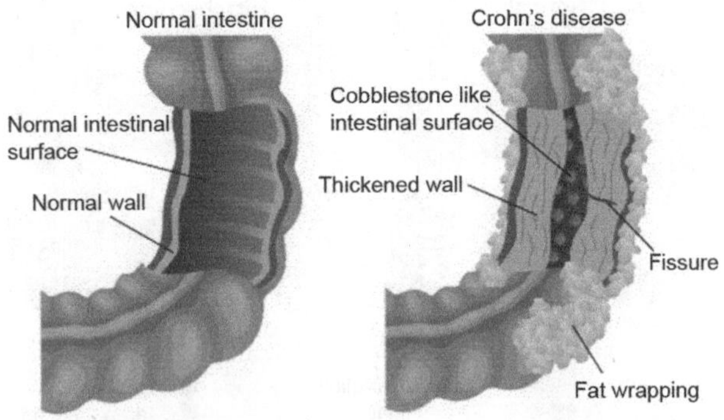

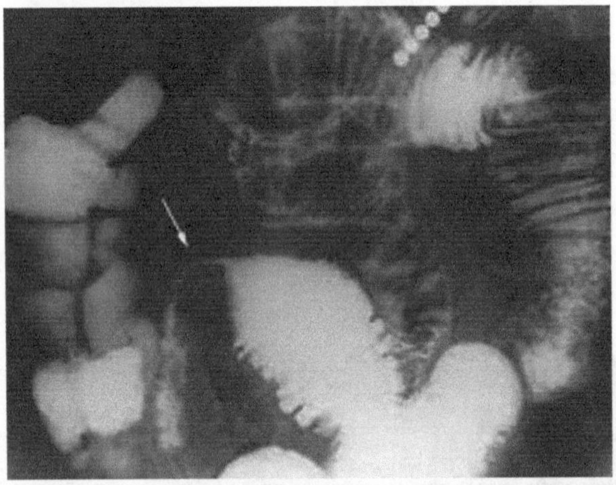

ULCERATIVE COLITIS

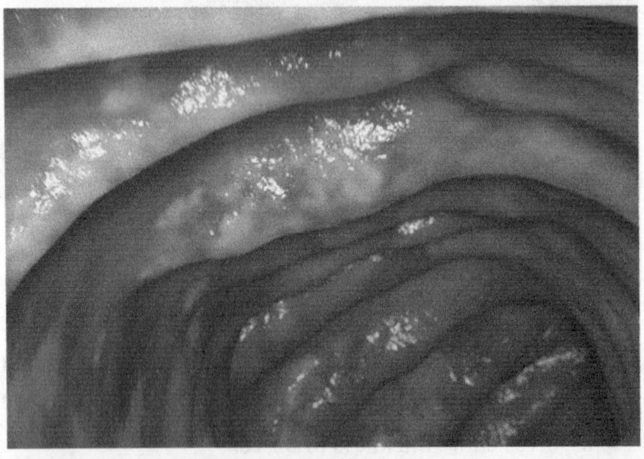

Features

- Pathologic process involving the mucosa and submucosa of the colon, without affecting muscularis
- Rectal involvement (proctitis) is the hallmark
- Pseudopolyps/inflammatory polyps

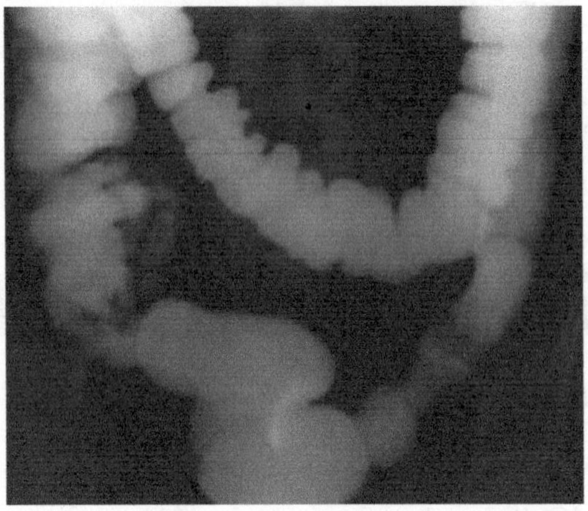

- Continuous uninterrupted inflammation of the colonic mucosa, beginning in distal rectum and extending proximally
- **Crypt abscess:** Neutrophils fill and expand the lumina of individual crypts of Lieberkühn
- p-ANCA positive
- Garden hose appearance
- **Pipestem** colon (ahaustral)

HEMORRHOIDS

Features

- **Internal hemorrhoids:**
  - o Located proximal to the dentate line
  - o **Painless**
  - o Can be ligated
  - o Banding is preferred
- **External hemorrhoids:**
  - o Located distal to dentate line
  - o 5-day self-curing lesion
  - o **Painful**
  - o Not ligated
  - o Excision is done

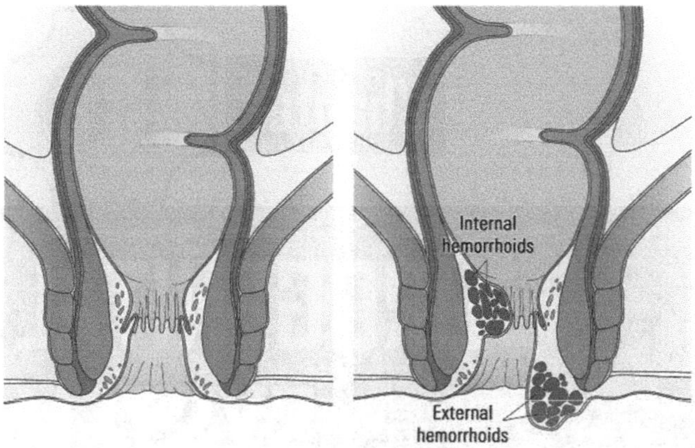

- **Degree of internal hemorrhoids:**
  - o **1st degree:** Painless bleeding, no prolapse
  - o **2nd degree:** Prolapse through the anus on straining but reduce spontaneously
  - o **3rd degree:** Prolapse through the anal canal but require manual reduction
  - o **4th degree:** Permanently prolapsed and **cannot** be reduced manually
- **Treatment:**
  - o Drugs (1st & 2nd)
  - o Rubber band ligation (1st & 2nd; selective 3rd)
  - o Operative hemorrhoidectomy (3rd & 4th)

FISTULA IN-ANO

Features

- A chronic abnormal communication, run outwards from the anorectal lumen to an external opening on the skin of the perineum or buttock
- Results from anorectal/cryptoglandular abscess

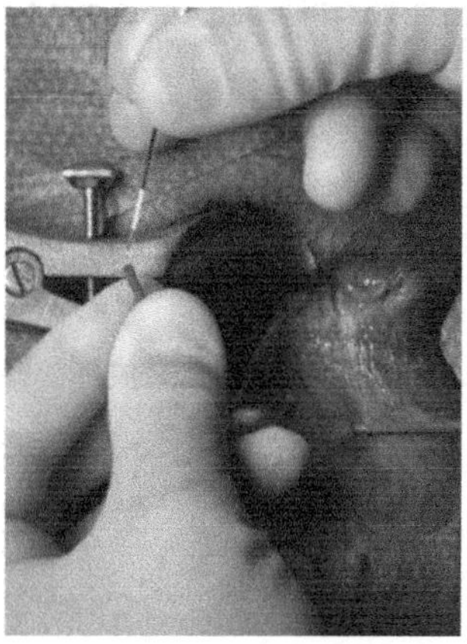

- **Types (with respect to internal opening above or below the anorectal ring):** High or low
- **Goodsall's rule:**
  - o Indicates the likely position of the internal opening according to the position of external opening
  - o Fistulas with external openings anterior to horizontal imaginary line drawn across the mid-point of anus connect to the internal opening by short **straight** track
  - o Fistulas with external opening posterior to the horizontal line run a **curvilinear** course and open internally into posterior midline

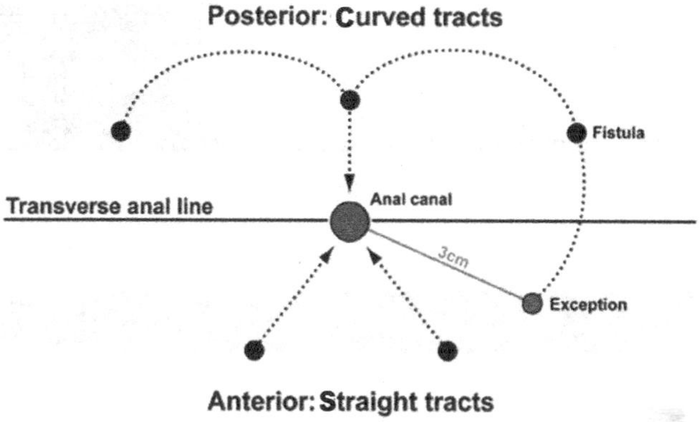

- MRI is the gold standard for fistula imaging

CARCINOMA ANAL CANAL

Features

- **MC** type is squamous cell Ca
- **MC complaint:** Bleeding per rectum
- Proctoscopy with biopsy is the investigation of **choice**
- CT scan of abdomen & pelvis is a must as all of the draining lymph nodes are not palpable
- **Treatment:**
  - o **Nigro regimen:** Chemoradiation
  - o **Chemotherapy:** 5-Fluorouracil + Mitomycin C/Cisplatin

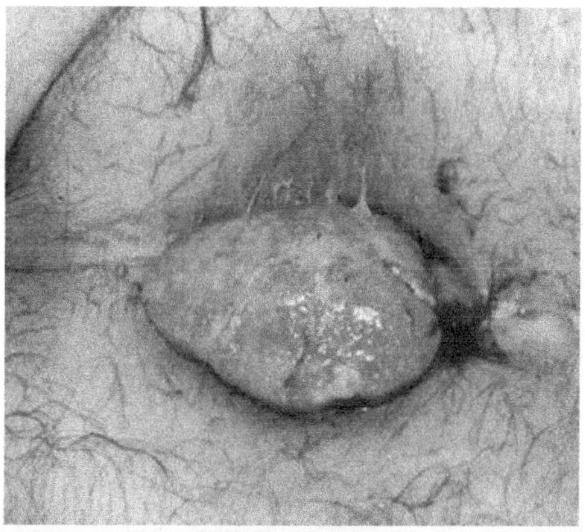

SECTION 2

SURGERY

Chapter 10

UROGENITAL SYSTEM

KIDNEY

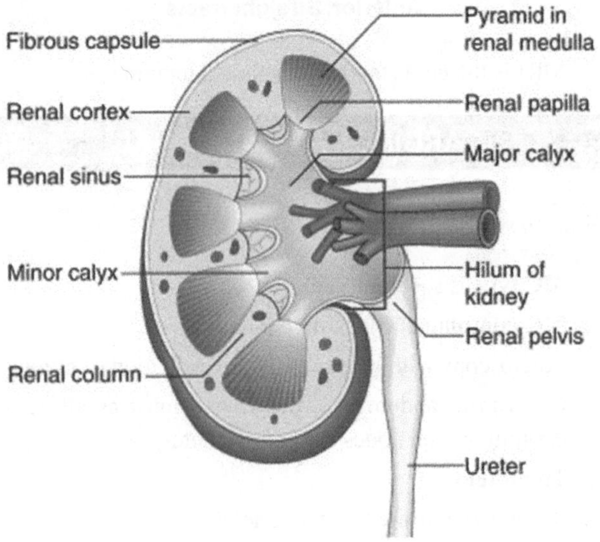

Kidney

- Kidney is situated retroperitoneally on the posterior abdominal wall
- **Structures at hilum (from anterior to posterior):**
    - o Renal vein
    - o Renal artery
    - o Renal pelvis

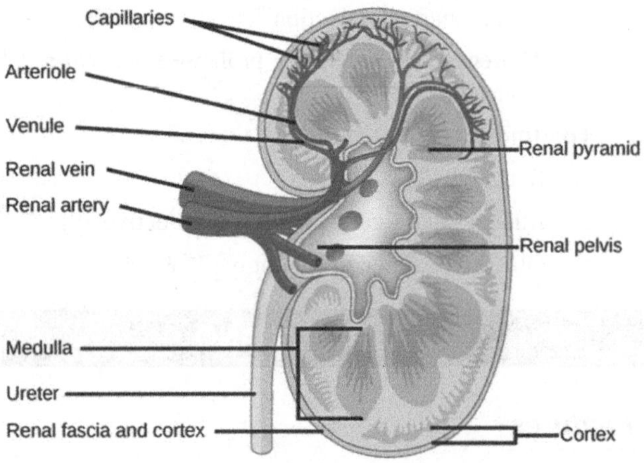

- **Kidney angle/Renal angle:**
    - o Angle between the **12th** rib & outer border of the sacrospinalis
    - o Pressure over this area elicits tenderness of kidney

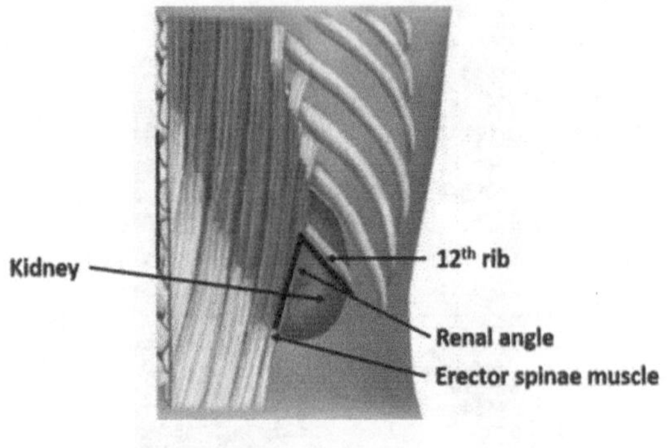

Coverings of kidney from inside outside are:

- Fibrous renal capsule
- Perirenal fat
- Renal fascia (fascia of Gerota; fascia of Zuckerkandl is the posterior layer of renal fascia)
- Pararenal fat

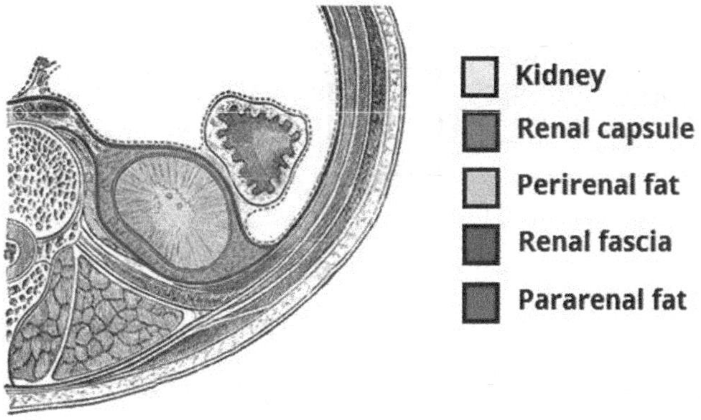

Tributaries of left renal vein

- Left gonadal vein
- Left suprarenal/adrenal vein
- Left inferior phrenic vein

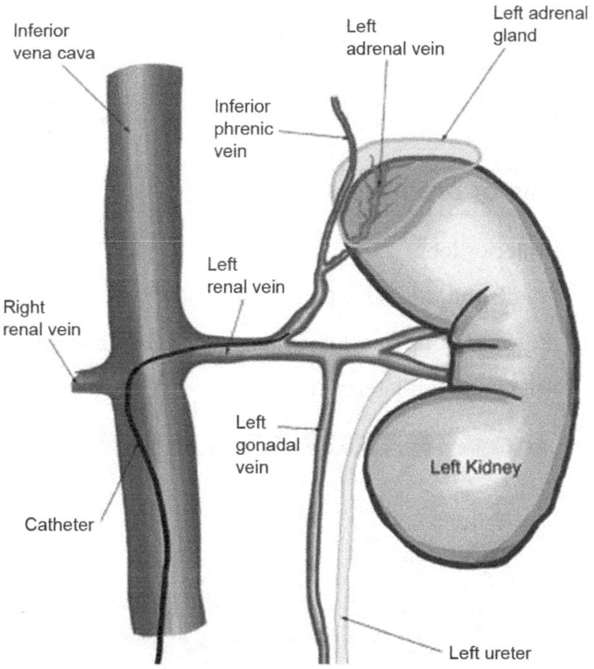

Renal transplantation

- Left kidney is selected for transplantation
- Iliac fossa is the preferred site for transplanted kidney

URETER

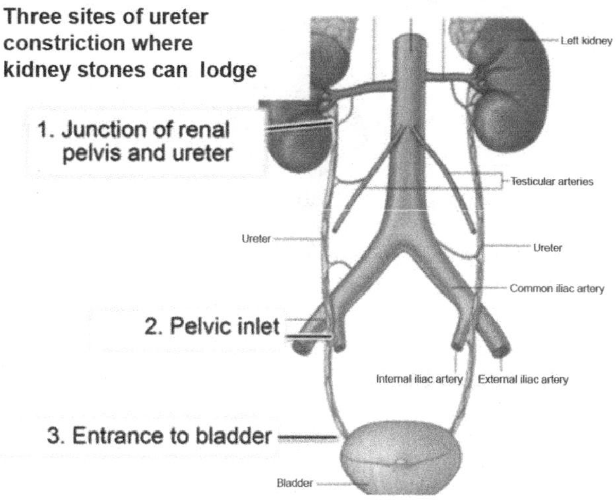

Anatomical features

- 25-30 cm long
- Begins within renal sinus as a funnel shaped dilatation called renal pelvis
- Enters the urinary bladder obliquely to open at the lateral angle of trigone
- **Normal constrictions:**
  - o PUJ/Pelviureteric junction
  - o At the brim of lesser pelvis
  - o Along its passage through the bladder wall

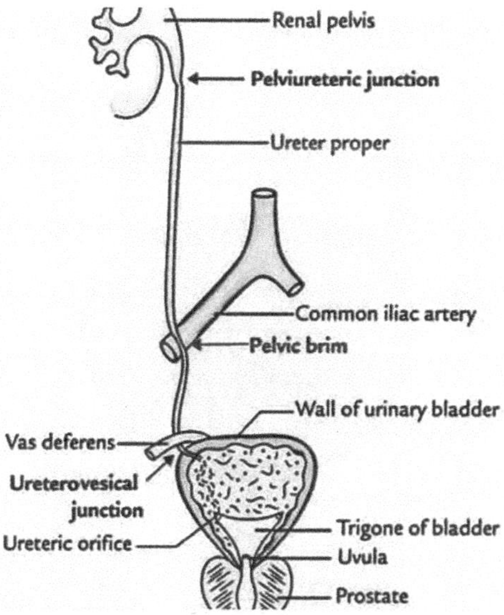

URINARY BLADDER

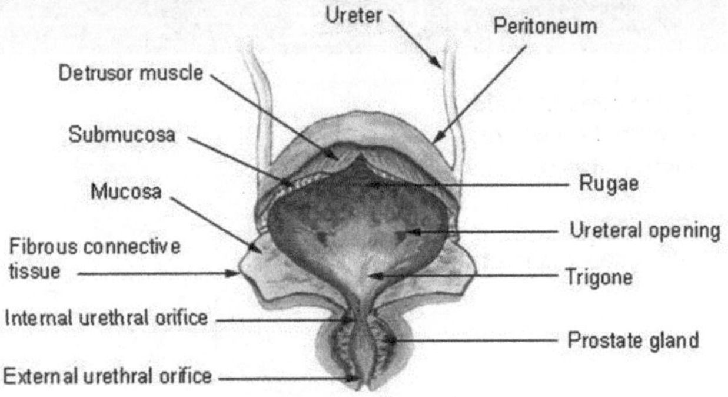

Figure: Urinary bladder

Urinary bladder

- Muscular reservoir of urine
- Situated posterior to pubic bones
- Size, shape, position depends on amount of urine in the bladder
- Lined by **urothelium**
- Trigone is a triangular area over the lower part of the base of the bladder
- Ureter opens into the posterolateral angle of the bladder
- **Sphincters:**
  - o **Internal:**
    - ♦ **Smooth** muscles
    - ♦ Innervated by autonomic nervous system
  - o **External:**
    - ♦ **Skeletal** muscles
    - ♦ Innervated by perineal branch of pudendal nerve

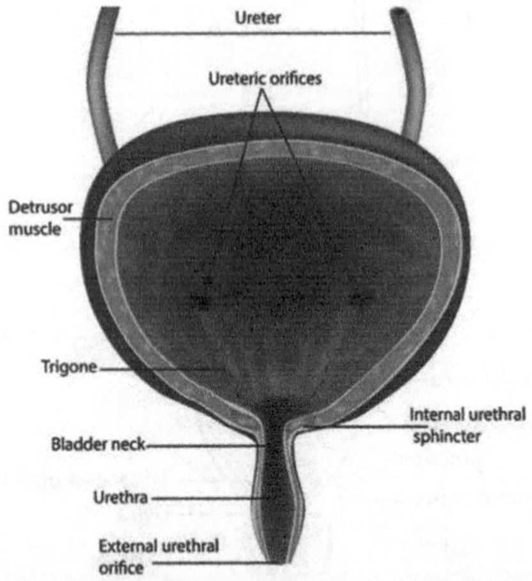

PROSTATE

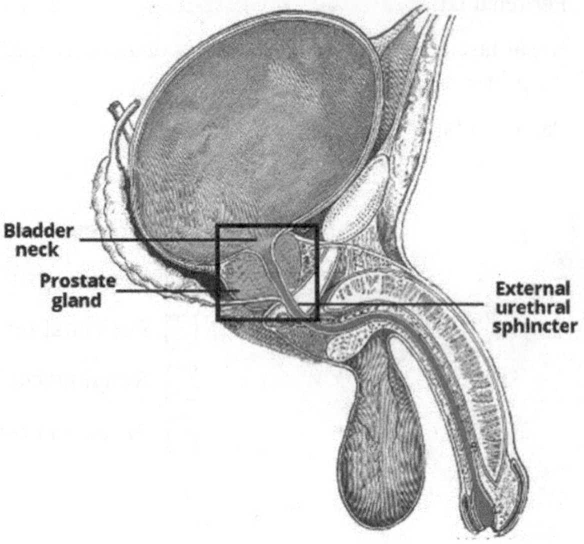

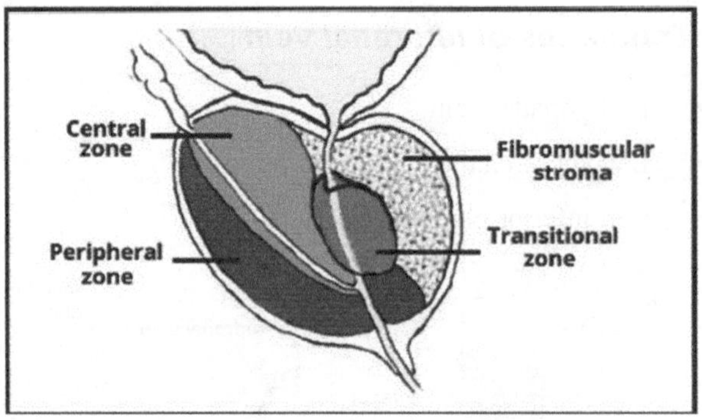

Lobes of prostate

- Anterior lobe
- Median/middle lobe (enlarged in BPH)
- Posterior lobe (most common site of malignancy)
- Right and left lateral lobes

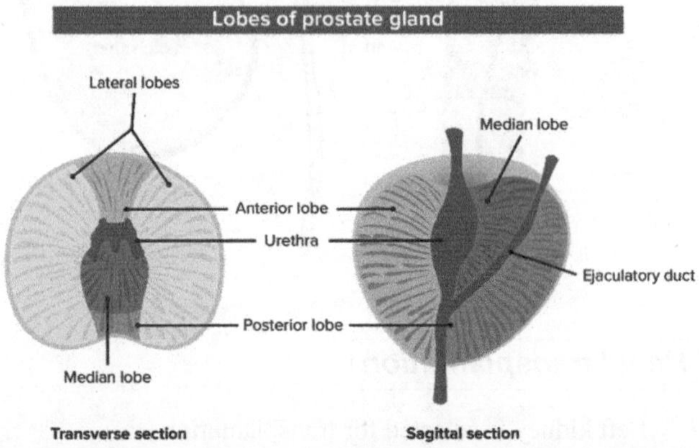

MALE URETHRA

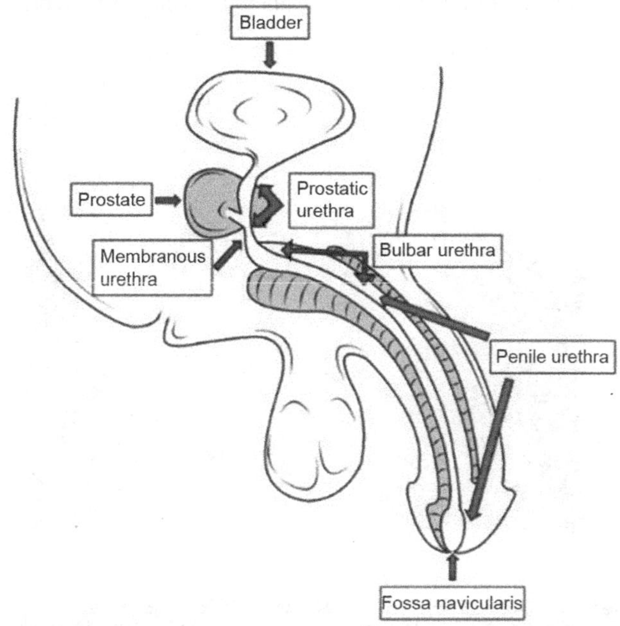

- **Anterior:**
  - o Penile
  - o Bulbar
- **Posterior:**
  - o Membranous
  - o Prostatic

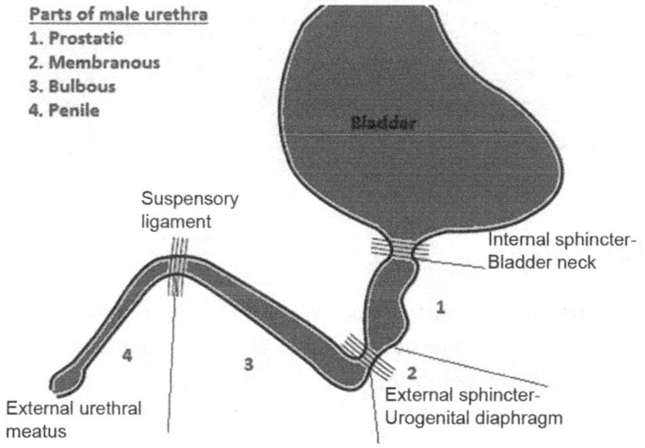

POLYCYSTIC KIDNEY DISEASE/PKD

Features

- **Adult PKD:** Autosomal **dominant**

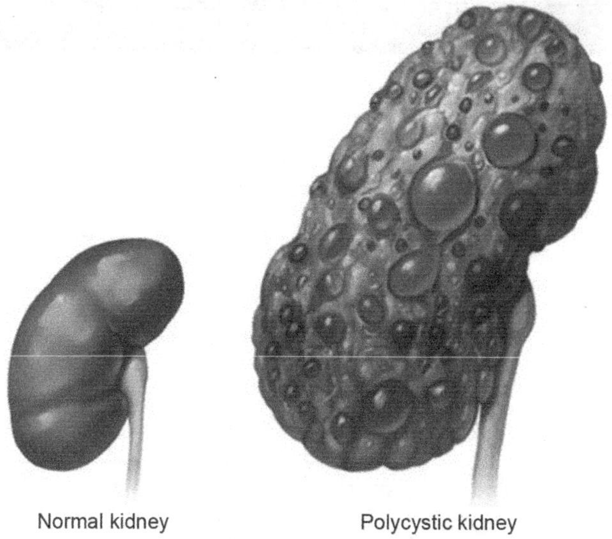

- **Infantile PKD:** Autosomal recessive
- Intravenous pyelography shows **spider** leg appearance

CONGENITAL PELVIURETERIC JUNCTION OBSTRUCTION

Features

- Most **common** cause of significant dilatation of the collecting system in the fetal kidney

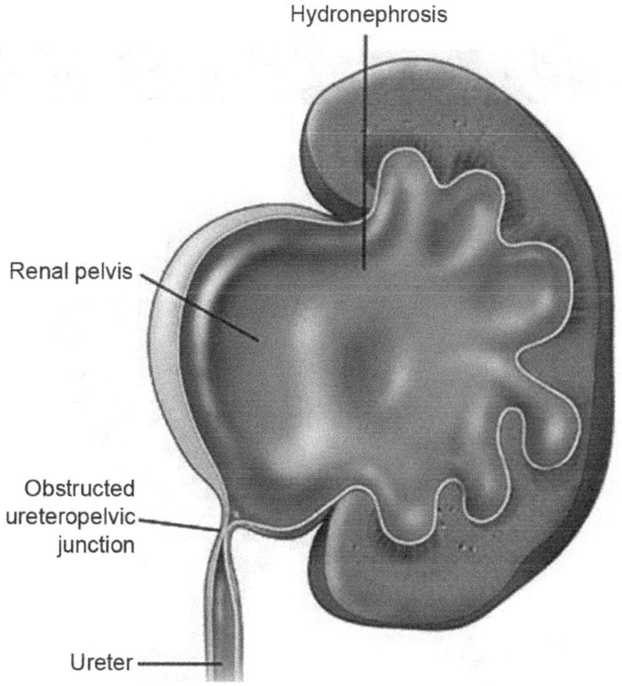

URETEROCELE

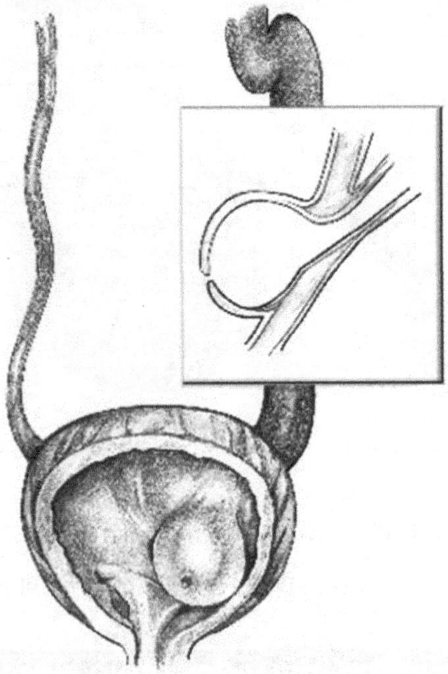

Features

- **Ballooning** of the distal submucosal ureters into the bladder
- **Adder** head or **Cobra** head appearance of excretory urography is noted

HORSESHOE KIDNEY

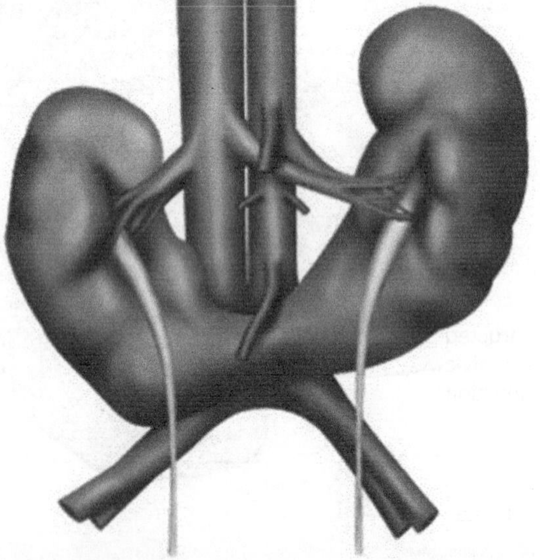

Features

- Fusion of lower poles of kidney opposite **L4** vertebra
- **Flower** vase appearance on intravenous pyelography

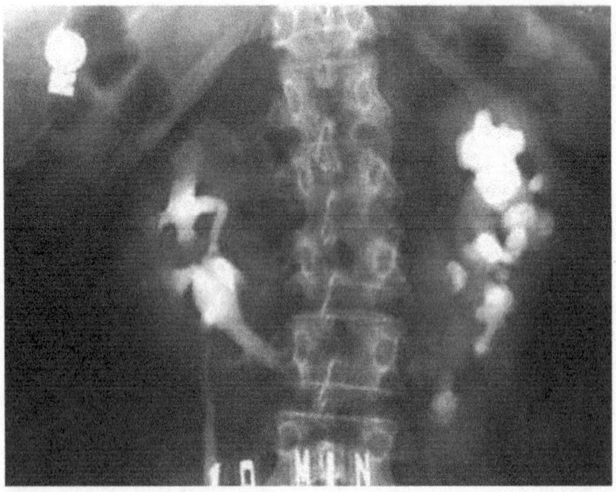

RENAL TUBERCULOSIS

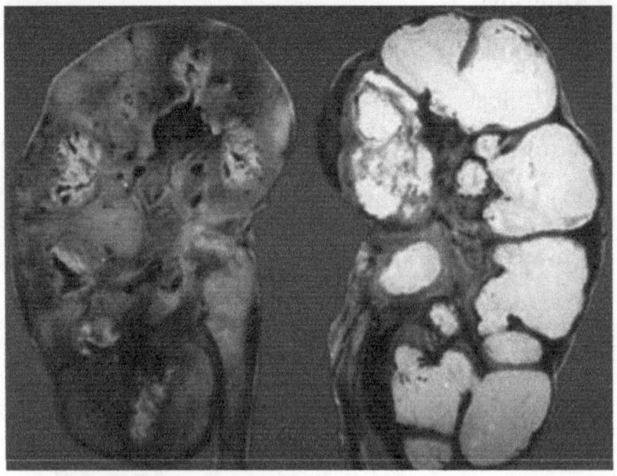

Features

- **Sterile pyuria:** Urine is pale and opalescent with presence of pus cells without organism in an acid urine (abacterial aciduria)
- Kidney is rarely palpable
- Caseous kidney/**putty** kidney/cement kidney (it goes for autonephrectomy)

Investigations

- Intravenous urography
- Three consecutive early morning samples of urine (EMSU) are collected and sent for microscopy (Ziehl-

Neelsen staining), culture (L-J media) or guinea pig inoculation

RENAL CALCULI

Types & features

- **MC stones:** Calcium stones (75-85%)
- **Radiolucent stones:** Uric acid
- **Stones MC in men:** Calcium
- **Stones MC in females:** Struvite stones
- **Stones MC in UTI with urease producing bacteria (proteus spp.):** Struvite stones
- **Stone which grows in alkaline urine:** Struvite stones
- **Stone which grow in infected urine:** Struvite stone
- **Stone hard to break in ESWL:** Cystine stones
- **Pain in ureteric calculi is due to:** Ureteric peristalsis

X-ray

- **Location of renal stone on lateral view of lumbar spine:** Renal calculi **overlies** spine in lateral view

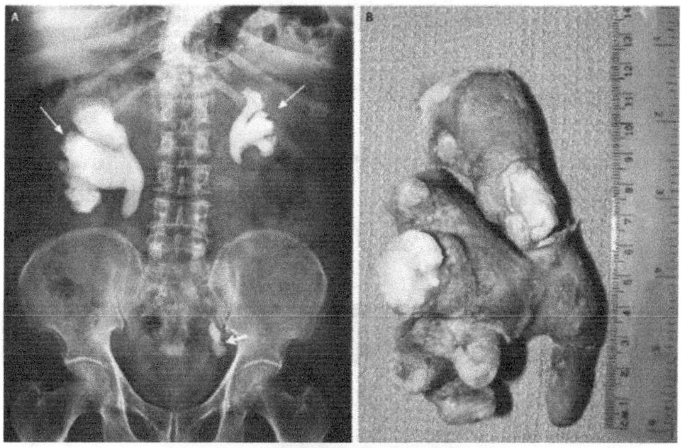

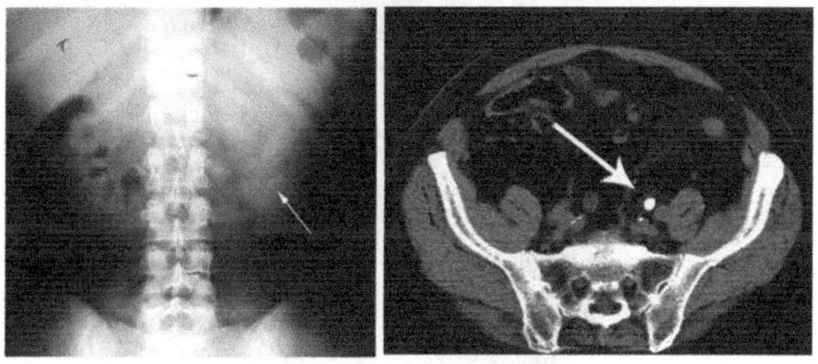

Dietel's crisis (Intermittent hydronephrosis)

- Renal colic is associated with swelling in loin
- Following **passage** of stone, large amount of urine is passed, swelling disappears and pain is relieved

Management

- ESWL/Extracorporeal shock wave lithotripsy
- Ureteroscopy
- Percutaneous nephrolithotomy/PCNL

WILMS' TUMOUR

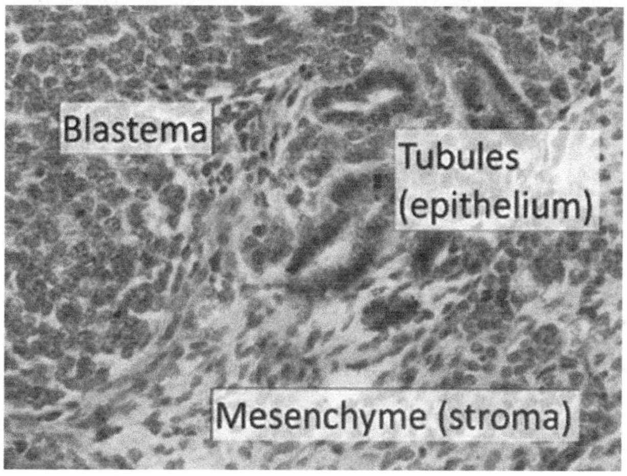

Features

- **Age group affected: 1-5** years
- Painless abdominal lump is the most **common** and earliest symptom
-

Triad

- Abdominal mass
- Pyrexia
- Hematuria

RENAL CELL CARCINOMA/GRAWITZ TUMOUR

Associated with

- Von Hippel Lindau syndrome
- Tuberous sclerosis
- Polycystic kidney disease

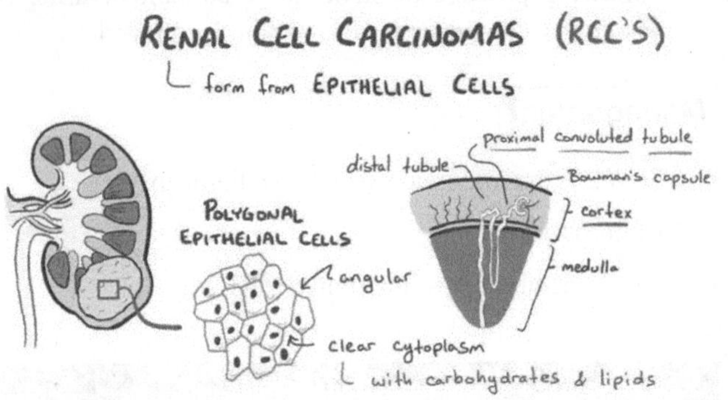

Classical triad of RCC

- Hematuria
- Flank pain
- Palpable flank mass

Features

- **Clear** cell Ca (60%)
- **MC site of metastasis: Lung** (cannon ball secondaries), followed by bone
- Can cause pulsatile skull metastasis
- **May cause:** Paraneoplastic syndromes (hypercalcemia, erythrocytosis, Cushing's syndrome etc.)

Management

- **Standard management of stage I or II, few cases of stage III:** Radical nephrectomy
- **Treatment of choice: Radical** nephrectomy

VESICOURETERIC REFLUX

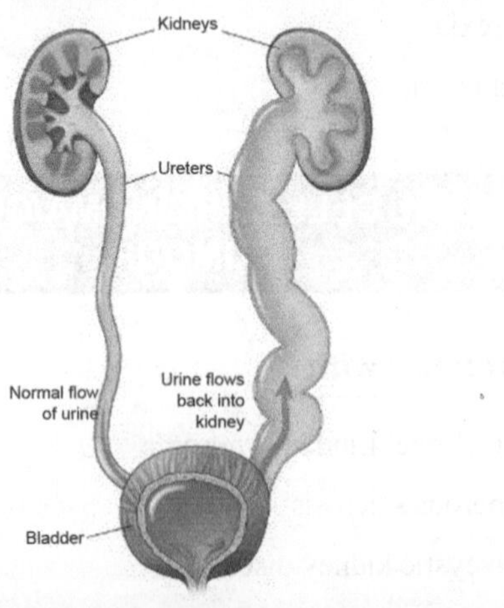

Features

- **Retrograde** flow of urine from the bladder into the ureters and to the renal pelvis
- Diagnosed after an attack of **UTI** (urinary tract infection)
- Reflux predisposes to renal infection (pyelonephritis)

EXOSTROPHY OF BLADDER/ECTOPIA VESICAE

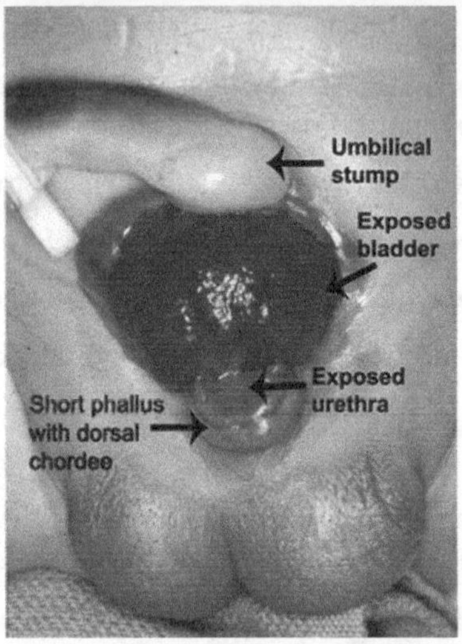

Features

- There is a **defect** in the infraumbilical part of the anterior abdominal wall, associated with incomplete development of the anterior wall of the urinary bladder

URINARY BLADDER CARCINOMA

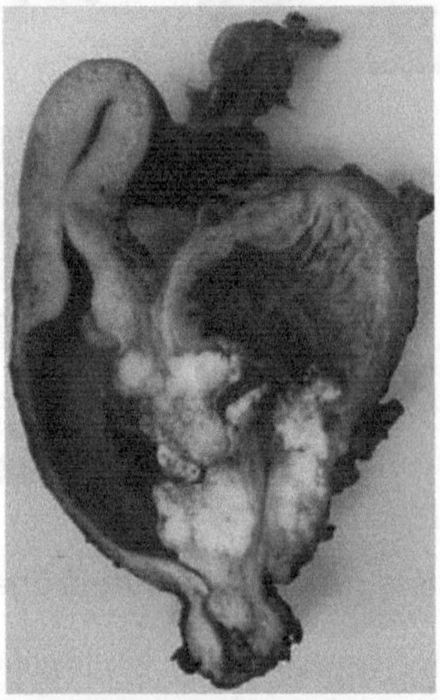

Features

- **Transitional** cell Ca (90%)
- **Risk factors:**
  - o Smoking
  - o 2-naphthylamine
  - o Occupations like painters, leather workers, dye workers etc.

Features

- **Squamous cell Ca:**
  - o Seen when squamous metaplasia or keratinisation has occurred
  - o Schistosomiasis (vesical bilharziasis)
- **Painless** hematuria
- **BCG** (intravesical) is used in treatment

BLADDER STONES

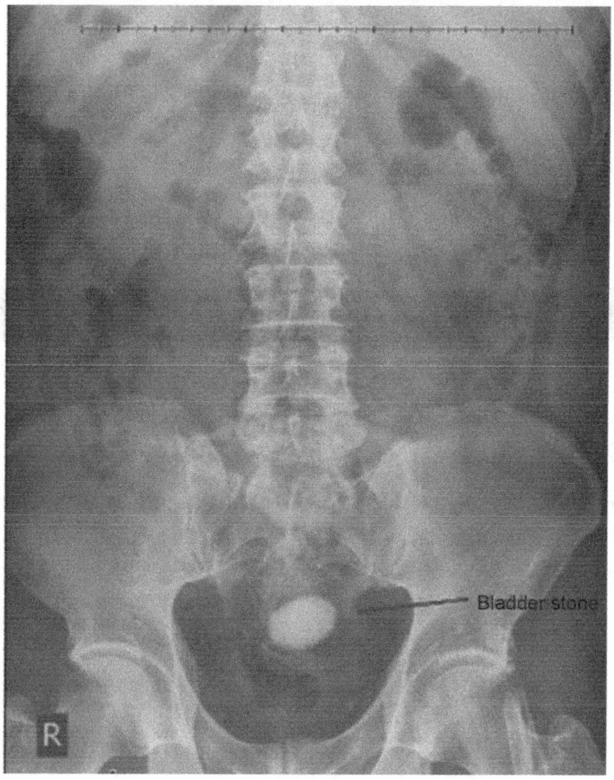

Features

- Seen in older men
- Most common type is ammonium urate stones

TB URINARY BALDDER

Features

- Cobblestone appearance
- Thimble bladder (long standing cases)
- **Golf** hole ureter

RUPTURE BLADDER

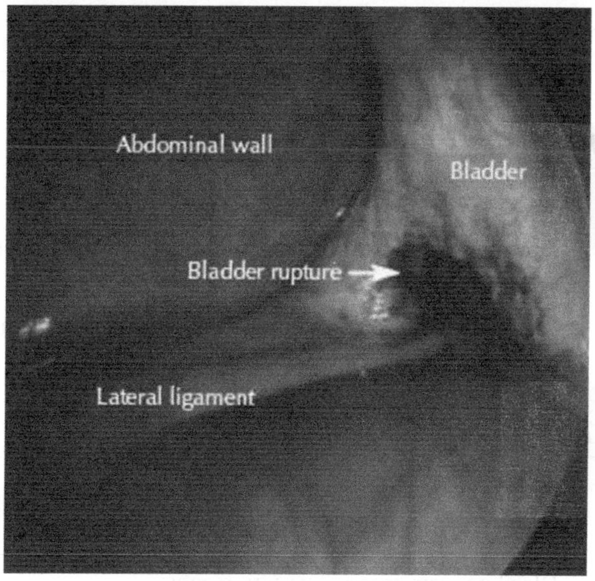

Features

- **Extraperitoneal:**
  - o Follows **pelvic** fracture leading to membranous urethral injury
- **Intraperitoneal:**
  - o Due to direct blow to lower abdomen
  - o Blood and urine will extravasate into the peritoneal cavity producing signs of peritonitis

URETHRAL RUPTURE

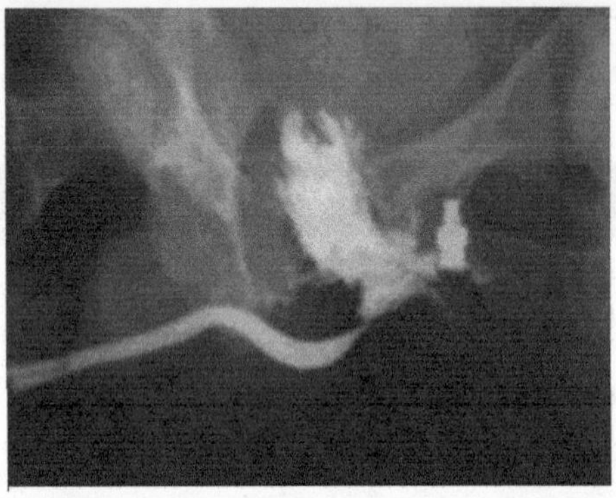

Figure: Complete Type II urethral injury. Large amount of contrast material extravasation without flow into the prostatic urethra or bladder. Fracture of the right pubic rami

Types

- Bulbar urethral injury (most common)
- Membranous urethral injury

Features

- **MC cause of urethra stricture:** Trauma
- **Part of urethra injured in pelvic fracture:** Membranous urethra
- **Mechanism of urethral injury:** Fall astride a projecting object (History of blow to perineum)

Triad of ruptured bulbar urethra

- Retention of urine
- Perineal hematoma
- Bleeding from external urinary meatus

Precaution in such cases

- **Avoid** catheterization

POSTERIOR URETHRAL VALVE

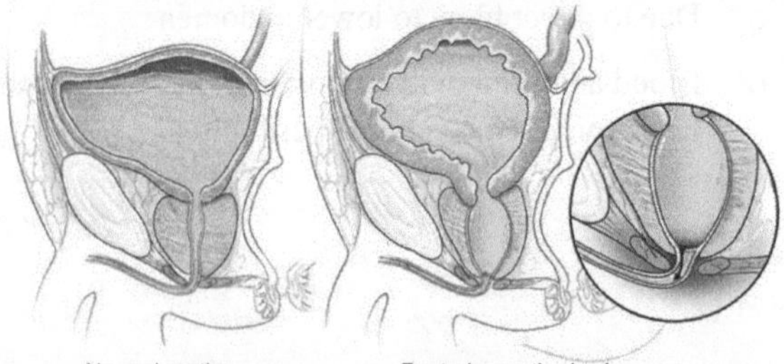

Features

- **MC** cause of obstructive uropathy in a male child
- Usually found distal to the verumontanum (Type I)

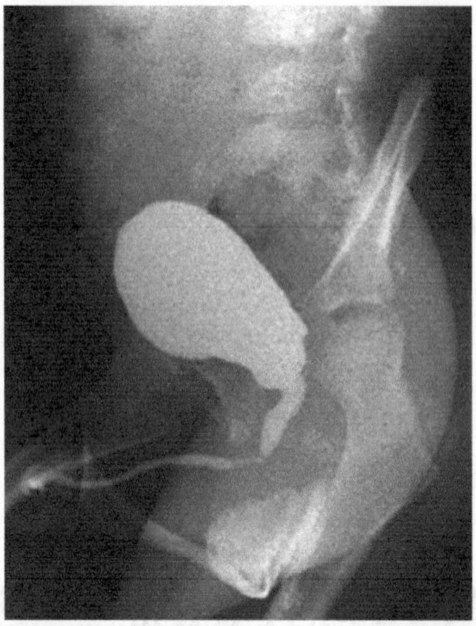

Feature

- MC cause of urinary **obstruction** in male infant

Diagnosis

- VCUG & endoscopy

HYPOSPADIAS

Features

- **MC** congenital anomaly of urethra
- Urethra opens on the underside (ventral surface) of penis/perineum

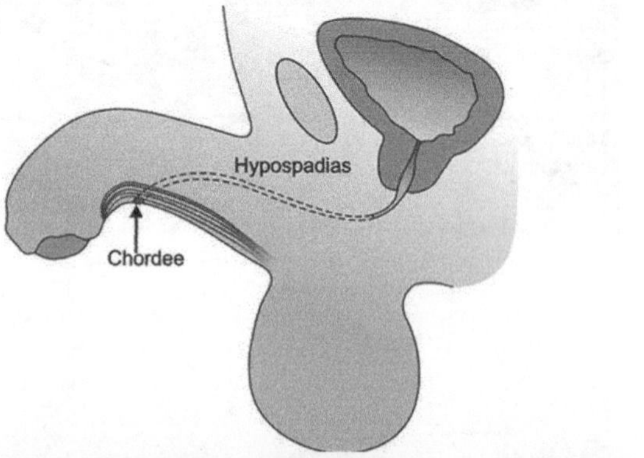

Associated terms

- Dorsal Hooded prepuce
- **Chordee:** Penis curved ventrally
- Meatal stenosis
- Bifid scrotum

Best time of surgery

- Circumcision is **not** done in patients with hypospadias as the prepuce can be later used in surgical repair
- **Stage I:** Managing chordee (Straightening of penis) at 18-24 months of age
- **Stage II:** Reconstruction of urethra at 5-7 years

INCOMPLETE DESCENT OF TESTES

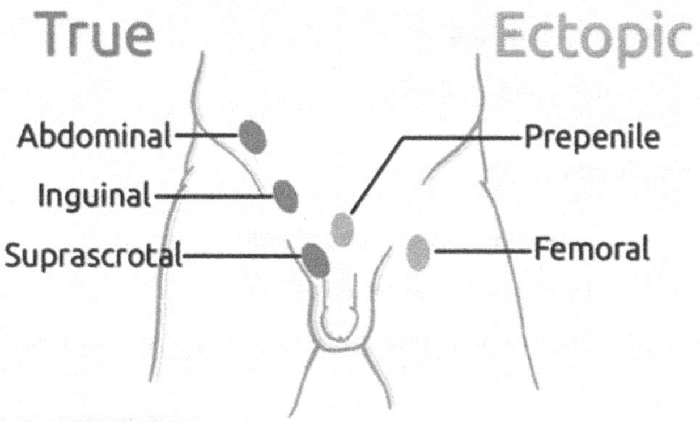

Features

- **Arrested** in normal path of descent
- Testis and scrotum **not** fully developed
- Malignant change/seminoma (even if the testes have been brought down surgically)
- Sterility (if bilateral)

Best time to operate

- **Orchidopexy** before 1 year

TESTICULAR TORSION

Features

- **MC** seen in adolescent

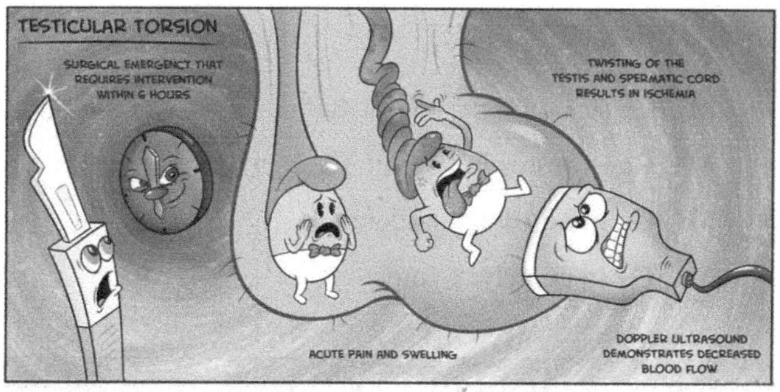

- Presents with sudden onset of pain in testis
- Follows vigorous activity before
- **Bell** clapper deformity is an important risk factor
- **Prehn's sign:**
    - o Elevation of testis by palm **increases** the pain in testicular torsion but the pain of epididymo-orchitis is relieved
- Surgery has to be done **within** 4 hours otherwise testis will undergo necrosis
- Both the affected and unaffected testis should go orchidopexy

TESTICULAR CARCINOMA

Features

- Bilateral in 10% of cases
- Abdominal cryptorchid testes are at higher risk as compared to inguinal cryptorchid testes

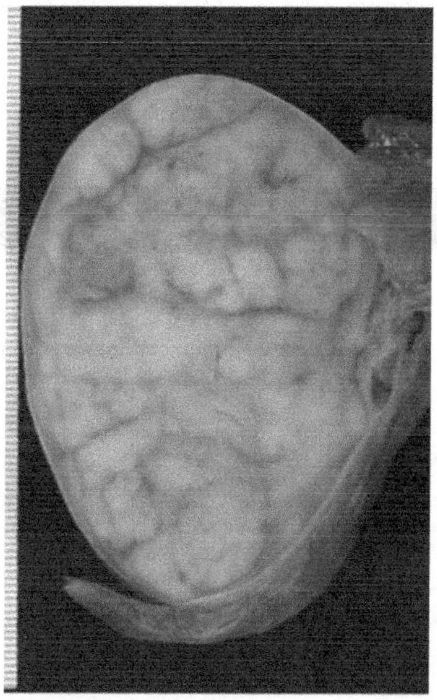

MC Types

- **MC Ca in infants:** Yolk sac tumour
- **MC Ca of testes in young:** Teratoma
- **MC Ca in adults:** Seminoma
- **MC Ca in elderly:** Lymphoma

SEMINOMA

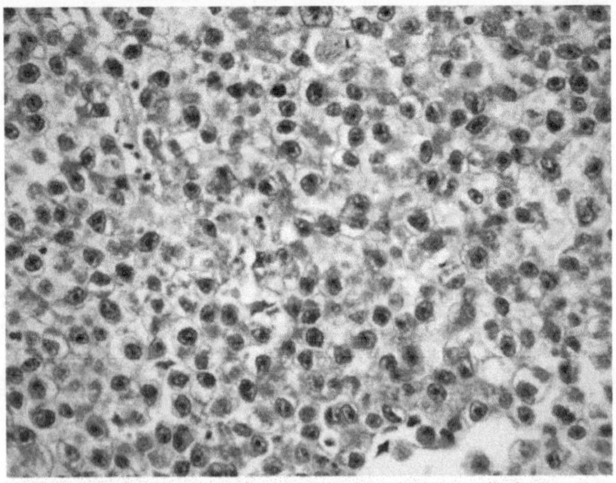

Demonstrating large cells with clear cytoplasm, distinct borders, squared off nuclei and prominent nucleoli. Admixed lymphocytes are present

Features

- **Most** seminoma presents with stage I disease (limited to testis)
- Radiosensitive
- Corresponds to dysgerminoma of ovary
- **Treatment of choice is:** Surgery

HYDROCELE

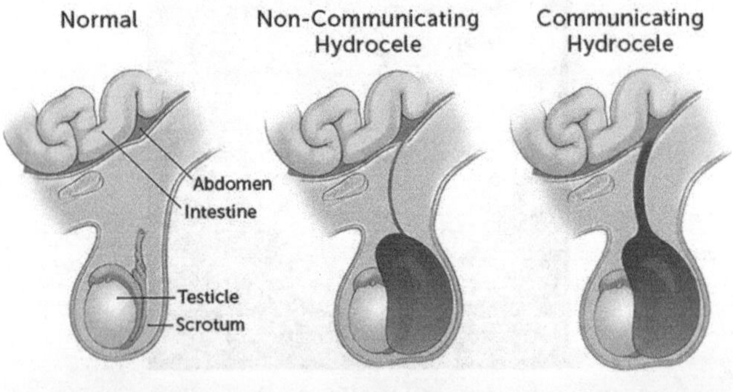

Features

- **Types:**
  - o **Vaginal hydrocele: MC** type
  - o Infantile hydrocele
  - o Congenital hydrocele
- Fluid is amber colored
- Shows transillumination
- **Surgeries:**
  - o **Lord's** plication
  - o Jaboulay's method

VARICOCELE

MC

- Seen on **Left** side
- Seen in young tall men

Features

- Bag of **worms** like feel on palpation
- May be secondary to renal cell Ca
- MC cause of male **infertility**, which is surgically treated

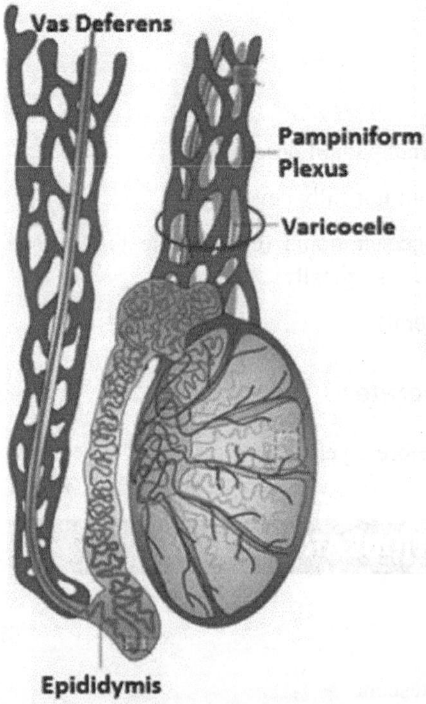

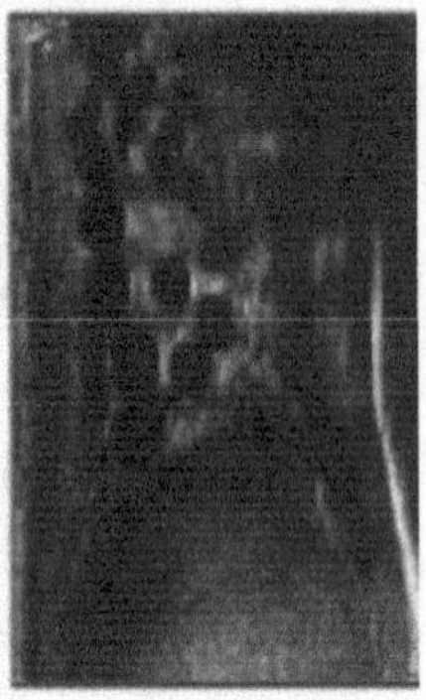

BENIGN PROSTATIC HYPERTROPHY

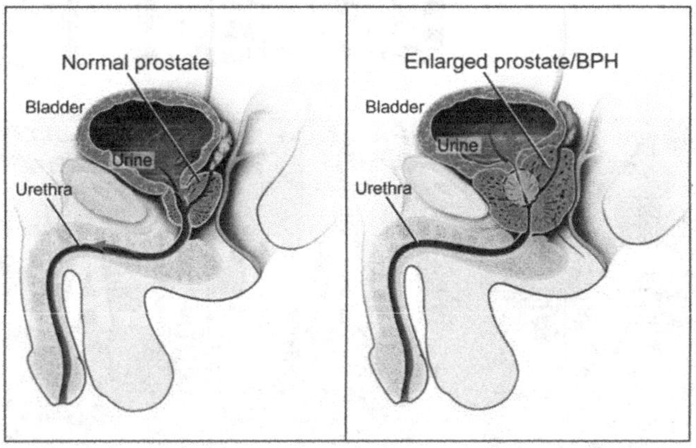

Pathology

- **BPH arises from: Periurethral** zone

Medical management

- **Alpha-adrenergic blockers: Prazosin**, Terazosin, Tamsulosin
- **5-alpha reductase inhibitors: Finasteride**

TURP

- Transurethral Resection of Prostate is the **gold** standard procedure for BPH
- **MC complication of TURP:** Retrograde ejaculation; due to injury to internal sphincter
- **Irrigation fluid used in TURP:** 1.5% isotonic glycine
- **Never** use Normal saline during TURP
- **Hyponatremia, drowsiness & altered sensorium after TURP may point toward:** Water intoxication/TUR syndrome (isotonic saline avoid such complication)

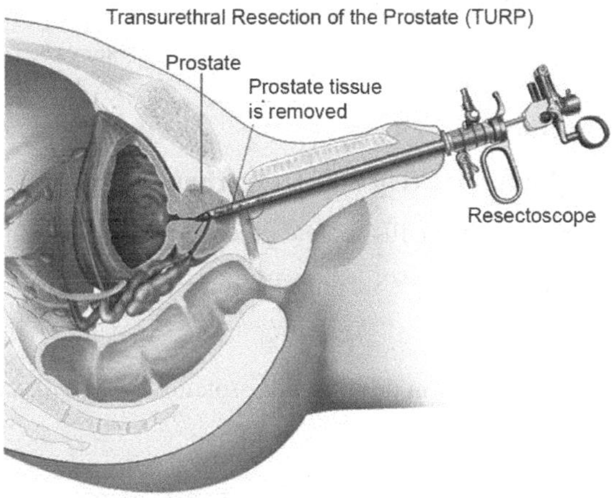

CARCINOMA PROSTATE

Features

- **MC** malignant tumour in men >65 years of age
- Bladder outlet obstruction and back pain **indicate** prostate carcinoma
- **MC nodes to be affected in lymphatic spread:** Obturator LN
- **Tumour markers:**
  - o Serum acid phosphatase
  - o PSA

Metastasis to vertebrae is via

- Batesons vertebral venous plexus
- **Order of metastasis:**
  - o Lumbar spine is the **MC** site
  - o Proximal femur

Staging system

- Gleason staging

Most effective screening protocol for prostate Ca

- Digital rectal examination
- PSA (Prostatic Specific Antigen)

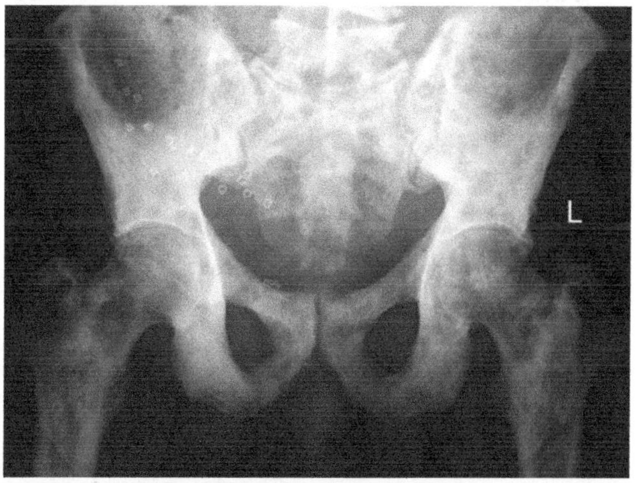

SECTION 2
SURGERY

Chapter 11

PANCREAS

ANATOMY

Anatomy

- Elongated retroperitoneal organ
- Lies against L1-L2 vertebrae, posterior to stomach

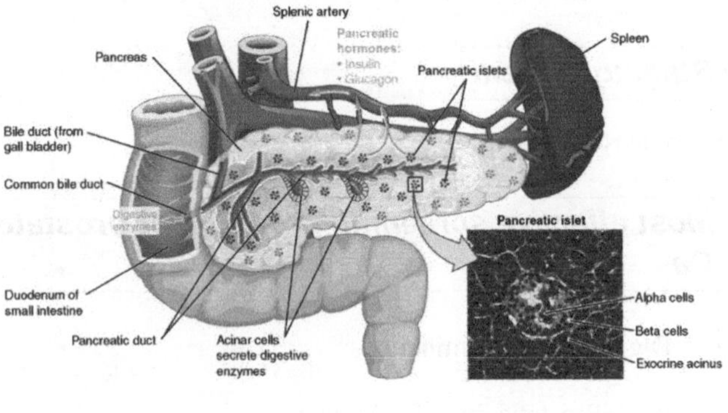

- **Parts:**
  - o **Head:**
    - ♦ Lies within concavity of duodenum
  - o Neck
  - o Body
  - o **Tail:**
    - ♦ Reaches hilum of the spleen
- **Ducts:**
  - o **Wirsung/Main:**
    - ♦ Joins with bile duct in the wall of 2nd part of duodenum to form hepatopancreatic ampulla of Vater & opens on the summit of major duodenal papilla
  - o **Santorini/Accessory:**
    - ♦ Opens into the duodenum at minor duodenal papilla

Anatomy of the Pancreas

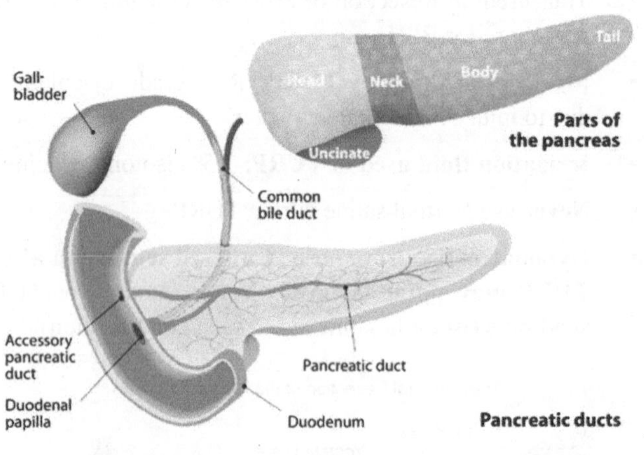

- **Functions:**
  - o **Endocrine (Islets of Langerhans):**
    - ♦ Alpha cells secrete glucagon
    - ♦ Beta cells secretes insulin
  - o **Exocrine:**
    - ♦ Helps in digestion of proteins, carbohydrates & fats

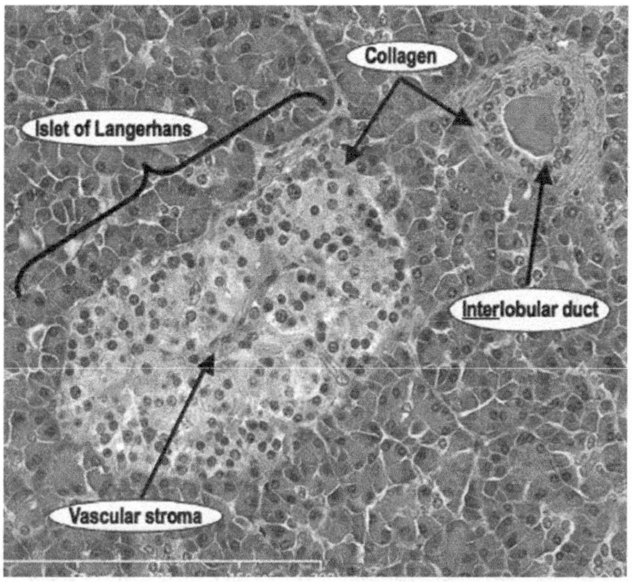

ANNULAR PANCREAS

Pathology

- 2nd part of duodenum is surrounded by a ring of pancreatic tissue

Management

- Duodeno**duodenostomy**
- Duodenojejunostomy

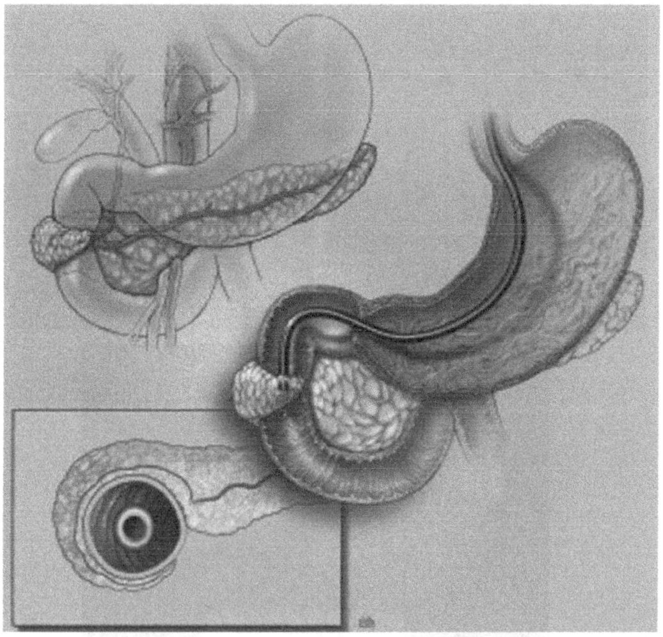

ACUTE PANCREATITIS

Causes

- **Gallstones**
- Alcoholism/Ethanol
- Trauma (MC cause in children)
- **Investigation which can cause acute pancreatitis: ERCP**

Abdominal signs

- **Cullen sign (umbilicus) & Grey Turner sign (around flanks):** Blue-red-purple or green-brown discoloration due to catabolism of hemoglobin
- **Mohammed prayer sign:** Sudden abdominal pain with partial relief on leaning forward

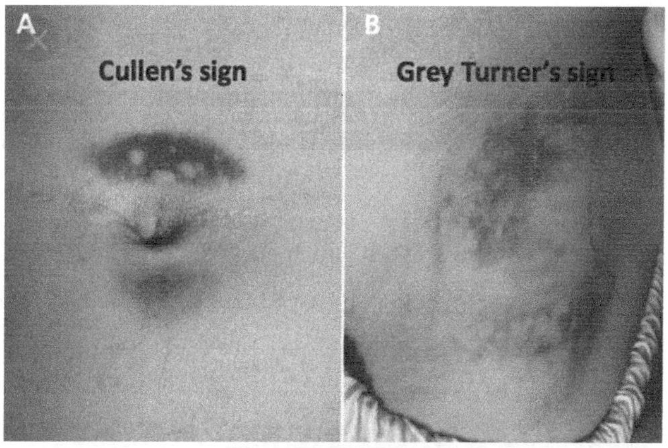

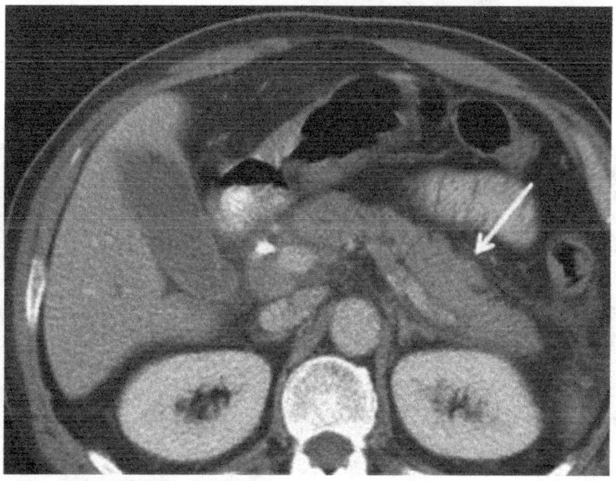

Investigations

- In initial 24-48 hours, serum **amylase** increases up to three-fold

- Serum lipase is most **specific**
- Acute gallstone pancreatitis may show increase in ALT (Alanine Transaminase)
- CT scan

Prognosis

- **Best prognosis:** Gallstone pancreatitis
- **Recurrent pancreatitis occurs in:** Methyl malonic acidemia

Conditions with raised serum amylase

- Pancreatitis
- Ruptured ectopic pregnancy
- Parotitis
- Biliary peritonitis (duodenal injuries)
- Mesenteric infarction

PANCREATIC PSEUDOCYST

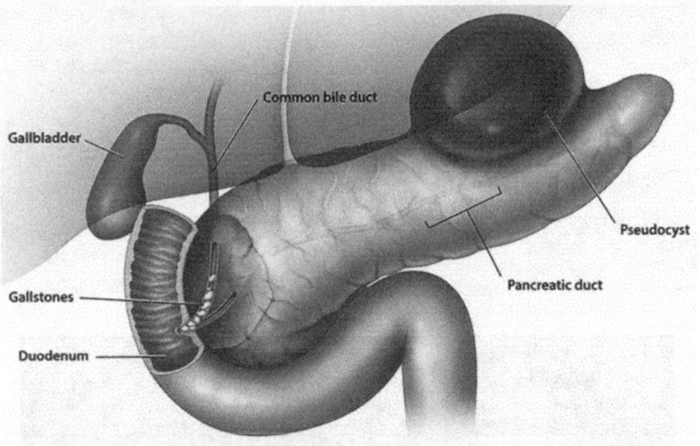

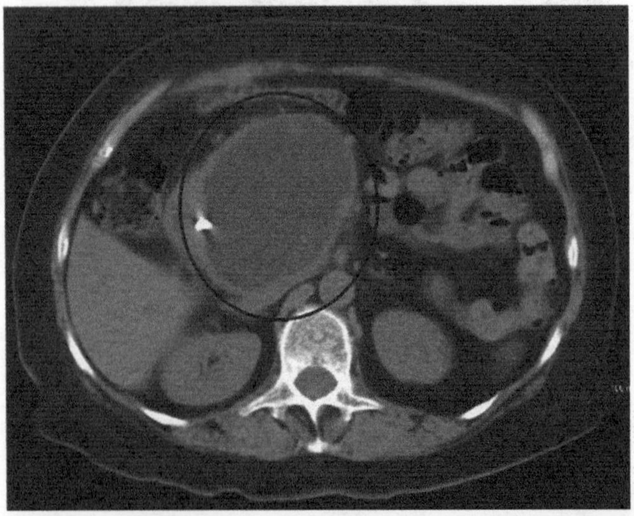

Causes

- **MC cause in children:** Trauma
- **MC cause in adults:** Pancreatitis

MC presentation

- Upper abdominal pain
- Infection is the **MC** complication

Management

- In 50% of cases, resolves spontaneously
- Internal drainage is the **best** treatment (cystogastrostomy)

CHRONIC PANCREATITIS

Causes

- **MC** cause is alcohol
- Trauma
- Pancreatic divisum

Classical triad

- Steatorrhoea
- Calcification
- Diabetes
- Pain is the **MC** symptom

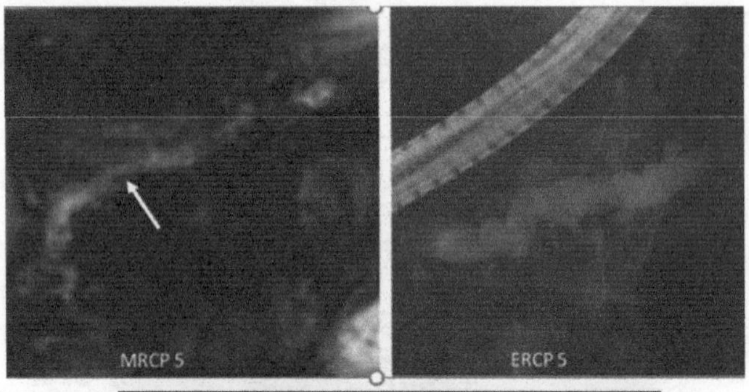

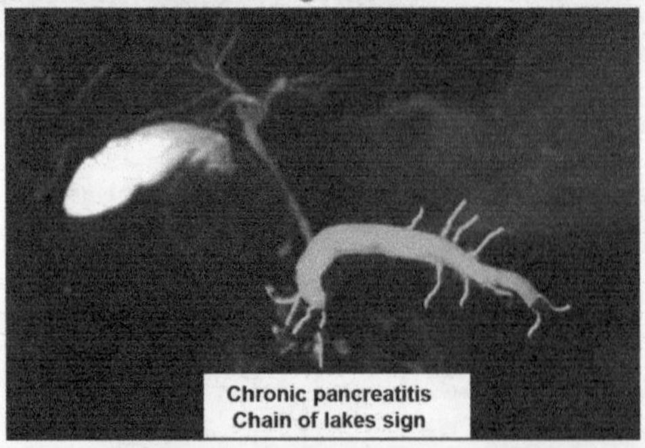

Chronic pancreatitis
Chain of lakes sign

Investigations

- MRCP is the **gold** standard
- Endoscopic USG
- ERCP shows **chain** of lakes appearance

PANCREATIC CA

Pathology

- **Most consistent risk factor:** Cigarette smoking
- **MC site:** Pancreatic head (70%)

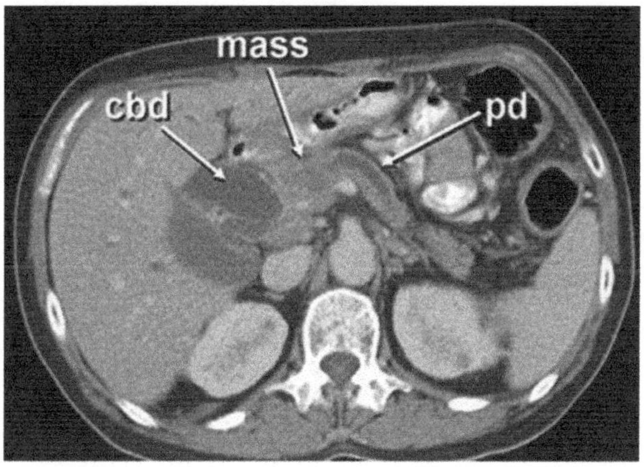

Features

- Weight loss & pain
- **Courvoisier's law:** Gallbladder is palpable in CBD obstruction due to malignancy (periampullary Ca), but not in CBD obstruction due to common bile duct stone
- CA19-9 is the **best** tumour marker
- CECT scan is the **IOC**
- **Whipple's** procedure is done

GASTRINOMA/ZES

MC site

- Duodenum
- **Passaros triangle:**
  - o Junction between the head & neck of pancreas
  - o Junction of cystic duct with CBD
  - o Junction between the 2nd part & 3rd part of duodenum

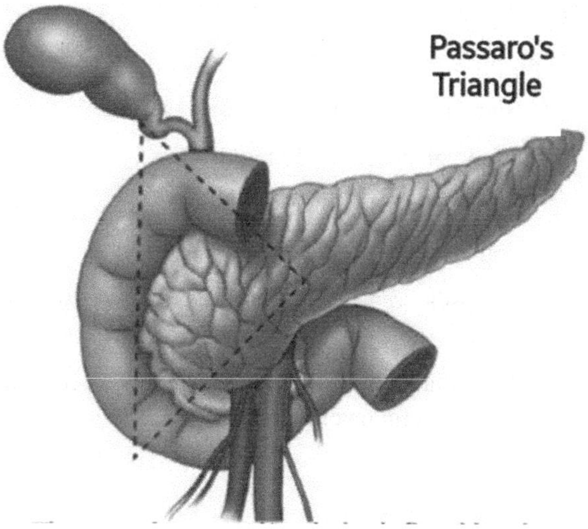

The gastrinoma triangle is defined by the junctions of the (1) cystic common bile duct (2) neck & body of pancreas (3) second & third portions of the duodenum. The vast majority (80%) of gastrinomas may be found within the anatomic confines of this triangle

Features

- Non beta cell tumour
- **It's a neuroendocrine tumour/NET secreting:** Gastrin
- **Triad:**
  - o Hypersecretion of gastric acid
  - o Severe peptic ulceration
  - o Non-beta cell tumour of pancreas/duodenal tumour

Most important investigation

- **Secretin injection test:** Increases gastrin value >200 pg/ml

DOC for ZES

- Proton pump inhibitors

Metastasis

- Hepatic metastasis occurs (33%)

INSULINOMA

Features

- **MC** endocrine tumour of pancreas (from beta cells)

- Usually, single
- **Whipple's triad:**
  - o Sign and symptoms of hypoglycemia
  - o Blood glucose <40-50 mg/dl
  - o Symptoms improve on administration of glucose
- Distributed equally throughout pancreas
- Total capsule removal is ensured to prevent tumour recurrence
- **Gold standard investigation:** 24 hours fasting blood sugar and Insulin level estimation

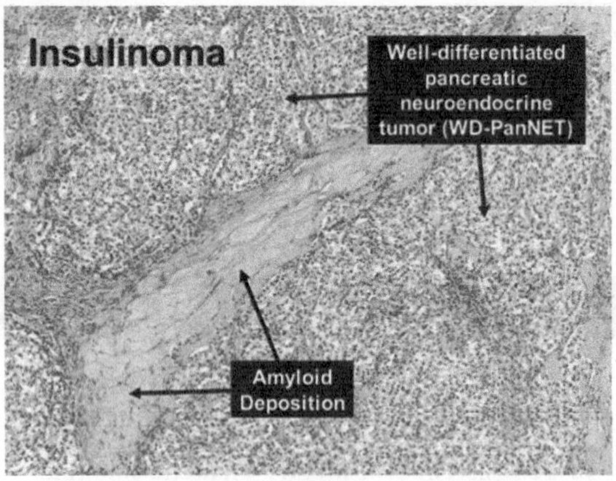

Chapter 12

SPLEEN

ANATOMY

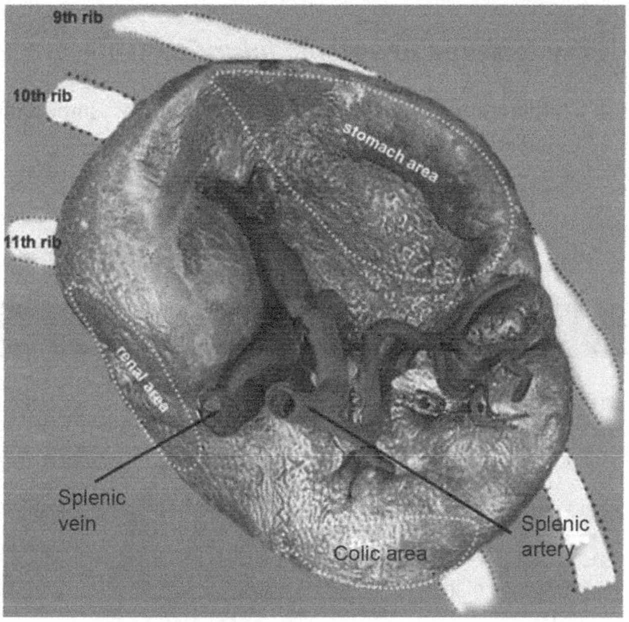

Features

- Wedge shaped structure in left hypochondrium
- Along the axis of 10th rib
- **Suspended by 2 ligaments:**
  - **Lienorenal/Splenorenal ligament:**
    - Transmits blood vessels to spleen
  - **Gastrosplenic ligament:**
    - Contains short gastric vessels which supplies the left half of greater curvature of stomach

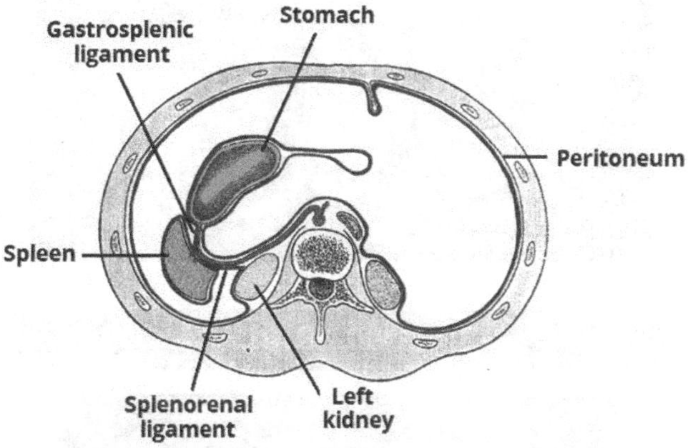

CYSTS OF SPLEEN

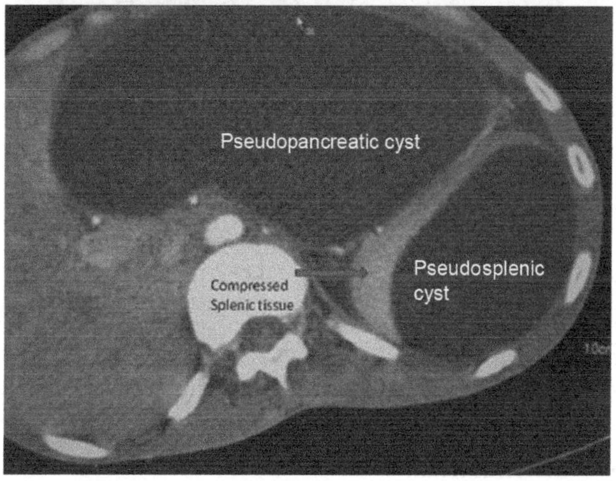

Cysts of spleen

- **MC cyst of spleen:** Pseudocyst
- **MC symptom of pseudocyst of spleen:** Left upper quadrant pain, radiating to shoulder

SPLENUNCULI

Features

- **MC** congenital anomaly of spleen
- Single/multiple accessory spleen
- Near the hilum of the spleen commonly (in **80%** cases)

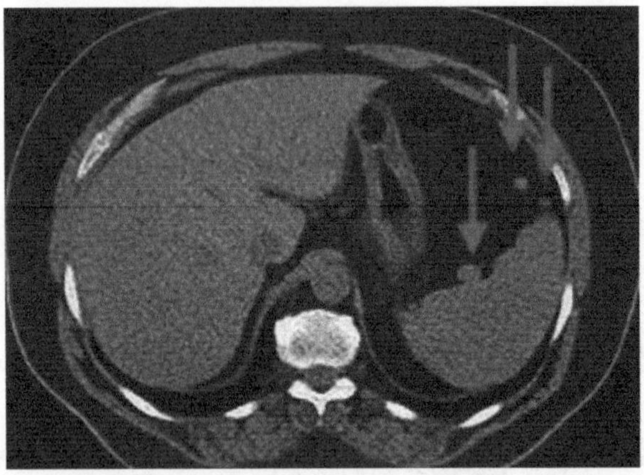

SPLENIC TRAUMA

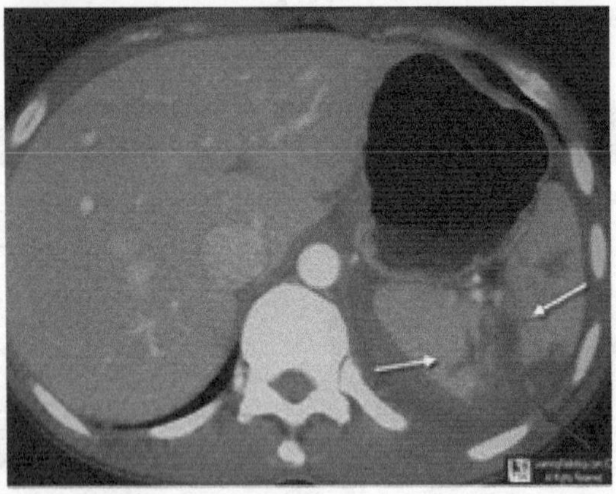

Features

- Spleen is the **MC** injured organ in blunt trauma to abdomen
- **Classical triad:**
  - o Elevated left hemidiaphragm
  - o Left lower lobe atelectasis
  - o Pleural effusion
- **Characteristic sign of splenic rupture: Kehr's** sign (referred pain) in left shoulder
- **Kehr's sign may also be seen in:**
  - o Diaphragmatic lesions
  - o Hemoperitoneum

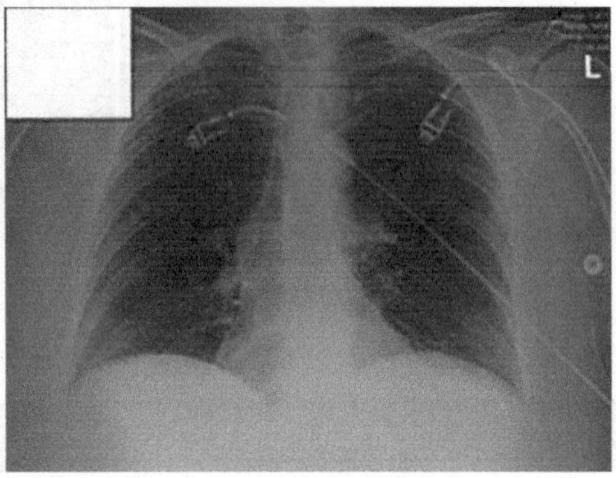

X-ray features of splenic injury

- Obliteration of splenic shadow (most important radiological sign)
- Obliteration of psoas shadow
- Elevation of left diaphragm

SPLENECTOMY

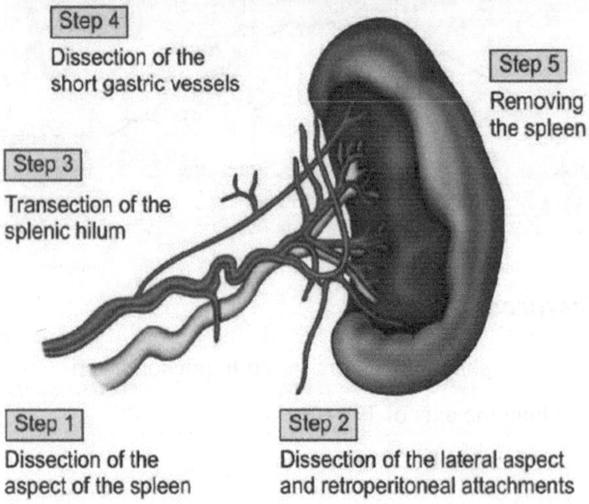

Indications

- Hereditary spherocytosis

- Hypersplenism
- Sickle cell anemia
- Splenic trauma (MC indication)

Splenectomy increases risk for

- **Pneumococcal** infections
- H. Influenzae type B infections

Overwhelming post-splenectomy infection/ OPSI

- **MC caused by:** Streptococcus pneumonia
- **MC complication:** Left lower lobe atelectasis

SECTION 2

SURGERY

Chapter 13

LIVER

ANATOMY

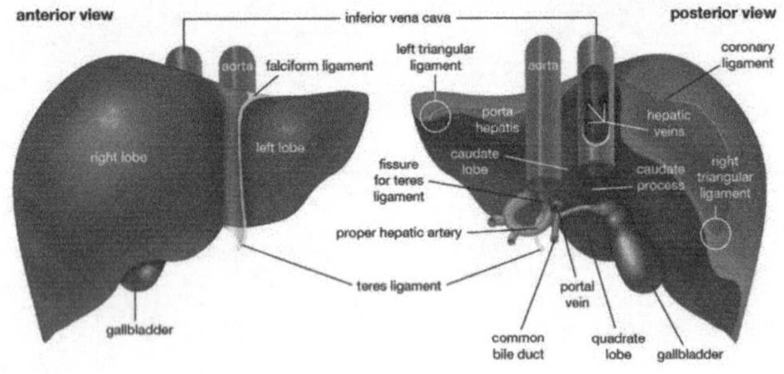

Features

- Liver is divided into right and left lobes by the attachment of the peritoneum of the falciform ligament
- The right lobe is further divided into a quadrate lobe and caudate lobe, by gallbladder, fissure for the ligamentum teres, the inferior vena cava and the fissure for ligamentum venosum
- **Dual blood supply:**
  - o **Portal vein:** 80%
  - o **Hepatic artery:** 20%
  - o Hepatic blood flow is around 1500 ml/minute
- **Couinaud's segments:**
  - o Eight segments
  - o Based on hepatic vein & portal vein division
- **Segment I is:** Segment I is caudate lobe
- **Segment IV is:** Segment IV is quadrate lobe

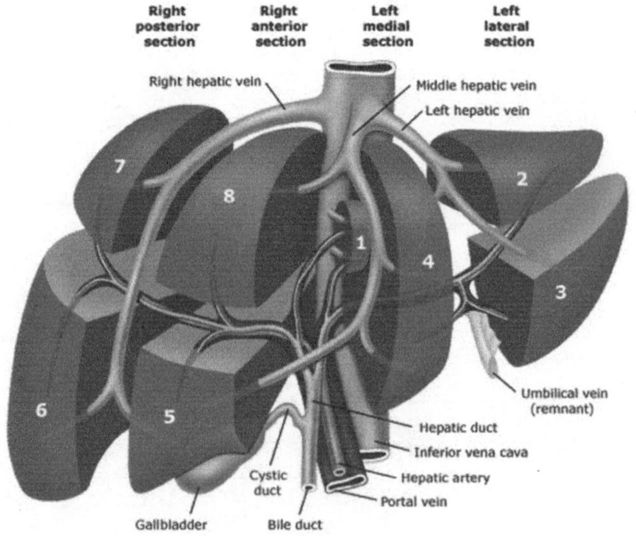

- **Vascular supply of segment I:** Independent vascular supply

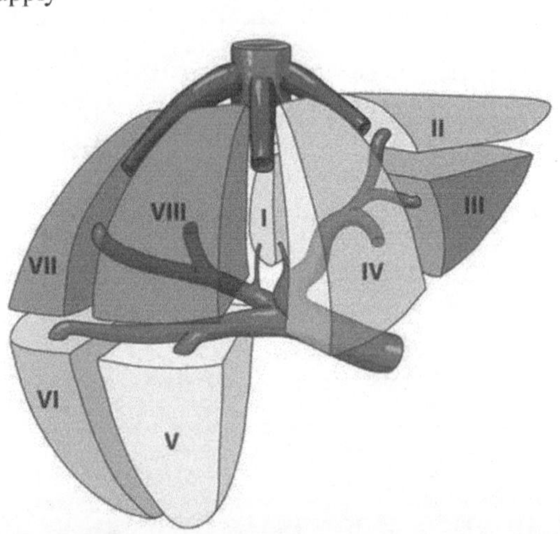

Portal vein

- **Formed** behind neck of pancreas by union of splenic vein & superior mesenteric vein
- **Normal pressure in portal venous system:** 5-10 mm Hg
- Portal **hypertension**: More than 12 mm Hg

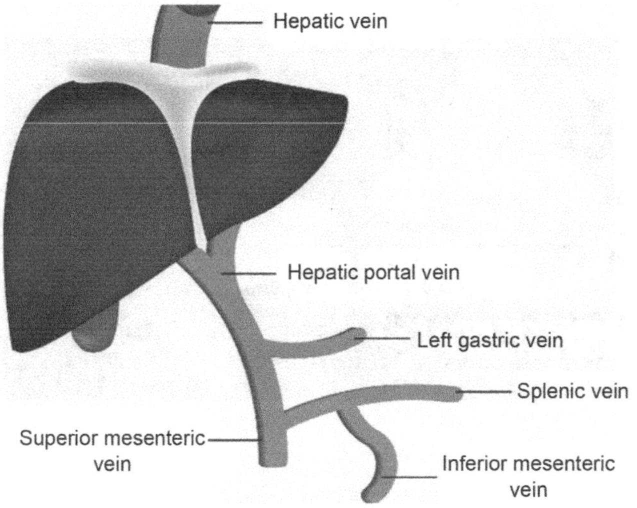

- **Portosystemic anastomosis:**
  - o **Anal canal:**
    - ♦ Systemic: Middle and inferior rectal vein
    - ♦ Portal: Superior rectal vein
  - o **Lower end of esophagus:**
    - ♦ Systemic: Accessory hemiazygous vein
    - ♦ Portal: Left gastric vein

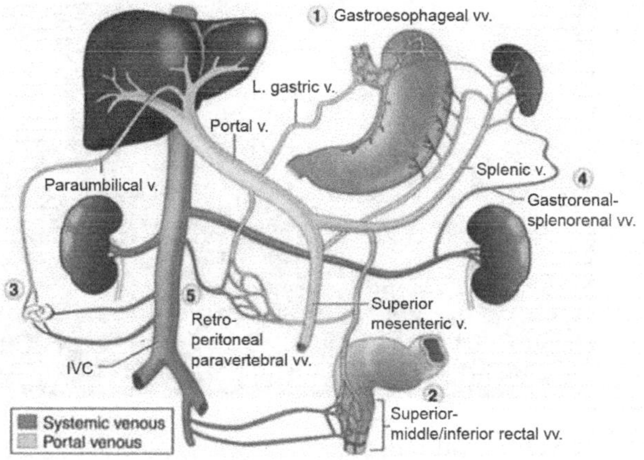

Portosystemic anastomoses. 1. Left gastric–azygos → esophageal varices. 2. Superior–middle/inferior rectal → hemorrhoids. 3. Paraumbilical–inferior epigastric → caput medusae (navel). 4. Gastrorenal-splenorenal. 5. Retroperitoneal paravertebral

  - o **Umbilicus:**
    - ♦ Systemic: Anterior abdominal wall veins
    - ♦ Portal: Left portal vein (via paraumbilical vein)

HEPATOCYSTIC TRIANGLE/HEPATOBILIARY TRIANGLE

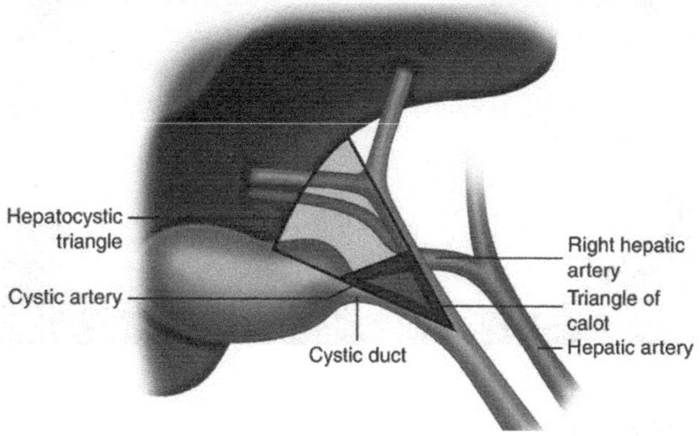

Bounded by

- Inferior surface of liver superiorly
- Cystic duct inferolaterally
- Common hepatic duct medially

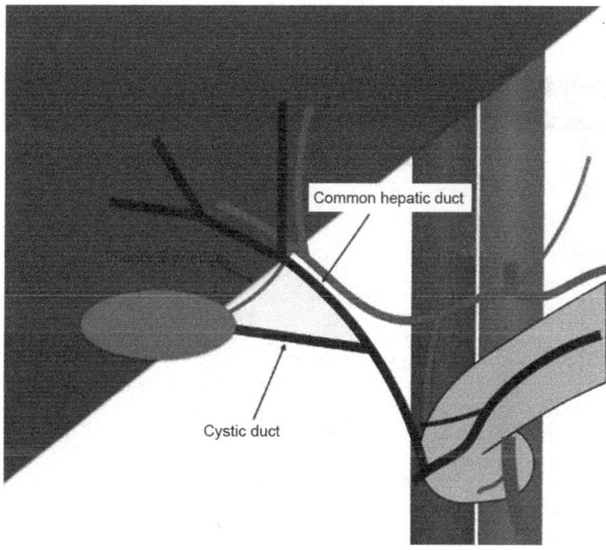

Content

- Cystic artery
- Lymph node of Lund
- Right hepatic artery

AMOEBIC LIVER ABSCESS

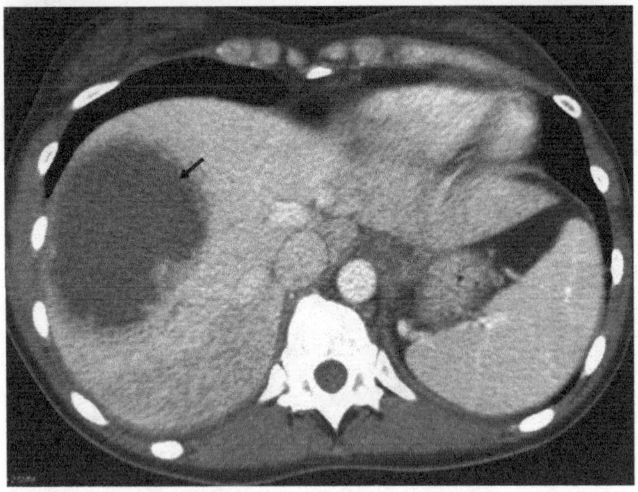

Features

- **Right** lobe (posterosuperior surface)
- **Anchovy sauce pus:** Due to liquefaction necrosis of liver and abscess
- Glisson's capsule is resistant to amoebic invasion
- Elevated prothrombin time

HYDATID CYST

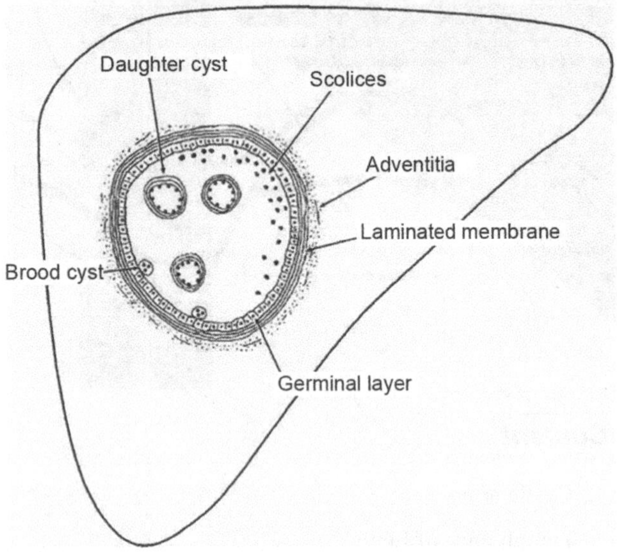

Features

- **MC** cause is Echinococcus granulosus
- **Definite host:** Dogs
- **Intermediate hosts:** Sheep
- **Accidental/End stage host:** Humans
- MC seen in **right** lobe
- Hepatomegaly
- Casoni's test

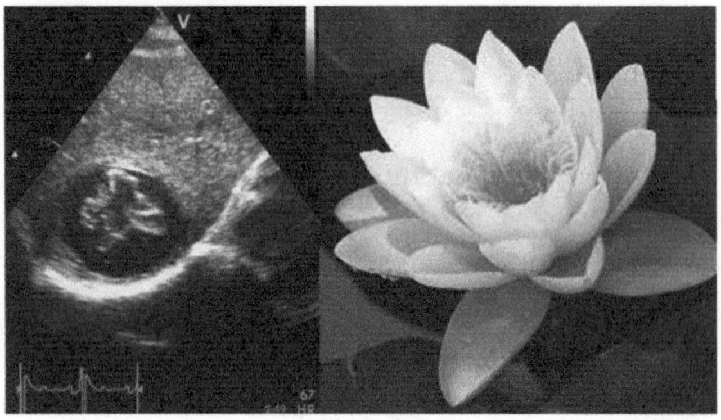

- **USG:**
  - o **Water** lily appearance
  - o Calcifications
- ELISA is sensitive
- No role of blood culture in diagnosis
- Crumbled **egg** appearance/white of a hard-boiled egg
- **Albendazole**/Mebendazole can shrink the cyst size

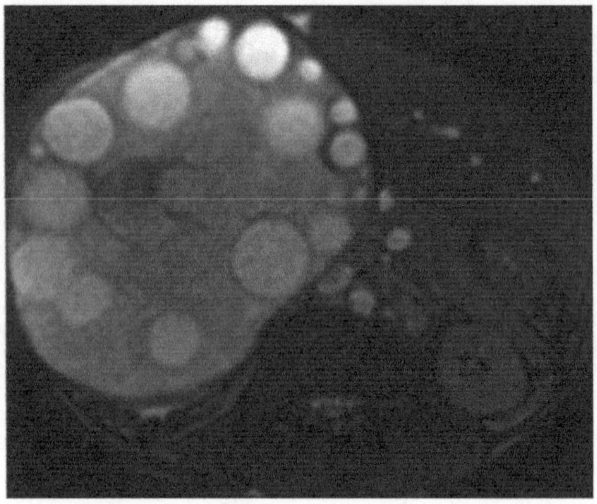

- **PAIR technique**
  - o Percutaneous aspiration
  - o Injection of scolicidal agent
  - o Reaspiration of cyst contents
- **Cystectomy**

PYOGENIC LIVER ABSCESS

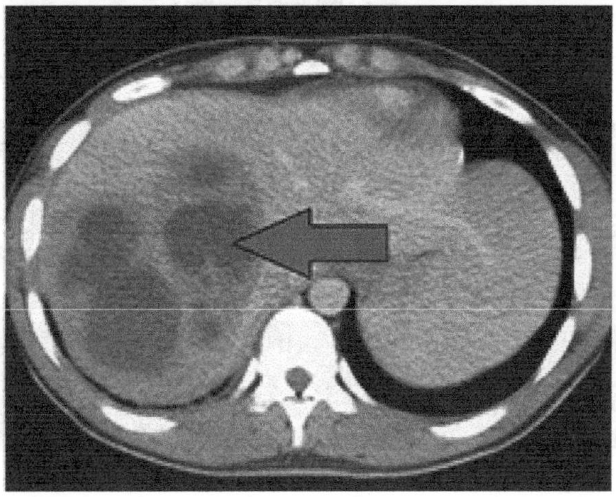

Features

- Usually single & large
- Infection through bile duct (**MC** route)
- Hematogenous route is 2nd MC route
- MC seen in **right** lobe
- Presents with fever, chills, abdominal pain

HEPATOCELLULAR CARCINOMA

Features

- **MC** primary malignant tumour
- **Risk factors:**
  - o HBV, HCV
  - o Alcoholic liver disease
  - o Aflatoxin
  - o Hemochromatosis

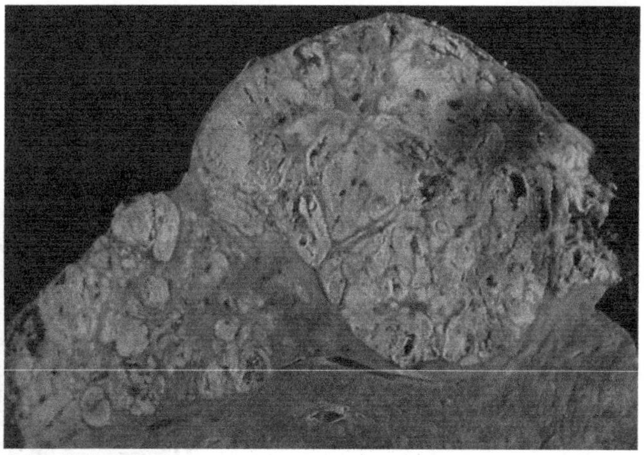

- Pain in right upper quadrant is the **MC** presentation
- **Tumour markers:**
  - o AFP value >400 mg/dL is **highly** suggestive
  - o PIVKA (Protein Induced Vitamin K Absence)
- **Screening**: USG, especially of high-risk population
- Complete excision of HCC (partial hepatectomy/total hepatectomy) is the treatment of **choice**

Fibrolamellar Ca

- Usually **not** associated with cirrhosis (5%)
- Slow growing, well circumscribed tumour
- Does **not** produce a fetoprotein but produces Neurotension
- **Good** prognosis, if treated

Indications for liver transplantation

- **Children:** Biliary atresia
- **Adults:**
  - o Primary sclerosing cholangitis
  - o Fulminant hepatitis etc.

SECTION 2
SURGERY

Chapter 14

GALLBLADDER

ANATOMY

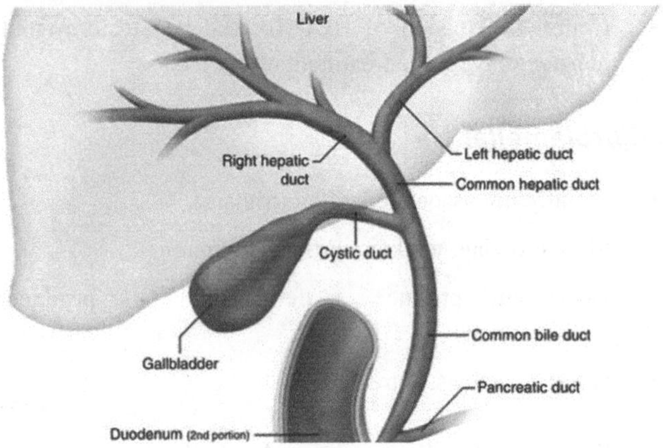

Features

- Pear shaped structure
- **Parts:**
  - o Fundus
  - o Body
  - o Infundibulum
  - o Neck
- Drains through cystic duct into common hepatic duct & forms common bile duct/CBD
- **Calot's triangle boundaries (purple coloured area):**
  - o **Above: Cystic artery**
  - o **Inferior:** Cystic duct and gallbladder
  - o **Medial:** Common hepatic duct

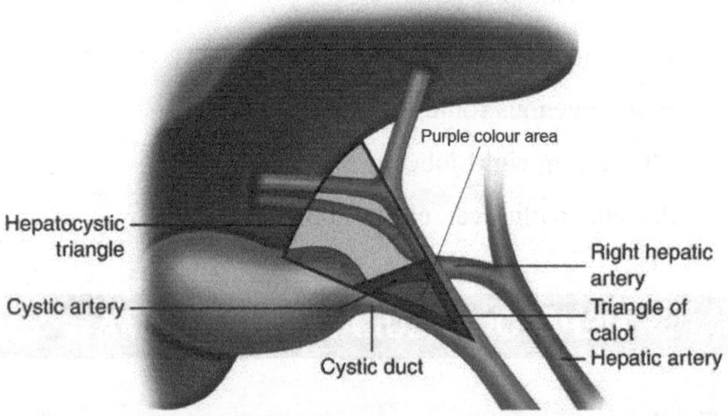

INVESTIGATIONS

Cholangiogram

- Can be done orally or intravenously

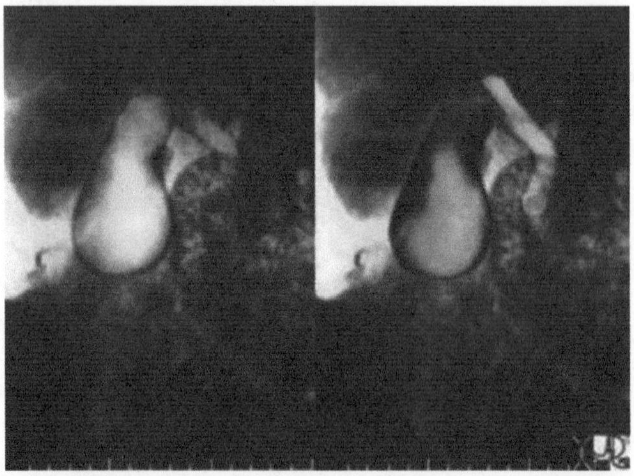

HIDA scan

- Gold standard in **diagnosing** acute cholecystitis

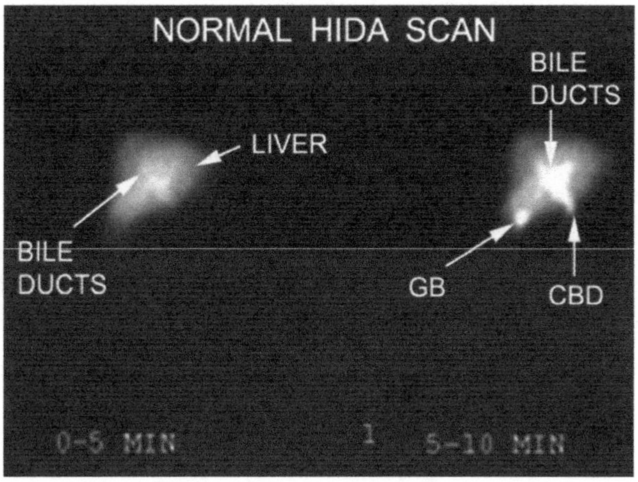

MRCP/Magnetic Resonance Cholangiopancreatography

- **Most** accurate
- Non-invasive investigation

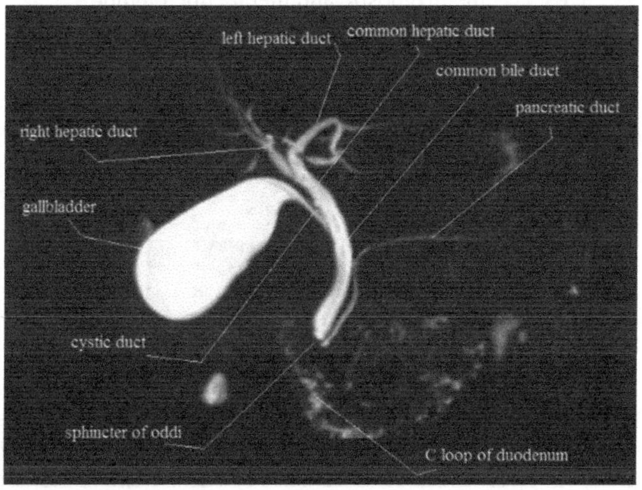

Endoscopic Retrograde Cholangiopancreatography/ERCP

- **Gold** standard in diagnosing common bile duct/CBD stones
- Replaced by MRCP nowadays
- Can **lead** to acute pancreatitis

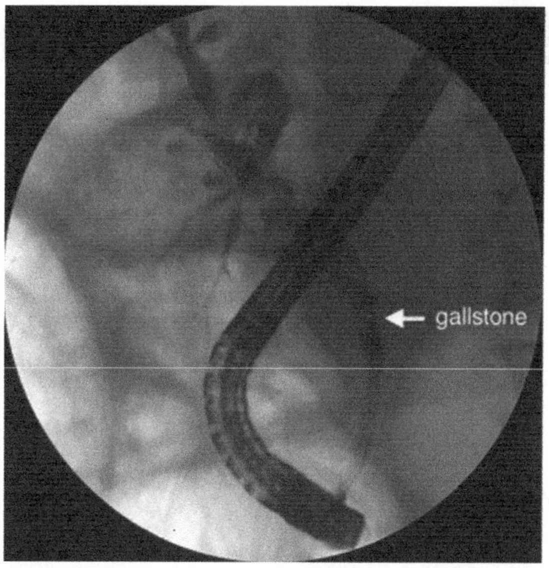

CHOLEDOCHAL CYST

Features

- It is defined as congenital **dilatation** of intrahepatic and extrahepatic ducts
- **Triad:**
  - o Pain
  - o Lump
  - o Intermittent jaundice

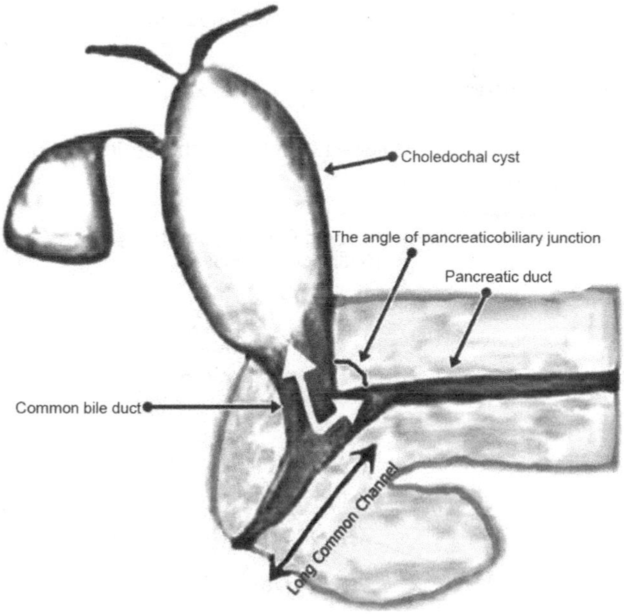

CHOLELITHIASIS

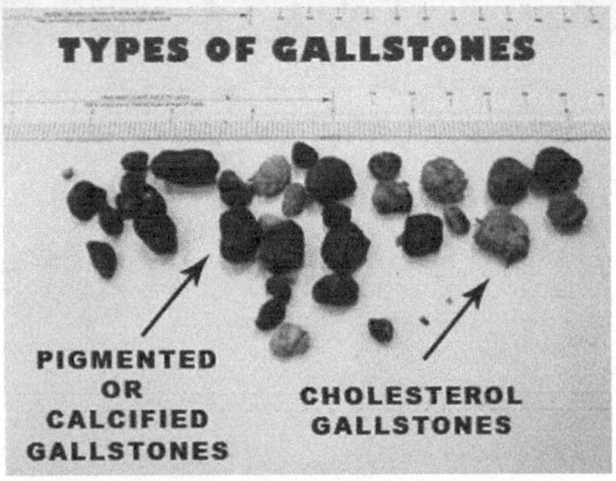

Type

- Cholesterol stones
- Brown pigment stones
- Black pigment stones
- Mixed

Pigment stones

- **Black:**
  - o Chronic hemolysis like hereditary spherocytosis, sickle cell anemia
  - o Liver cirrhosis
- **Brown:**
  - o Forms due to bile stasis and infection

Treatment

- Laparoscopic cholecystectomy is the **gold** standard surgery for gallstones

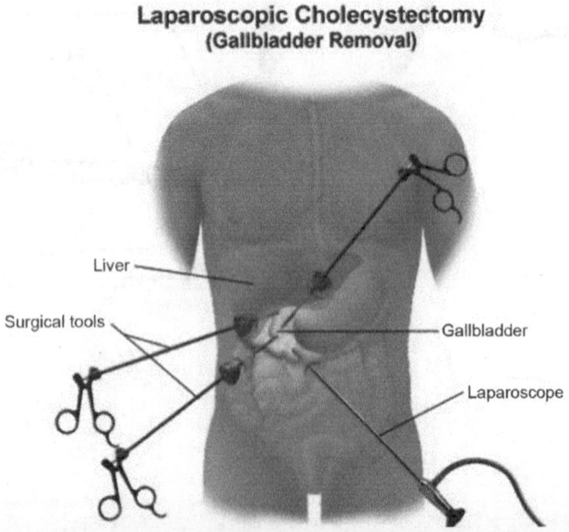

Complications of gallstones

- Acute & chronic cholecystitis
- Carcinoma of gallbladder
- Acute pancreatitis
- Cholangitis
- Gallstone ileus (acute intestinal obstruction)
- Gallbladder carcinoma

COMMON BILE DUCT STONE

Features

- **Types:**
  - o **Primary:** Forms in the CBD
  - o **Secondary:** Formed in GB and then enters CBD
- **MC cause of obstructive jaundice:** CBD stone
- Dilated CBD of more than **8 mm**, strongly suggest CBD stones
- **Sign seen in cholangiography: Meniscus** sign
- **ERCP** is the diagnostic and therapeutic method

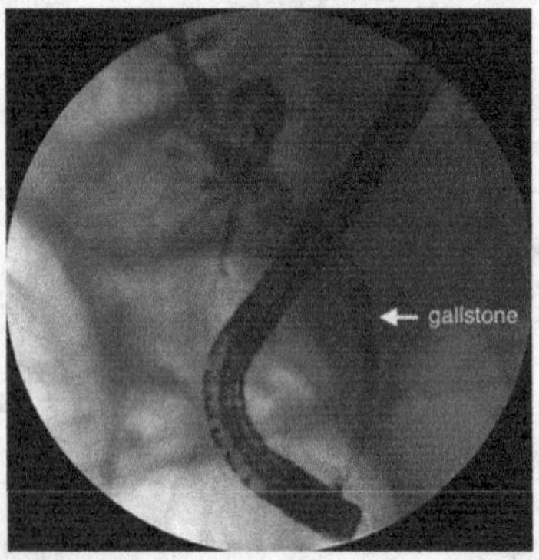

GALLSTONE ILEUS

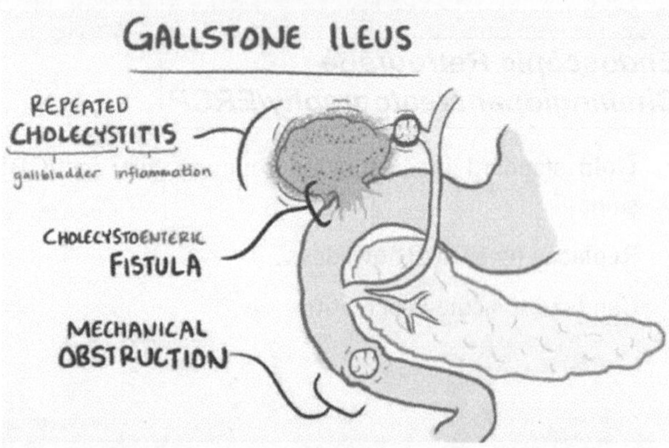

Features

- **MC site of obstruction:** Terminal ileum
- There is intermittent small intestine obstruction by the gallstone which has passed via the choledochoduodenal **fistula**
- **Rigler's triad:**
    - o Cholecystoenteric fistula
    - o Pneumobilia
    - o Intestinal obstruction

Management

- **Enterotomy** & removal of stone with closure of fistula and cholecystectomy

ACALCULOUS CHOLECYSTITIS

Features

- Acute inflammation of the gallbladder **without** gall-stones
- Highest mortality
- Commonly seen in patients on long-term total parenteral nutrition/recovering from major surgery
- USG is the investigation of **choice**

CALCULOUS CHOLECYSTITIS

Features

- One of the important complications of GB stones

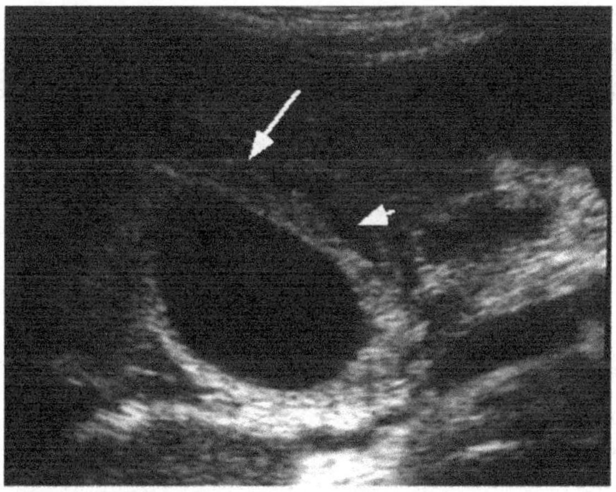

Acute cholecystitis Ultrasound of the right upper quadrant in a patient with acute cholecystitis reveals marked thickening of the gallbladder wall (arrow) with fluid surrounding the distended gallbladder (arrowhead) Courtesy of Jonathan Kruskal, MD

- **Clinical signs:**
    - o **Murphy's sign:** There is inspiratory arrest on deep palpation in right upper quadrant due to pain
    - o **Boas sign:** There is hyperesthesia below right scapula
- **Treatment:** Early cholecystectomy

CHOLANGITIS

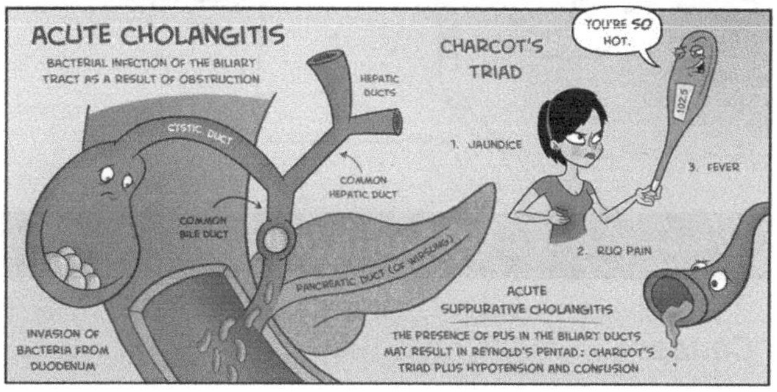

Features

- **Causes:**
    - o ERCP
    - o CBD stone is the **MC** cause
- Commonly presents with fever with chills and rigors
- **Charcot's triad:**
    - o Pain
    - o Jaundice
    - o Fever/rigors
- **Reynold's pentad:**
    - o Charcot's triad
    - o Septic shock
    - o Mental status changes

PRIMARY SCLEROSING CHOLANGITIS

Features

- Fibrosing cholangitis of bile ductules leading to inflammatory stricture and obliteration of extrahepatic and intrahepatic ducts
- Presents with intermittent jaundice, fatigue, pruritis
- May **result** in cholangiocarcinoma
- ERCP is the **gold** standard investigation

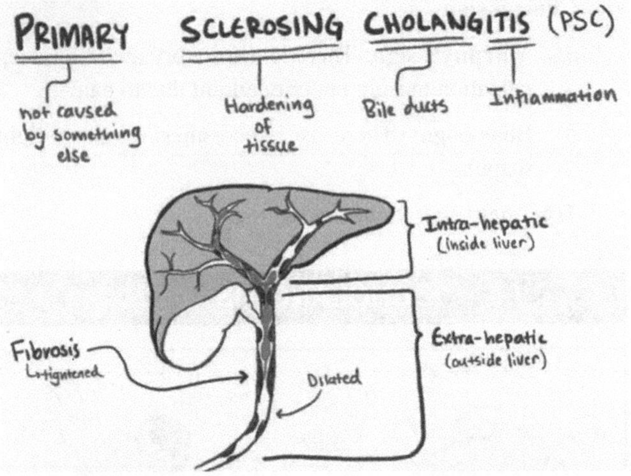

HEMOBILIA

Causes

- Trauma
- Gallstones

Triad of hemobilia

- Abdominal pain
- Obstructive jaundice
- Melena

CARCINOMA OF GALLBLADDER

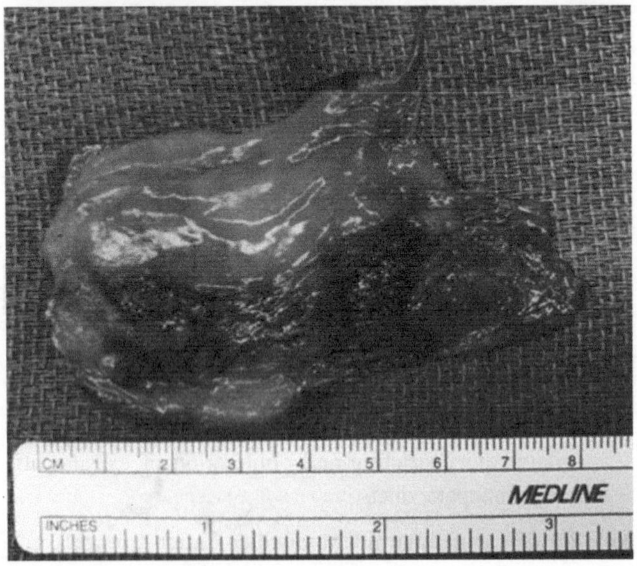

Features

- **MC** malignancy of biliary tract
- **75%** are gallstones associated
- Fundus and body are the **MC** site of Ca
- **Presentation:**
  - o Pain
  - o Weight loss
  - o Jaundice (a **poor** prognostic sign)
  - o Fever
  - o Palpable mass
- **MC** type is adenocarcinoma
- USG shows excessive localized thickening of GB
- FNAC is **contraindicated** in inoperable cancers

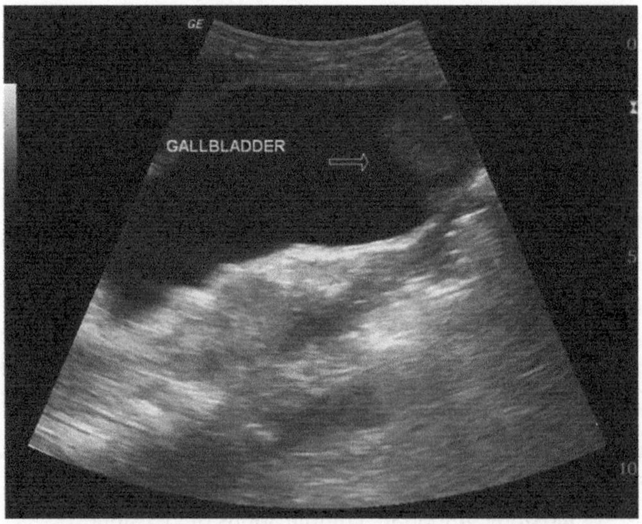

CHOLANGIOCARCINOMA

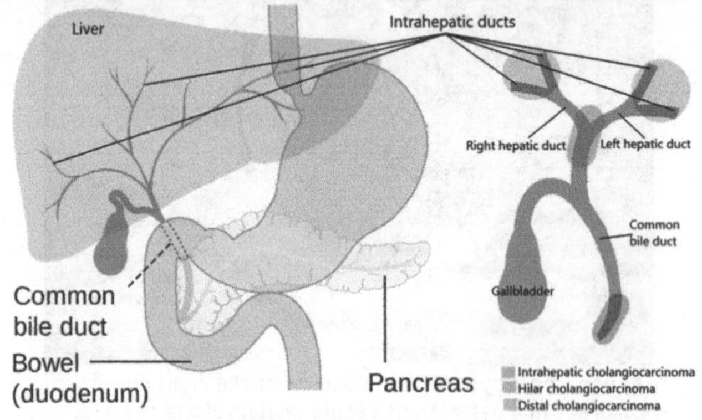

Features

- **MC** site is hilum of bile duct (Klatskin tumour)
- **Risk factors:**
  - Primary sclerosing cholangitis
  - Clonorchis sinensis
- Painless jaundice followed by pruritis
- CA19-9 (**prognostic** importance)

SECTION 2

SURGERY

Chapter 15

HERNIA

ANATOMY

Inguinal canal

- **3.75** cm long, extending from deep inguinal ring to superficial inguinal ring
- **Superficial inguinal ring:**
  - o Defect in external oblique **aponeurosis**
  - o Lies immediately above pubic tubercle
- **Deep inguinal ring:**
  - o Defect in **fascia** transversalis
  - o Situated 1.25 cm above the inguinal ligament, midway between the anterior superior iliac spine and pubis symphysis

Inguinal canal

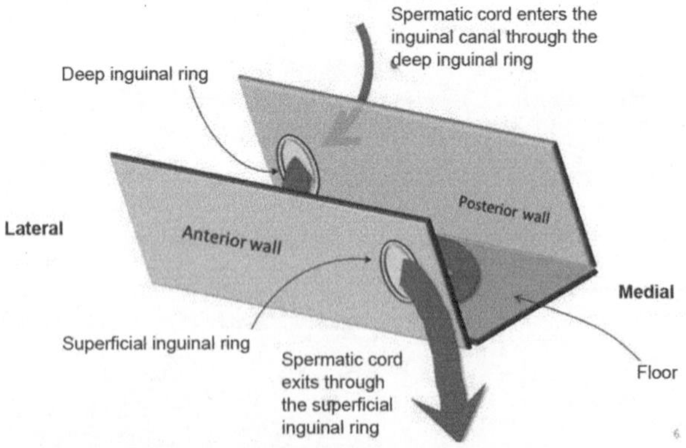

- **Structures passing through inguinal canal:**
  - o **Male:**
    - ♦ Spermatic cord
    - ♦ Ilioinguinal nerve
  - o **Female:**
    - ♦ Round ligament of uterus
    - ♦ Ilioinguinal nerve

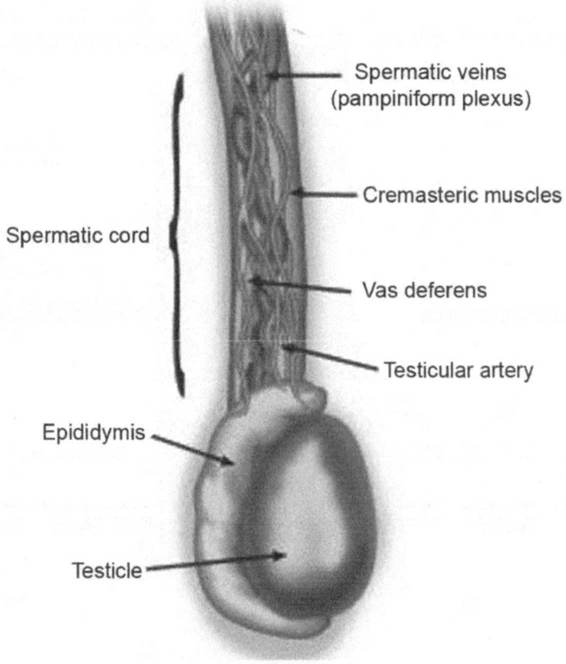

- **Contents of spermatic cord:**
  - o Remains of processus vaginalis
  - o Ductus deferens
  - o **Arteries:**
    - ♦ Artery to ductus deferens

  - ♦ Testicular artery
  - ♦ Cremasteric artery
- o Pampiniform plexus of veins
- o Genital branch of genitofemoral nerve

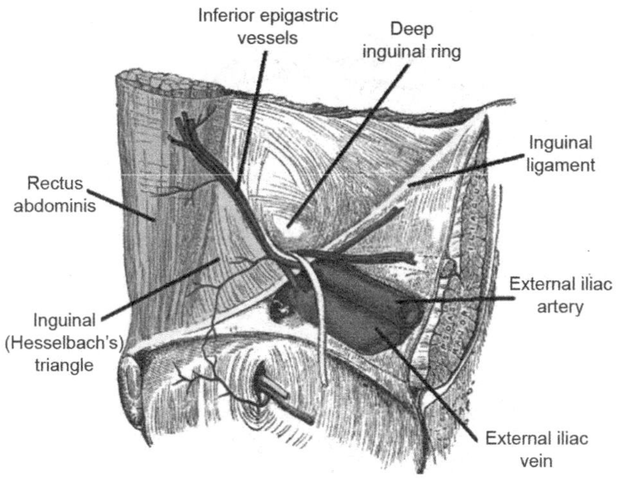

- **Hesselbach's triangle:**
  - o **Medial:** Outer border of rectus abdominis
  - o **Lateral:** Inferior epigastric vessels
  - o **Below:** Medial part of inguinal ligament
- **Boundaries of Femoral canal:**
  - o **Medial:** Lacunar ligament
  - o **Lateral:** Femoral vein
  - o **Base:** Femoral ring
  - o **Anterior:** Inguinal ligament
  - o **Posterior:** Cooper's ligament

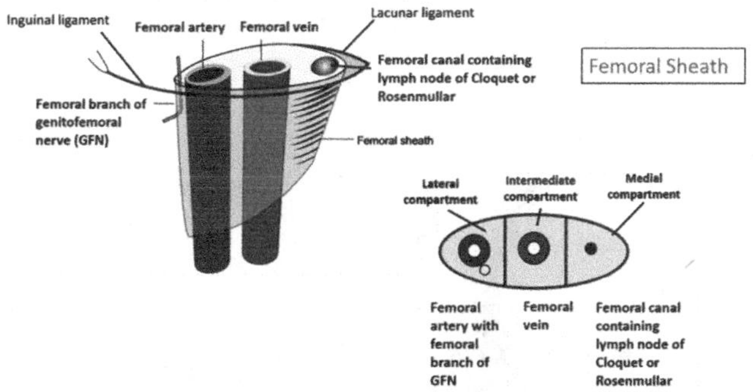

HERNIA

Features

- It is defined as an abnormal protrusion of an organ or tissue through a defect in its surrounding walls

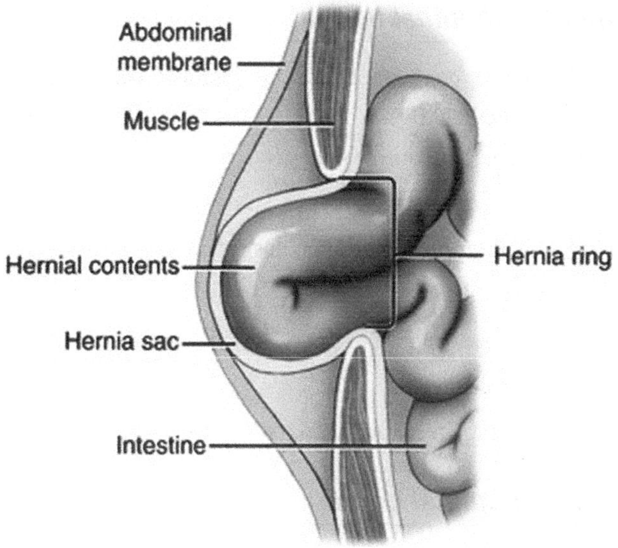

- **Nyhus classification:**
  - o **Type I:** Indirect inguinal with normal internal ring
  - o **Type II:** Indirect inguinal with enlarged internal ring
  - o **Type IIIA:** Direct inguinal hernia
  - o **Type IIIB:** Indirect inguinal hernia enlarged enough to encroach upon the posterior inguinal wall
  - o **Type IIIC:** Femoral hernia
  - o **Type IV:** Recurrent hernia
    - ♦ **A:** Direct
    - ♦ **B:** Indirect
    - ♦ **C:** Femoral
    - ♦ **D:** Combined

INGUINAL HERNIA

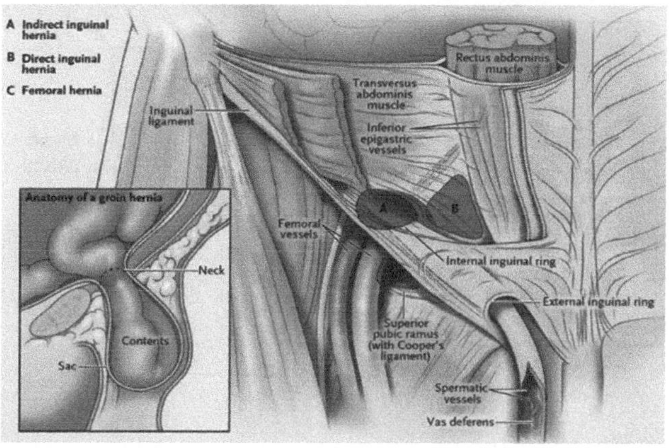

Indirect inguinal hernia

- Herniated content enters into inguinal canal through **deep** inguinal ring
- **MC** type of hernia in both genders
- MC in the **young**
- Sac is **lateral** to inferior epigastric artery
- **Types:**
  - o Bubonocele
  - o Funicular
  - o Complete/scrotal

Direct inguinal hernia

- 35% cases of inguinal hernia in adults are of direct type
- Always **acquired**
- Seen in **elderly**
- Sac passes through a weakness or defect of transversalis fascia in the posterior wall of the inguinal canal/ Hesselbach triangle (**not** through the deep inguinal ring)
- Direct hernia does **not** attain a large size or do not reach up to scrotum
- Sac lies **medial** to inferior epigastric artery
- Obstruction/strangulation is rare

Surgeries

- **Herniotomy:**
  - o Ligation of hernia sac
- **Hernioplasty:**
  - o Herniotomy +
  - o Strengthening of the posterior wall using exogenous material like prolene **mesh**

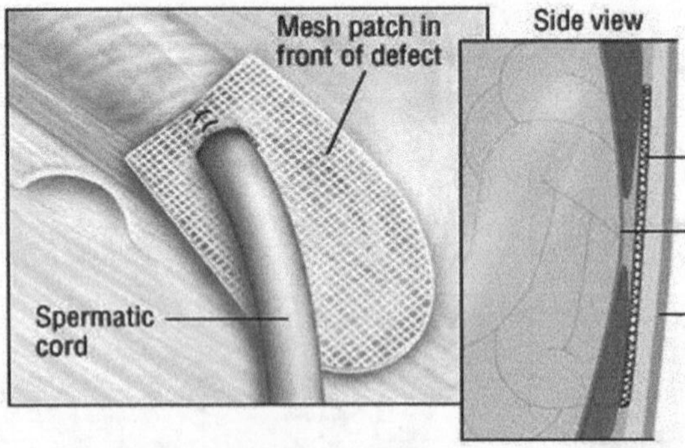

- **Herniorrhaphy:**
  - o Herniotomy +
  - o Posterior wall **repair** using in situ structures

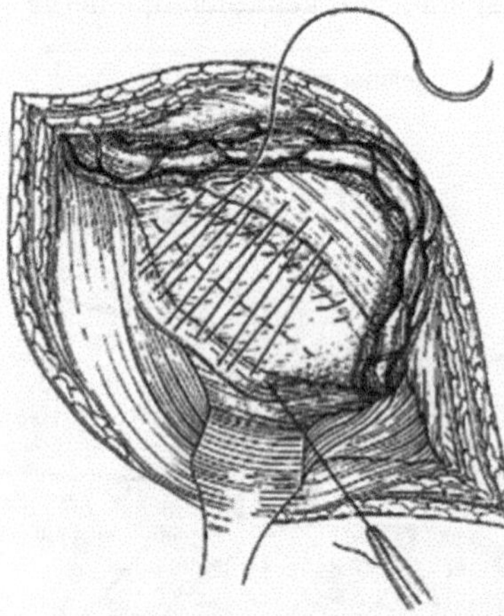

Figure: The completed 4-layer sutured shouldice repair (Kingsnorth and LeBlanc, 2003; p. 1563)

HERNIA EN GLISSADE/SLIDING HERNIA

Features

- Hernia in which posterior wall of the sac is also formed by a **viscus** (retroperitoneal structure) in addition to the peritoneum
- Viscera is liable to be injured if the hernia sac is resected during surgery
- **Left side are:**
  - o Sigmoid colon & mesentery
- Sigmoid colon is the **MC** content overall
- **Right side are:**
  - o Cecum

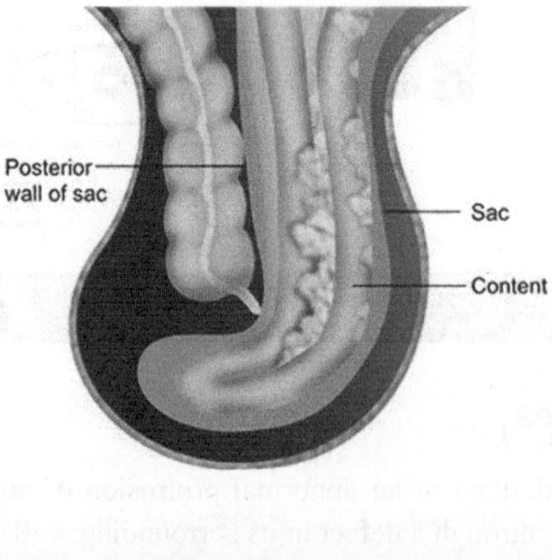

FEMORAL HERNIA

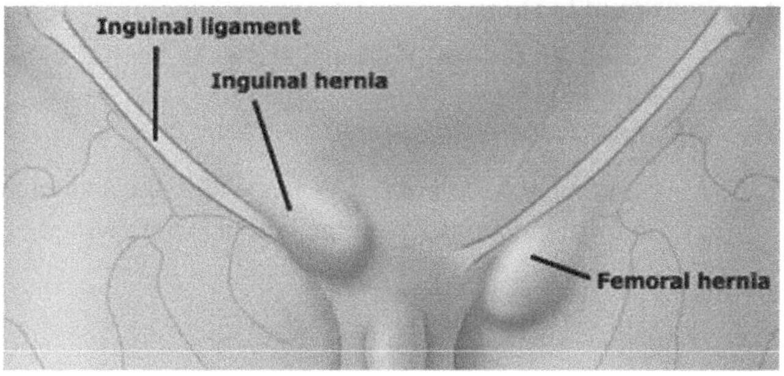

Features

- **MC** in female, but the MC type of hernia in females is indirect inguinal hernia
- **MC** on Right side
- **MC** strangulates
- Rare before puberty
- Mass or bulge **lateral & below** to pubic tubercle

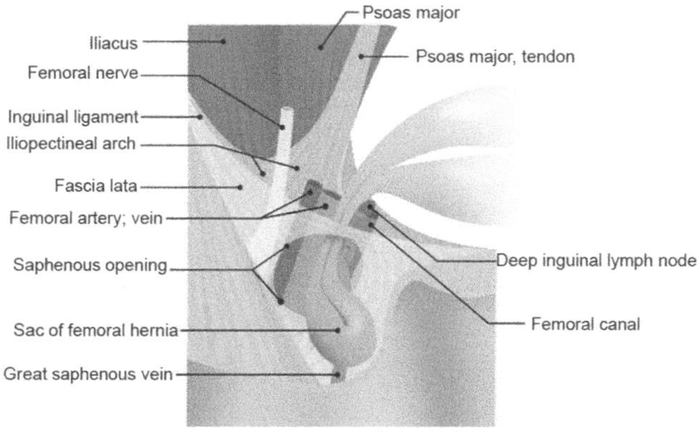

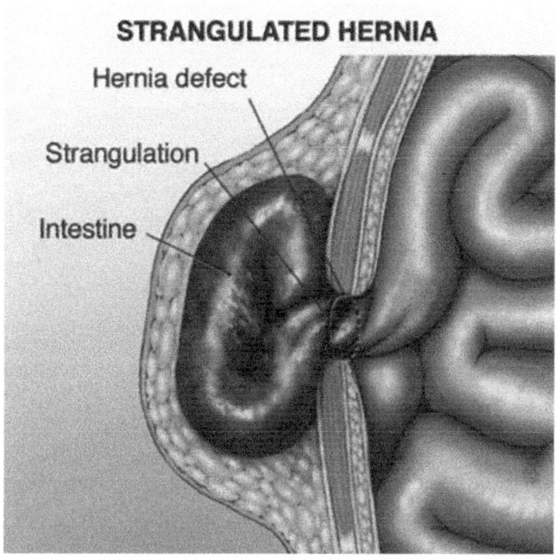

OTHER TYPES OF HERNIA

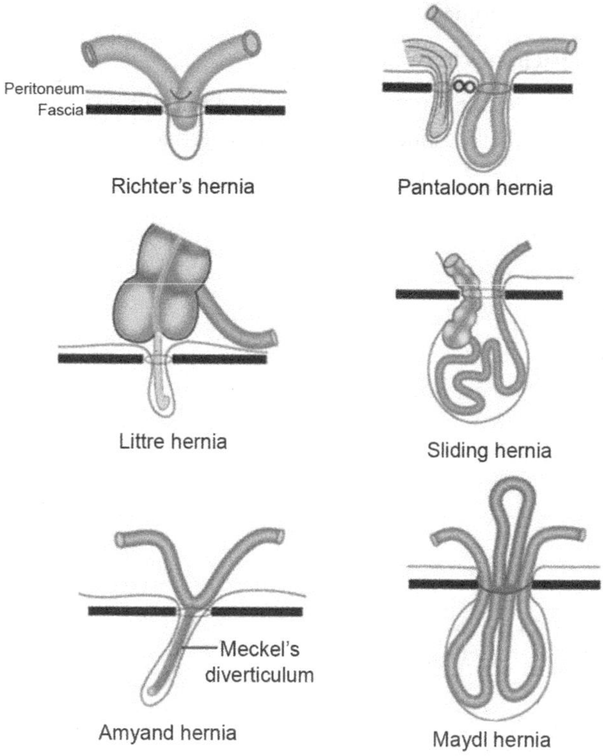

Figure: Types of hernias

Types

- **Spigelian hernia:**
  - o Interparietal hernia (subumbilical/level of **arcuate** line)
- **Littre's hernia:**
  - o Hernia of **Meckel's** diverticulum
- **Morgagni's hernia:**
  - o Hernia between costal & sternal parts of **diaphragm**
- **Obturator hernia:**
  - o More common in females because of larger and more oblique design of the **obturator** canal
- **Umbilical hernia:**
  - o Are seen in infants & quite common
- **Exomphalos/Omphalocele:**
  - o Due to **failure** of all or part of the midgut to return to the coelom during early fetal life

- **Epigastric hernia:**
  - o Located between the xiphoid process and the umbilicus
- **Richter's hernia:**
  - o Sac contains only a portion of the **circumference** of the intestine (usually small intestine)
- **Dual/Saddle bag/Pantaloon hernia:**
  - o Consists of **2 sacs** that straddle the inferior epigastric artery. One being medial and other lateral
- **Incisional hernia:**
  - o Result of **failure** of fascial tissue to heal & close following laparotomy
- **Maydl's hernia/Hernia-in-W:**
  - o Strangulated loop of the **W** lies within the abdomen so local tenderness over the hernia is not marked

SECTION 2

SURGERY

Chapter 16

NEUROSURGERY

GLASGOW COMA SCALE

Components

- **Eye opening:**
  - o **4:** Spontaneous eye opening
  - o **3:** Eye opening to loud voice
  - o **2:** Eye opening on painful stimuli
  - o **1:** Do not open eye

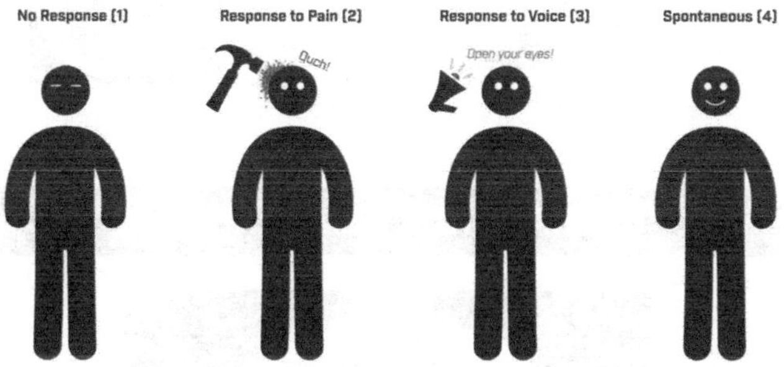

- **Verbal response:**
  - o **5:** Normal, oriented
  - o **4:** Confused
  - o **3:** Inappropriate words
  - o **2:** Sounds only
  - o **1:** No sounds
- **Motor response:**
  - o **6:** Obeys command
  - o **5:** Localizes pain

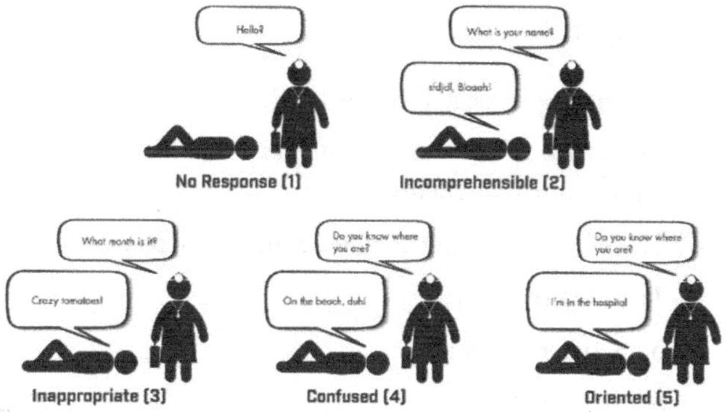

  - o **4:** Withdrawl in flexion
  - o **3:** Abnormal flexion
  - o **2:** Extension
  - o **1:** No motor response

GCS and head injury

- **GCS 15 with no loss of consciousness:** Minor head injury
- **GCS 14-15 with loss of consciousness:** Mild head injury
- **GCS 9-13:** Moderate head injury
- **GCS 3-8:** Severe head injury
- **Remember:**
  - o Minimum score for each component is 1, so minimum GCS possible is 3 (**never** 0)
  - o Components can be remembered as **EVM-456** (**E**lectronic **V**oting **M**achine; E for eye opening, V for verbal response and M for motor response) and maximum scoring for each component as **456** (4 for eye opening, 5 for verbal response and 6 for motor response)

- o Best response is counted. For example, if the motor response in the right limb is 4 and that in the left limb is 5, then motor response would be counted as 5

SUBARACHNOID HEMORRHAGE

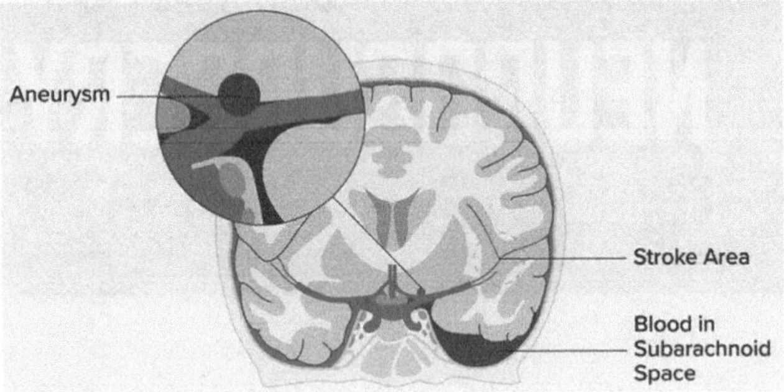

Features

- Hematoma is located **below** arachnoid mater
- **MC** cause of spontaneous subarachnoid hemorrhage is rupture of Berry aneurysm
- There is excruciating **headache** and loss of consciousness
- **Triple H therapy:**
  - o Hypervolemia
  - o Hypertension
  - o Hemodilution

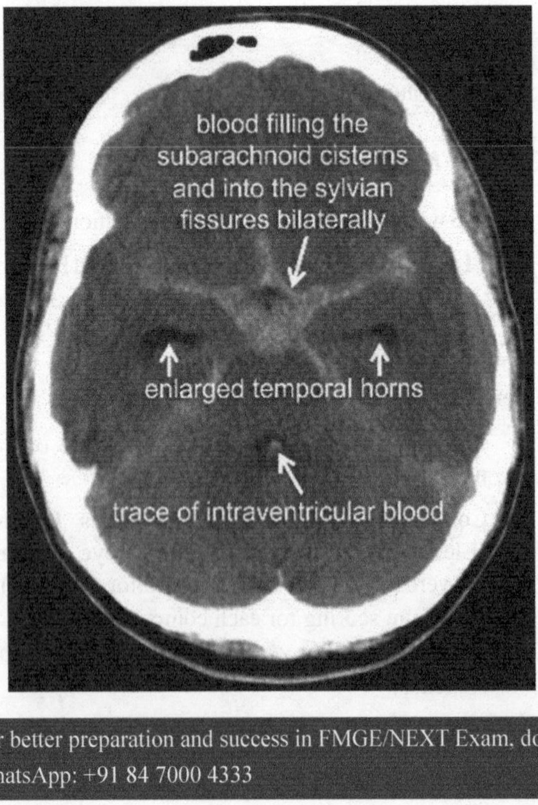

SUBDURAL HEMORRHAGE

Features

- **Classification:**
  - o **Acute:** <3 days
  - o **Subacute:** 4-21 days
  - o **Chronic:** >21 days
- Hematoma is **located** between dura mater and arachnoid mater
- Source of bleeding is bridging veins/emissary **veins**
- There is impaired consciousness from the impact time
- **CT** scan shows concavoconvex appearance

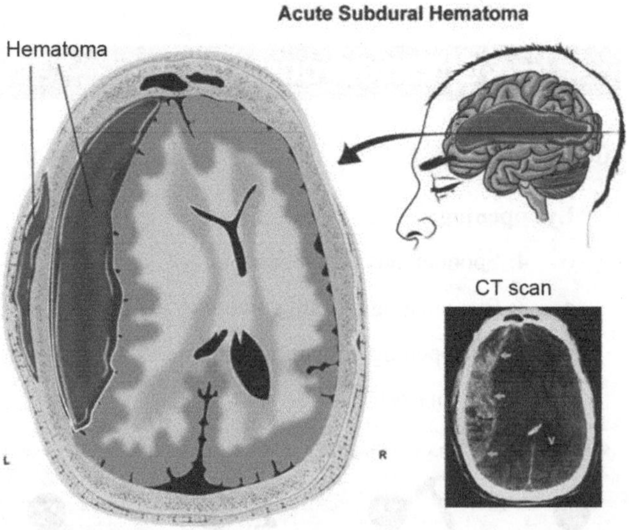

EXTRADURAL HEMORRHAGE

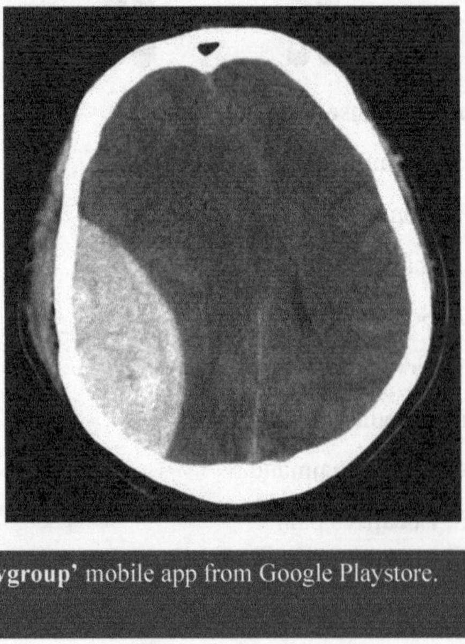

Features

- Hematoma is located **between** dura mater and skull bone
- Usually associated with skull fractures
- Middle meningeal artery is the **source** of bleeding
- Pterion (temporal bone) is the **MC** site of fracture
- **Lucid internal is seen:**
  - o Initially headache only
  - o After some time, contralateral hemiparesis, low consciousness level and pupillary dilatation (same side) because of herniation
- **CT** scan shows biconvex/lens shaped/lentiform hyper-dense lesion
- Craniotomy and surgical evacuation are to be done as **early** as possible

HYDROCEPHALUS

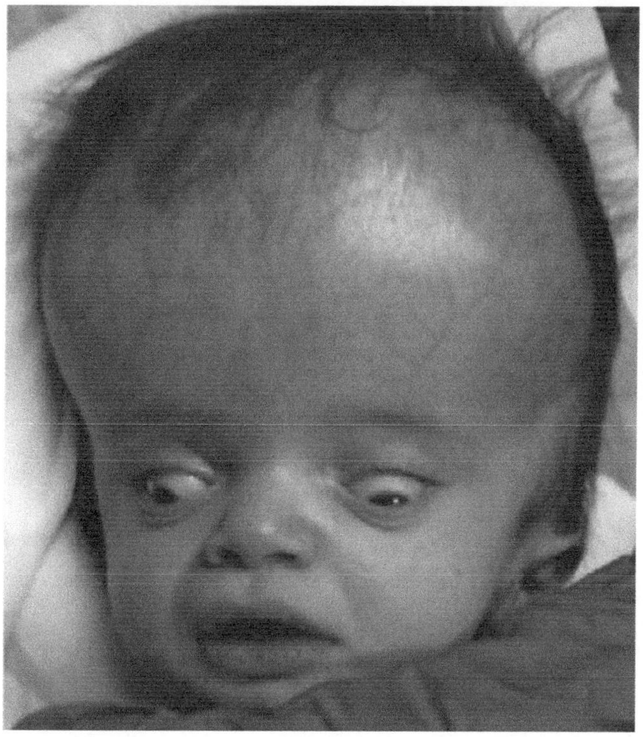

Features

- Increase in CSF pressure
- **Types:**
  - o Obstructive
  - o Communicating
- Do **not** perform lumbar puncture, especially in obstructive type. This can result in tonsillar herniation and death
- Managed by **VP** shunt (Ventriculoperitoneal shunt)

NEURAL TUBE DEFECTS

Features

- **Meningocele:**
  - o There is protrusion of dura mater and arachnoid mater only and the neural tissue remain inside
  - o **MC** seen in lumbar region
  - o **No** neurological deficit as there is no protrusion of neural elements

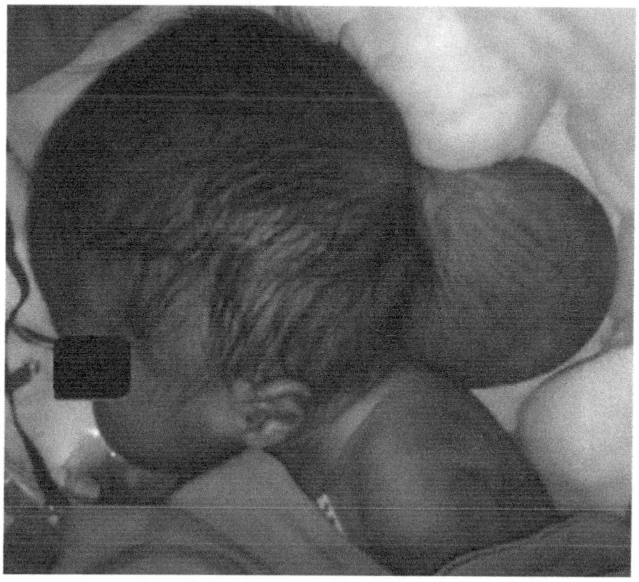

- **Meningomyelocele:**
  - o Commonly due to **folic** acid deficiency in mother
  - o Usually associated with hydrocephalus
  - o Neurological **deficit** present as the neural tissue is protruded along with meninges
  - o Amount of deficit depends on the site of protrusion
    - ♦ Hydrocephalus and deficits are more if the site of protrusion is thoracic region and low in lumbar region
  - o Surgery **must** be done within 24 and 28 hours to avoid CNS infection

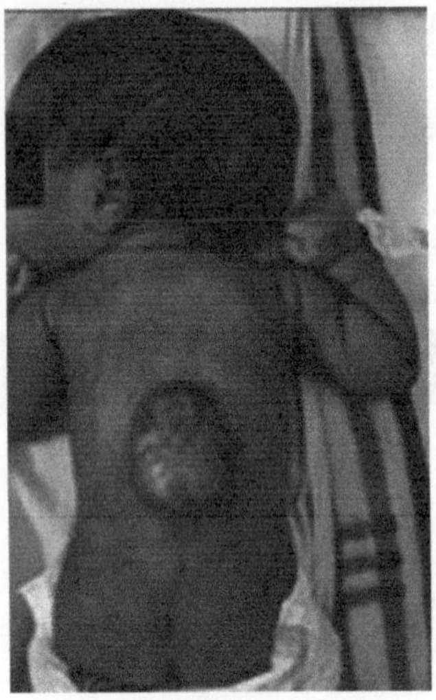

Figure: Child with lumbar meningomyelocele

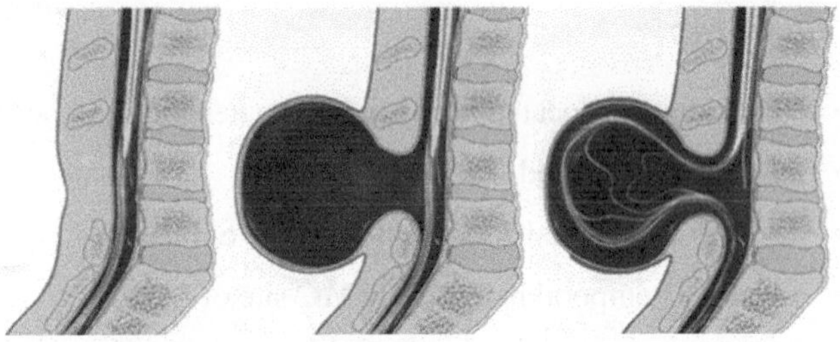

Chapter 17
TRAUMA

FLAIL CHEST

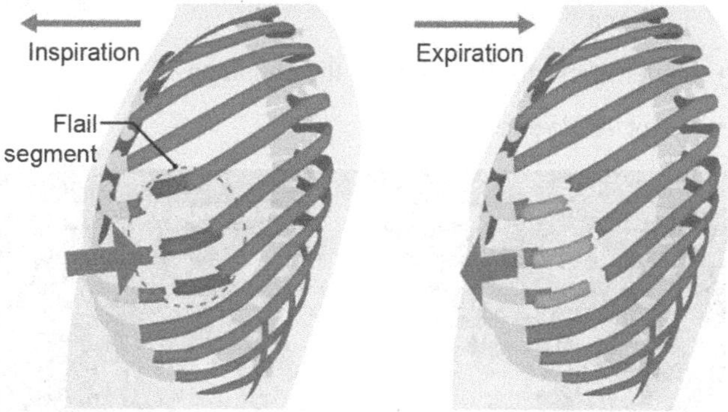

Features

- **Three** or more adjacent ribs are fractured at **two** or more locations
- So, a segment of chest wall becomes independent of the rest of thoracic wall
- On inspiration, **paradoxical** movement of the chest wall occurs

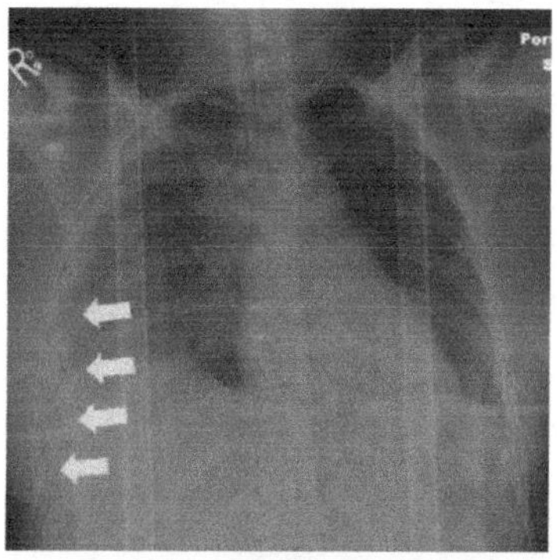

TENSION PNEUMOTHORAX

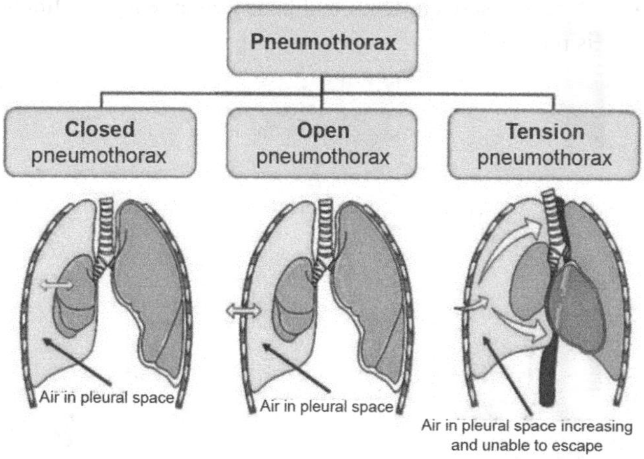

Features

- During inspiration, air is pumped into the pleural cavity, through a valvular opening in the visceral pleura and underlying injured lung
- Lung **collapse** first and as air continuously collects in the pleural cavity, **mediastinum** shifts towards the opposite side, further decreasing the volume of the functioning lung
- Further increase in the intrapleural pressure, reduces the venous return, atrial filling and ventricular filling and so cardiac **output** and cardiac function
- **Clinical presentation:**
  - o Tachypnoea
  - o Tachycardia

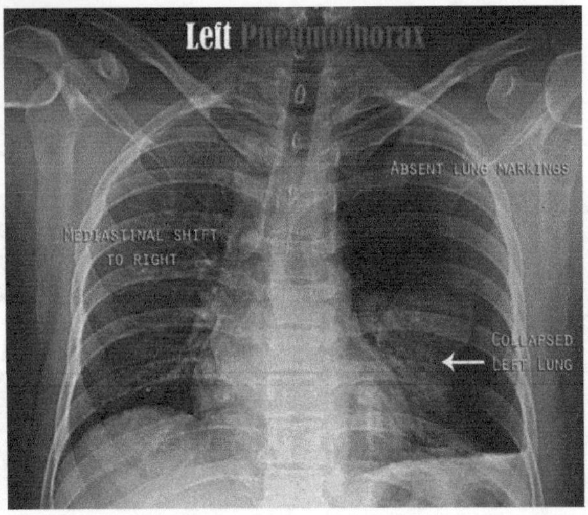

- o Decreased/**Absent** breath sounds
- o **Resonant** on percussion with severe mediastinal/ tracheal shift
- o Cyanosis and hypotension

- It causes sudden death and hence emergency treatment is required

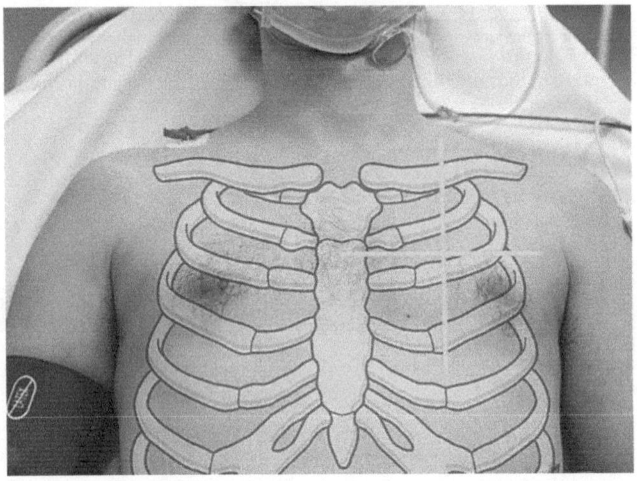

- Once clinically diagnosed, a wide bore needle is immediately placed in the **second** intercostal space in mid-clavicular line and a sterile glove is kept on the hub (blunt) end of the needle to create a valve so as to prevent inward sucking of air from outside

ABDOMINAL TRAUMA

Features

- **MC organ injured in blunt injury:** Spleen
- **MC organ injured in penetrating trauma:** Liver
- **Intra-abdominal injuries and investigations:**
  - o **Stable patient:** CT scan
  - o **Unstable patient:** USG

FAST

- **F**ocused **A**ssessment with **S**onogram for **T**rauma
- Particularly used in unstable patients of abdominal trauma
- Identifies any **free** fluid in the abdomen
- Not 100% sensitive

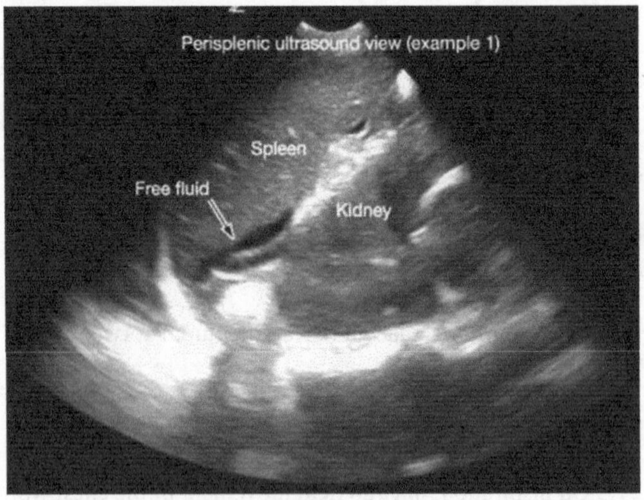

SECTION 2
SURGERY

Chapter 18

MISCELLANEOUS

ANATOMY OF SKIN

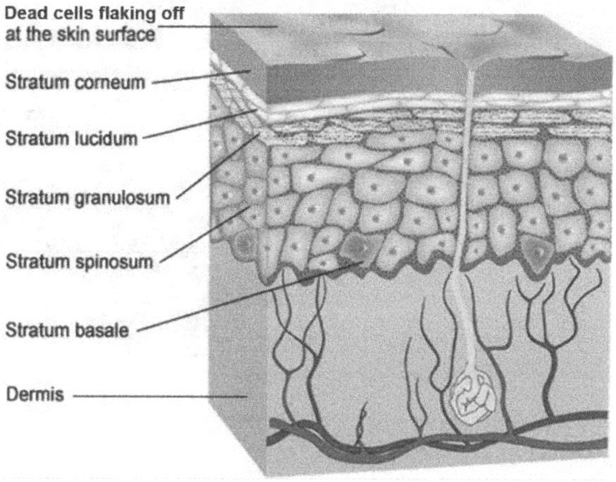

Layers of epidermis

- **Stratum corneum:** One-third of epidermis

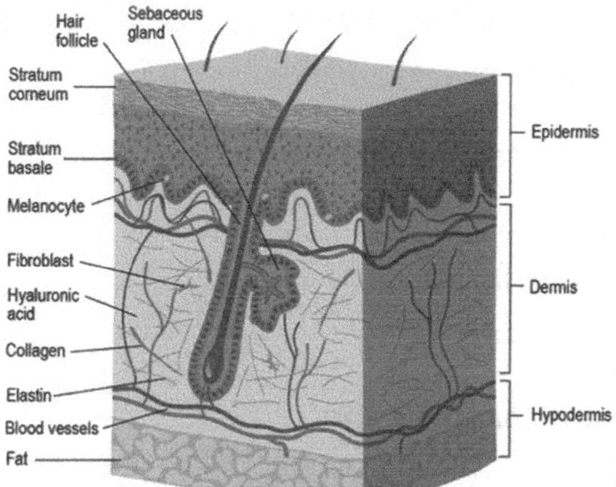

- **Stratum lucidum:** Seen only in palms & soles
- Stratum granulosum
- Stratum spinosum
- Stratum basale

Dermis

- 95% of skin
- 15-40 times thicker than epidermis
- Contains collagen fibres, elastic fibres, capillaries, venules, arteriole, lymphatics, nerves, erector pili muscle, sweat glands, sebaceous glands etc.

BASAL CELL CARCINOMA/RODENT ULCER

Features

- Arises from epidermal basal cells
- Locally invasive (no lymphatic/blood stream dissemination)
- Most common form of skin Ca
- Sunlight is predisposing factor
- Usual site is face, usually above a line joining the ear lobule to the angle of the mouth
- **MC site:** Face/Inner canthus of eyes
- White races
- Unknown in black
- Noduloulcerative type is the MC type

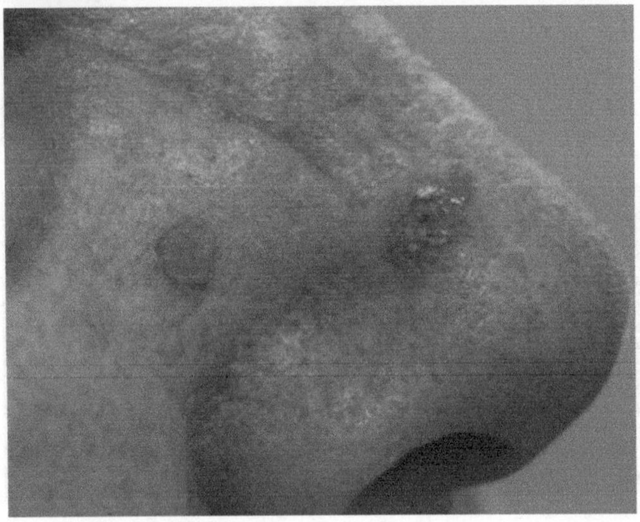

Mode of spread

- Direct
- Very slow growing
- MC low grade malignancy of head & neck region

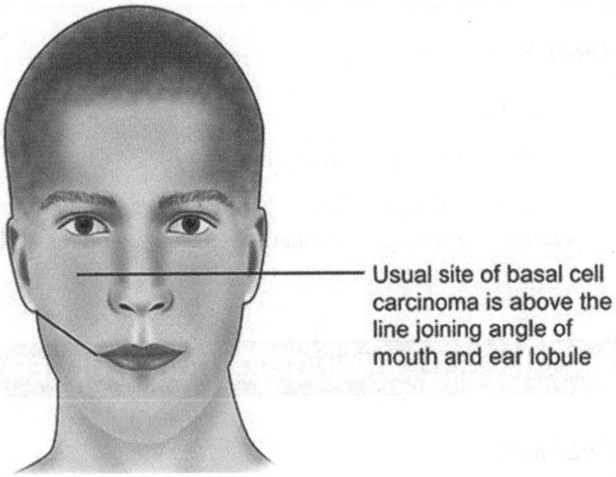

Management

- Moh's micrographic excision
- Highly radiosensitive
- Excision with healthy margin can be done

MALIGNANT MELANOMA

Mode of spread

- Lymphatic channels (regional LN are MC site of metastasis; by embolism; local satellite or in-transit lesions may be seen)
- Hematogenous (lungs, liver)
- MC tumour which metastasizes to breast

Non-cutaneous MM

- Conjunctiva (managed by radiotherapy)
- Choroid (enucleation is done)
- Mouth & tongue

Cutaneous MM

- Arises from epidermal melanocytes
- Exposure to sunlight (decreased ozone layer)
- MC site is trunk (males) & lower limbs (females)

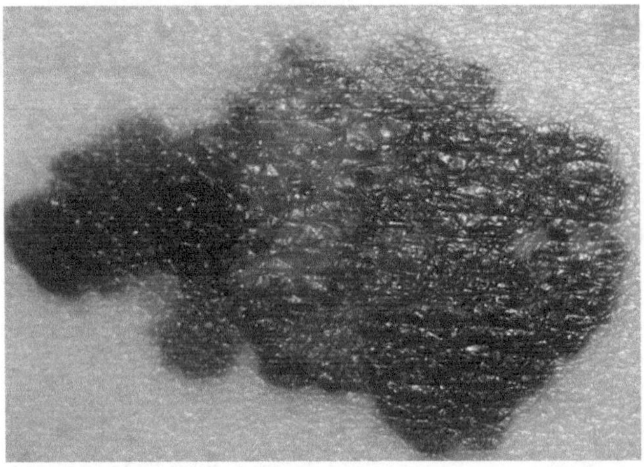

Types

- Lentigo maligna melanoma
- Superficial spreading melanoma
- Nodular melanoma
- Acral lentigenous melanoma
- Amelanotic

Lentigo maligna melanoma

- Least common
- Least malignant
- Seen on face

Superficial spreading

- MC type

- Irregular edges and variegated color pattern is characteristic

Nodular melanoma

- Most malignant
- Poor prognosis
- Younger age group

Acral lentigenous melanoma

- Occurs in palms and soles
- Poor prognosis

Amelanotic

- Lesions are usually pink
- Poorest prognosis (worse than even nodular form)
- Treatment varies as per stage of tumor
- Tumor thickness is a better measure of prognosis than level of invasion
- Lesions <0.76 mm in thickness has a very favorable prognosis

RHABDOMYOSARCOMA

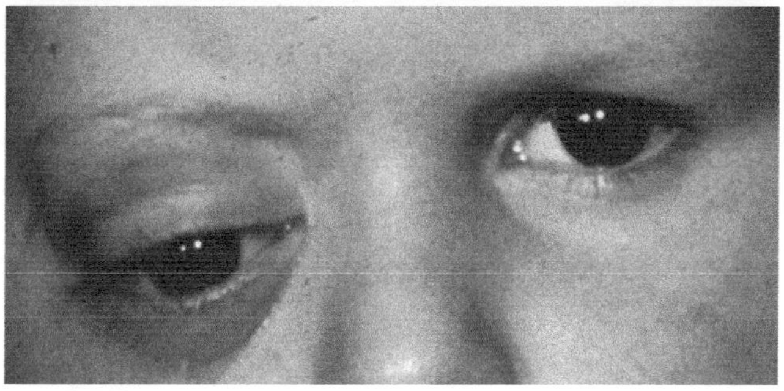

Features

- **MC soft tissue tumour in a child:** Rhabdomyosarcoma
- **MC type of RMS:** Embryonal RMS
- **Mode of spread of embryonal RMS:** Lymphatic
- **Prognosis depends upon:** Grade of tumour

TOTAL PARENTERAL NUTRITION

TPN is used as a primary therapy in

- Indicated in patients with compromised gut functions who require nutritional therapy for > 10 days

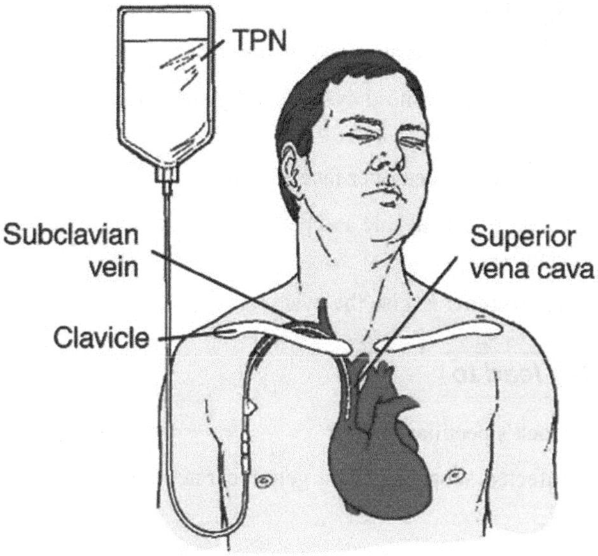

- Severe burns
- Short bowel syndrome

Complications of TPN

- Air embolism (most fatal)
- Weight loss in 7 days

Metabolic changes in TPN

- Essential fatty acid deficiency
- Electrolyte disorder (hyperkalemic hyperchloremic metabolic acidosis) etc.

SEBACEOUS CYST

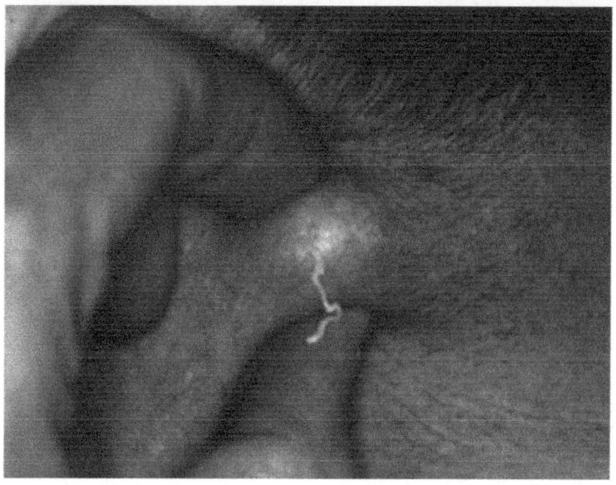

Features

- Due to obstruction of a sebaceous duct

- Retention cyst
- Contents are keratin (and its breakdown product)
- Type of epidermoid cyst (lined by superficial squamous cells)
- Commonly seen over face & scalp
- Never occurs at sole and palm (as there are no sebaceous glands)
- **Treatment:** Excise the cyst

May lead to

- Cock's peculiar tumour
- Infected sebaceous cyst gets ulcerated and the ulcer is covered by excessive granulation tissue resembling a fungating epithelioma

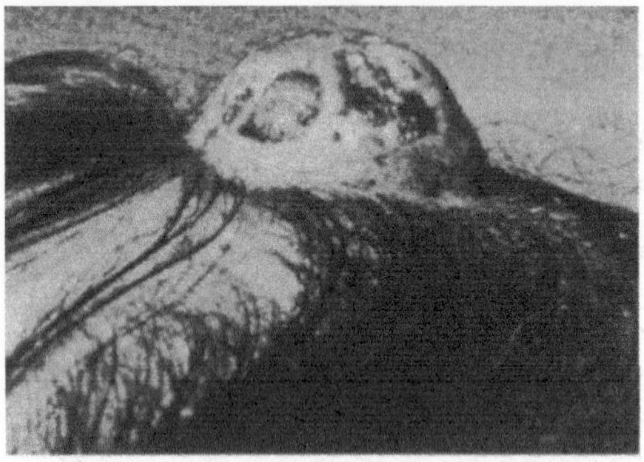

Figure: Cock's 'peculiar tumour' (an infected, ulcerated sebaceous cyst)

SECTION 3

OBSTETRICS

Chapter 1

Embryology

EMBRYOLOGY

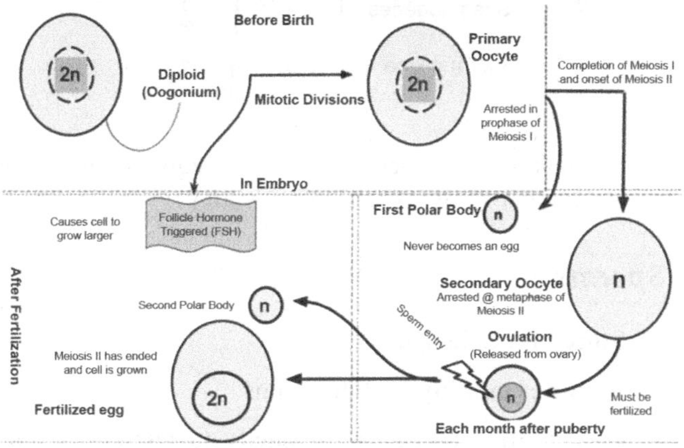

Oogenesis

- The female gonad is the ovary
- Oogenesis is the process involved in the development of mature ovum
- **Oogonia (primitive germ cells) are derived from:** Yolk sac
- **Number at oogonia is maximum at 20th week:** 7 million
- Oogonia enter into prophase of the 1st meiotic division to become primary oocyte
- **Total number of primary oocytes at birth:** 2 million
- **At puberty:** 4 lakhs primary oocytes are left behind
- Out of this, some 400 are likely to ovulate during the entire **reproductive** period
- Primary oocyte has 22 pairs of autosomes (body characteristic) & 1 pair of sex chromosome (XX)
- Primary oocyte undergoes first meiotic division to form secondary oocyte (23,X) and one polar body (23,X)
- Ovulation occurs soon after the formation of secondary oocyte
- Secondary oocyte completes the second meiotic division only after fertilization, forming mature ovum & the second polar body
- In the absence of fertilization, the secondary oocyte does not complete the second meiotic division and degenerates

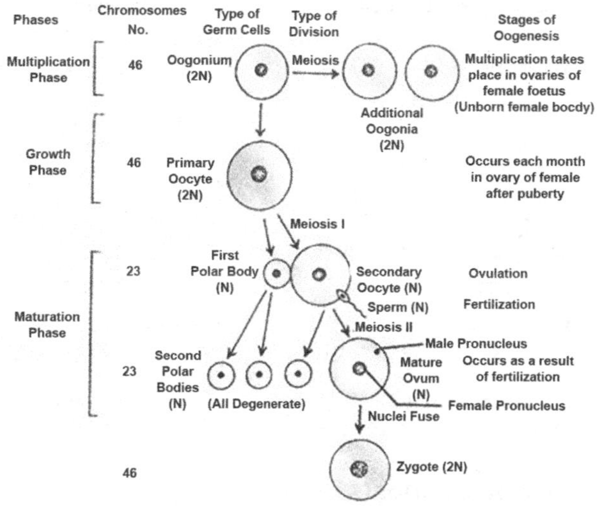

- **Steps:**
  - o Oogonia → Primary oocytes (by mitosis)
  - o Primary oocyte **remains** in prophase of first meiotic division (diplotene phase) from 5 months until puberty. Oogonia are around 40,000 in number

- o At puberty (just before ovulation) → First meiotic division is **completed** → Secondary oocyte + 1st polar body
- o When the primary oocyte divides, almost all its cytoplasm goes to the daughter cell, which forms the secondary oocyte
- o The other daughter cells (first polar body), receives half the chromosomes of the primary oocyte, but almost no cytoplasm
- o The first polar body is, therefore formed merely to get rid of unwanted chromosomes
- o Secondary oocyte immediately undergoes second meiotic division but this is **arrested** at the end of metaphase
- o This second meiosis is completed only **if** there is fertilization by sperm
- o Secondary oocyte completes **second** meiotic division only after fertilization by the sperm
- o 2nd polar body is formed at the time of fertilization
- o If there is no fertilization, then secondary oocyte degenerates 12 hours after ovulation (at LH **peak**)

- First polar body is released 24 hours **prior** to ovulation
- **Second polar body is released at the time of:** Fertilization
- **Oogonia & germ cell are derived from:** Yolk sac
- **1st polar body is formed during:** Oogenesis

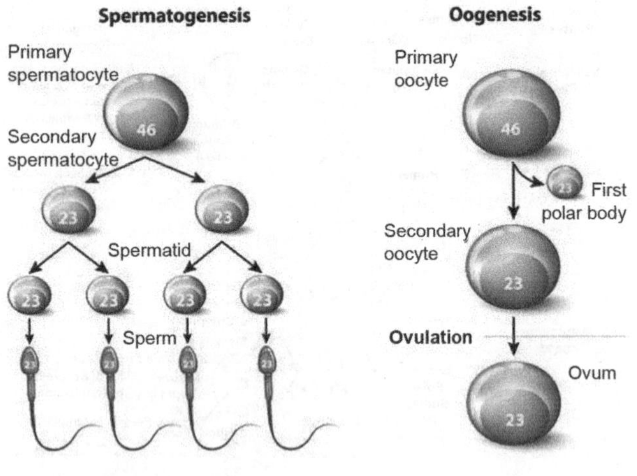

Spermatogenesis

- Formation of sperm (spermatozoa) from primordial germ cells (spermatogonia) only after puberty
- Occurs in seminiferous tubules of the testes
- Occurs at a 5 degrees Celsius **lower** temperature than the core temperature (testes hangs from the body)
- **Time: 74** days
- Spermatogonia → Primary spermatocytes (by mitosis)
- Primary spermatocytes → Secondary spermatocytes (by **first** meiotic division)
- Secondary spermatocytes → Spermatids (by **2nd** meiotic division)

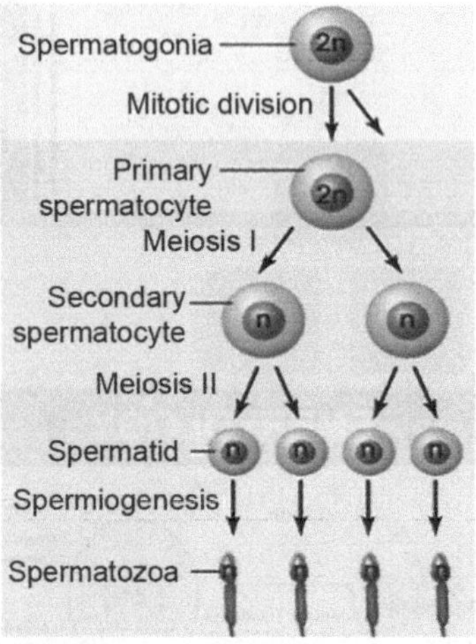

- Spermatids → Spermatozoa (undergo morphologic changes; no division; **spermiogenesis**)

Sperms

- **Stored in:** Epididymis
- **Acquires motility in:** Epididymis
- **Capacitation (acquiring capacity to fertilize ovum) occurs in:** Fallopian tube
- Only the capacitated sperms can fertilize ovum
- Capacitated sperm reaches ampulla of fallopian tube (which is the site of fertilization)
- **Length of mature sperm:** 50 – 60 microns

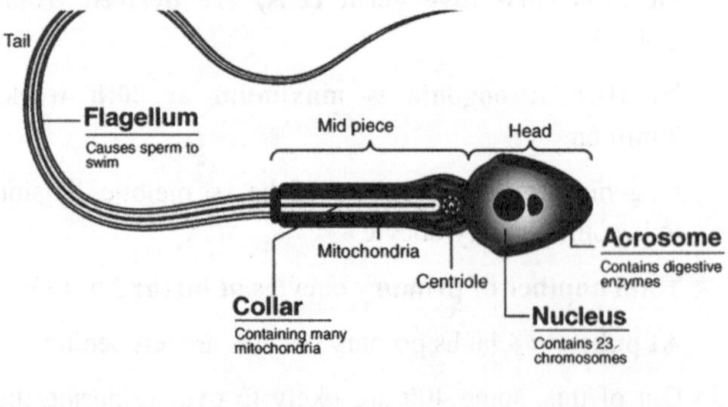

- **Parts:**
  - o **Head:**
    - ♦ Head is covered by **acrosome**, that helps in penetration of the spermatozoon into the ovum during fertilization
    - ♦ It is derived from Golgi apparatus (contains lysosomal enzymes hyaluronidase & acrosin)
  - o **Neck:** Contains spherical centrioles
  - o **Middle piece:** Formed by **Mitochondria**, also known as power house of sperm ***(Mnemonic: M for M)***
  - o **Principal piece:** Tail
  - o **End piece:** Formed by centrioles & tubules (provides motility)

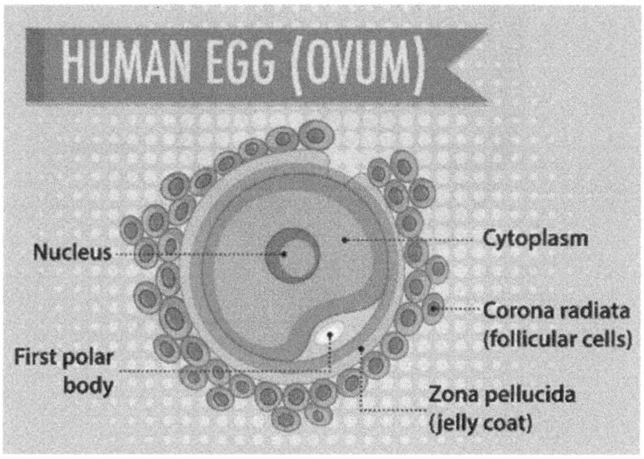

Fertilizable life span

- **Oocyte:** 12-24 hours
- **Sperm:** 48-72 hours

FERTILIZATION

Events after first day of menstrual cycle

- **Secondary oocyte extrusion:** On day **14th**
- Secondary oocyte reaches tube
- **Fertilization with extrusion of second polar body:** Day **14th to 16th**
- Formation of zygote, 2-cell stage & 4-cell stage
- **Early morula:** Day 17th
- **Late morula:** Day **18th**
- **Early blastocyst stage with disappearance of zona pellucida:** Day **19th to 20th**
- **Early phase of implantation:** Day **20th to 21st**

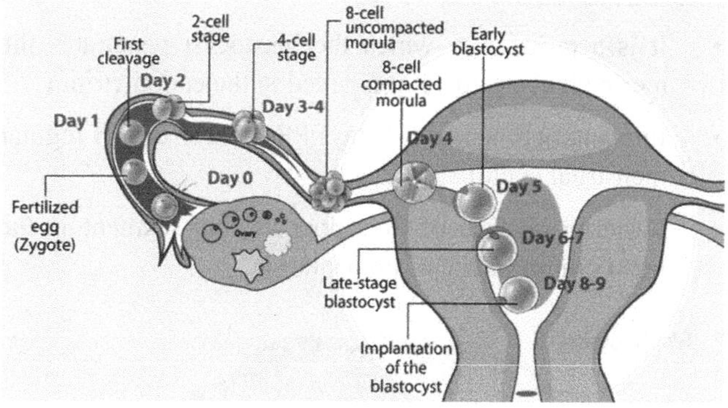

Fertilization & post-fertilization (PF) events

- Acrosomal reaction occurs after sperm binds to zona pellucida
- Fusion of male and female pronucleus to form the zygote is known as fertilization
- **MC site of fertilization:** Ampulla of fallopian tube
- Then zygote undergoes cell division and becomes – 2 cell, 4 cell, 8 cells and 16 cell stage
- Zygote **stays** in fallopian tube for 3 days post-fertilization (PF)
- **Zygote reaches uterine cavity in which stage:** 16 celled stage/morula on **4th** day PF (18th day of cycle)
- As the morula enters the uterine cavity, fluid enters it and morula gets **converted** to Blastocyst
- **Blastocyst cells differentiate into:**
  - o Trophoblast (cells arranged in periphery)
  - o Inner cell mass
- **Normally** implantation occurs in posterior wall of the body of the uterus near the fundus

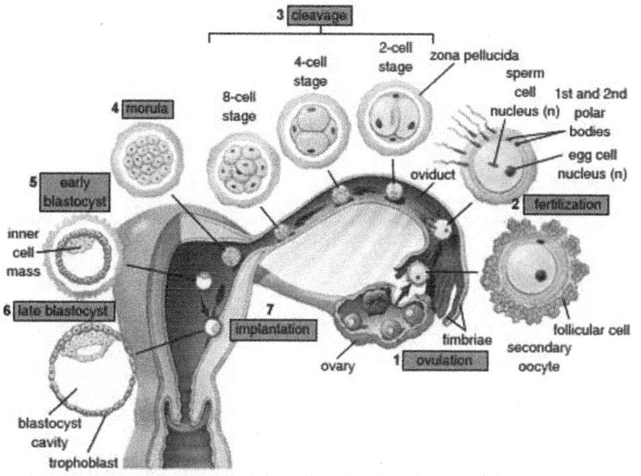

Implantation

- It is a process by which the blastocyst penetrates the uterine mucosa to get implanted in the endometrium
- Implantation begins **6-7** days PF (**20-21**[st] day of regular menstrual cycle)
- Posterior surface of the upper uterine segment is the **most common** site of implantation

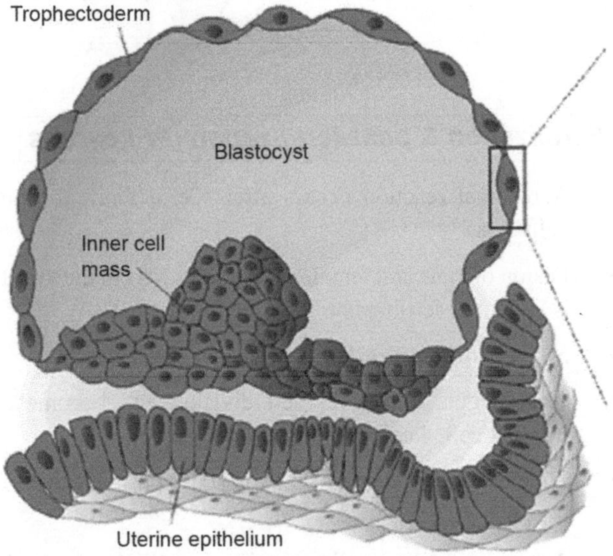

Decidua

- It is the endometrium of pregnancy
- **D. basalis/serotina:**
  - o In contact with base of blastocyst; between the embryo and myometrium
- **D. capsularis/reflexa:**
  - o Covering the blastocyst; between the embryo and uterine cavity
- **D. vera/parietalis:**
  - o Rest of the decidual lining outside the site of implantation; lines the remaining uterine cavity

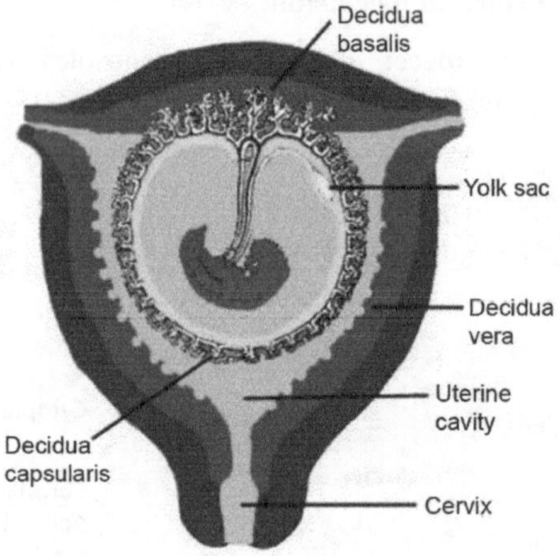

SECTION 3 OBSTETRICS

Chapter 2

Placenta, Fetal Membranes and Umbilical Cord

PLACENTA

Placenta

- Discoid
- Hemochorial (direct contact of the chorion with maternal blood)
- Deciduate (some maternal tissue is shed at parturition)
- **2 sources:**
  - o Chorion frondosum (**fetal** surface)
  - o Decidua basalis (**maternal** surface)

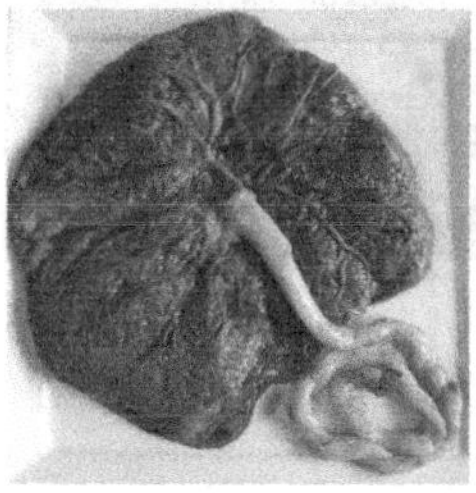

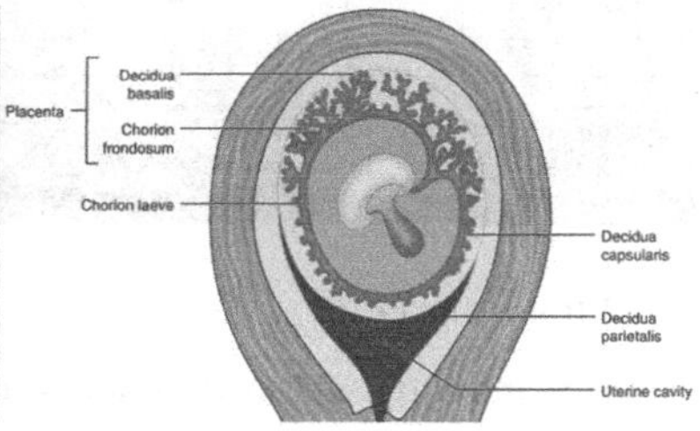

- **Placenta at term:**
  - o **Weight:** 500 grams
  - o Ratio of weight of placenta to weight of baby is 1:6
- **Nitabuch's membrane:**
  - o Zone of fibrinoid deposition; where trophoblasts & decidua meet (in placenta)
  - o It limits the further invasion of the decidua by the trophoblast
  - o Absence of Nitabuch's membrane result in placenta accreta, increta and percreta

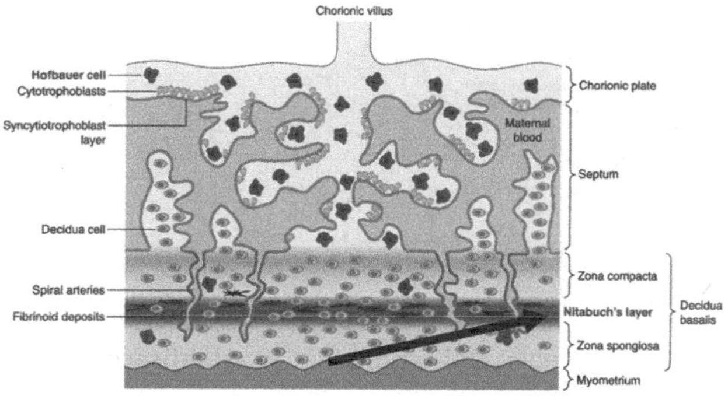

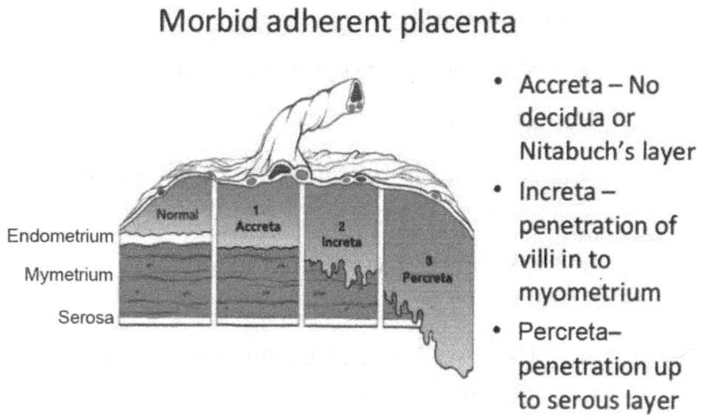

- **Placental circulation:**
  - o Placenta has villi and intervillous spaces

- o **Villi** carry fetal blood
- o **Intervillous** space has maternal blood
- o Both maternal and fetal blood are present in placenta but they do **not** mix
- o **It means, there are two independent circulations in placenta:** Uteroplacental and Fetoplacental
- o **Uteroplacental circulation is established on: 10-11th** day

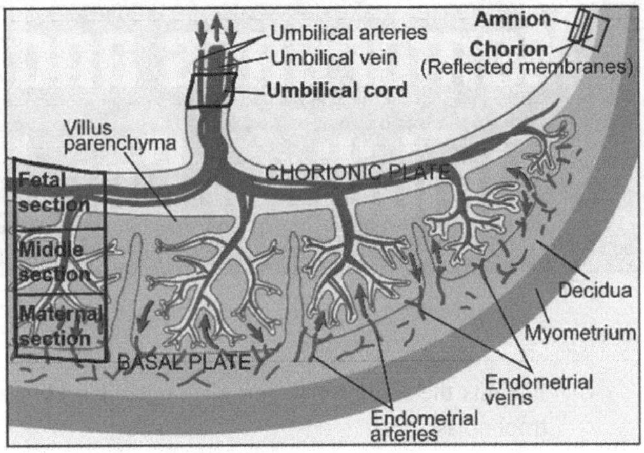

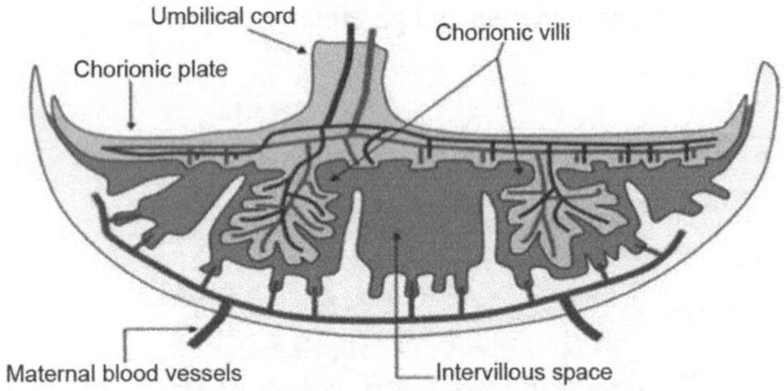

- o **Fetoplacental circulation is established on: 21-22nd** day
- o **Uteroplacental:**
  - ♦ Spiral arterioles open into the intervillous space
- o **Fetoplacental:**
  - ♦ It is via umbilical veins (UV) and umbilical arteries (UA)
  - ♦ UV carries **oxygenated** blood from placenta to fetus
  - ♦ The two UA carries **impure** blood from the fetus to the placenta

Placental pathologies

- **Placental infarction:**
  - o **MC** placental lesion
  - o Can lead to placental abruption or pre-eclampsia

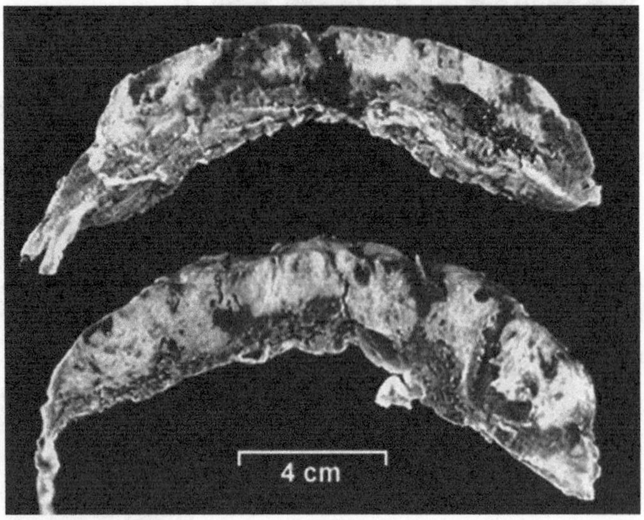

- **Placentomegaly:**
  - o Placental thickness is more than **40 mm** at term (normally 30 mm)
  - o May occur due to gestational diabetes, hydrops fetalis etc.

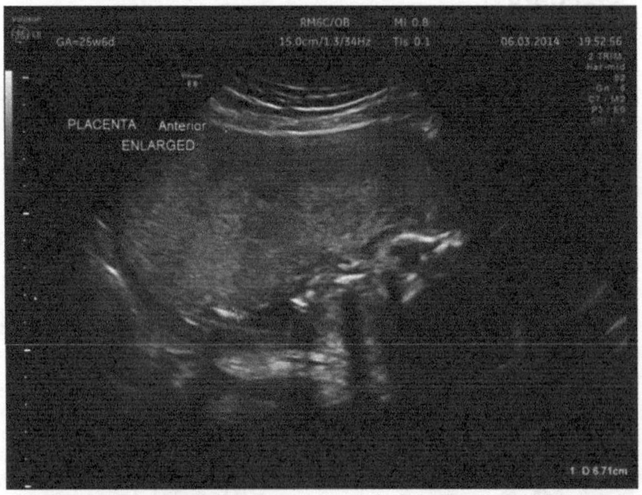

- **Small placenta:**
  - o Intrauterine growth retardation/IUGR
  - o Post-datism
- **Succenturiate placenta:**
  - o Small part of placenta is separated from rest of the placenta
  - o Leash of blood vessels connects the main placenta to this extra lobe
  - o This can lead to postpartum hemorrhage/**PPH**

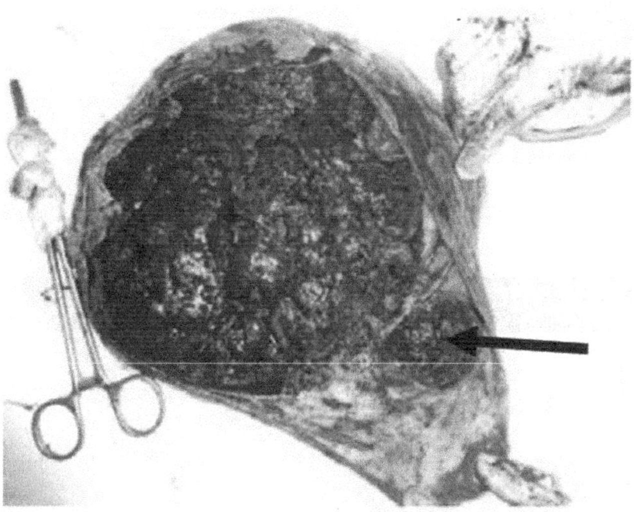

- **Extrachorial placenta:**
    - o Chorionic plate normally extends to the periphery of the placenta
    - o The diameter of chorionic plate is similar to basal plate
    - o In extrachorial placenta, the chorionic plate is smaller than the basal plate
    - o **Circumvallate placenta** is a variety of extrachorial placenta
    - o In circumvallate placenta, chorionic plate is covered by a double fold of amnion and chorion

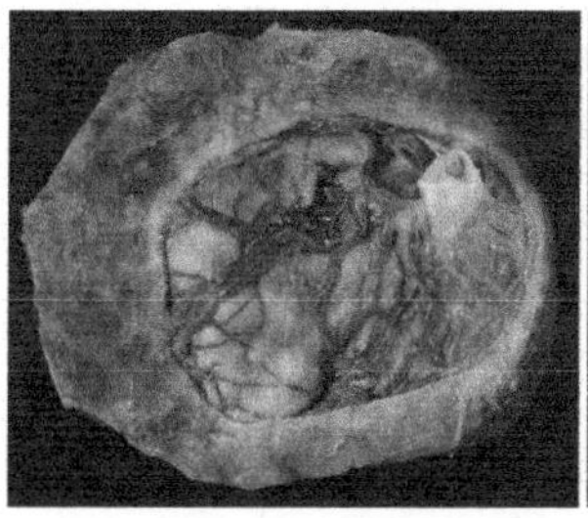

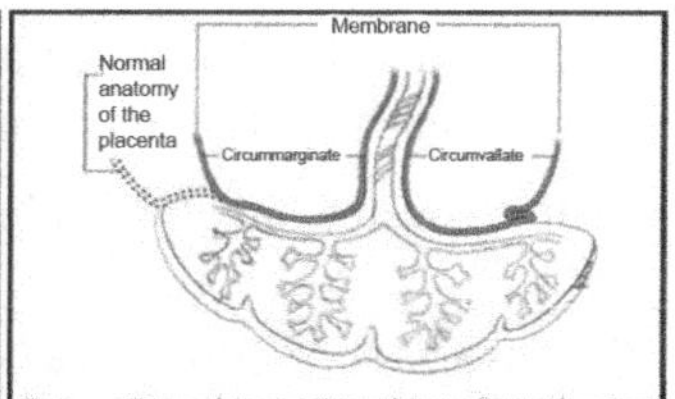

Figure : Diagram of circummarginate and circumvallate membrane insertion. In both, the fetal membranes do not insert at the edge of the placenta but rather at some point inwards. In circumvallation there is a plication of the membranes evident as a fibrin ridge on gross examination. In circummargination, the membrane insertion is flat and a ridge is not present

Placental hormones

- Progesterone
- Estrogen
- HPL (Human Placental Lactogen)
- HCG (Human Chorionic Gonadotropin)
- Main site of hormone synthesis in placenta is **synctiotrophoblast**

Progesterone

- Main hormone during pregnancy
- Converts endometrium to decidua
- **Source:**
    - o **Initial 6-7 weeks:** Corpus luteum
    - o **At 8-10 weeks:** Placenta

Estrogen

- Fetal adrenal gland produces **DHEA** (**De**Hydro-**E**pi**A**ndrostenedione), which is utilized by placental enzymes to synthesize estradiol and estriol
- Estrogen cannot be synthesized by placenta alone

HPL

- Conserve glucose so that it is utilized by fetus

HCG

- **Function:** Rescue & maintenance of corpus luteum till 6 weeks of pregnancy
- **HCG is secreted by:** Synctiotrophoblast (principal site of protein & steroid hormones in pregnancy)
- Structurally HCG is a Glycoprotein with molecular weight of 36000-40000
    - o **2 subunits (alpha & beta):**
        - ♦ Alpha subunit is biochemical similar to LH, FSH and TSH (non-specific)
        - ♦ Beta subunit is relatively **unique** to HCG

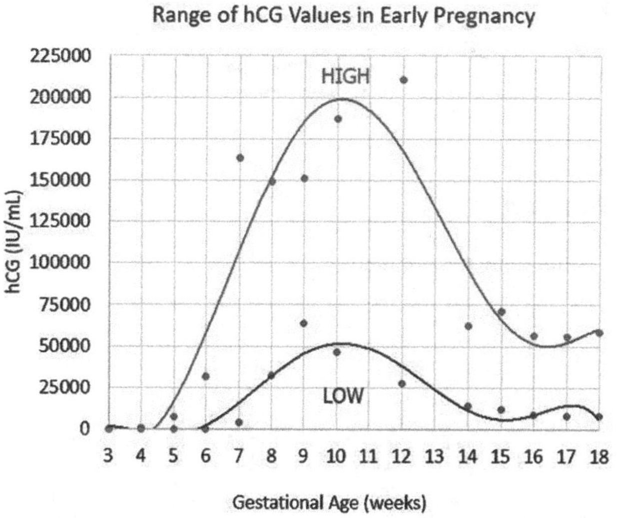

- Act as a stimulus for secretion of progesterone by the corpus luteum of pregnancy
- **Plasma half-life**: 24-36 hours

- Can be detected in maternal serum as early as 8-9 days post fertilization/22nd day of menstrual cycle/5-6 days before missed period
- **Doubling time:** 1.4-2 days
- **Maximum blood & urine levels:** 1,00,000 IU/L between 60-70 days (8-10 weeks)
- Disappears from circulation within 2 weeks following delivery

High HCG levels

- Multiple pregnancies
- H. mole/choriocarcinoma
- Down syndrome

Low HCG levels

- Ectopic pregnancies
- Spontaneous abortion

FETAL MEMBRANES

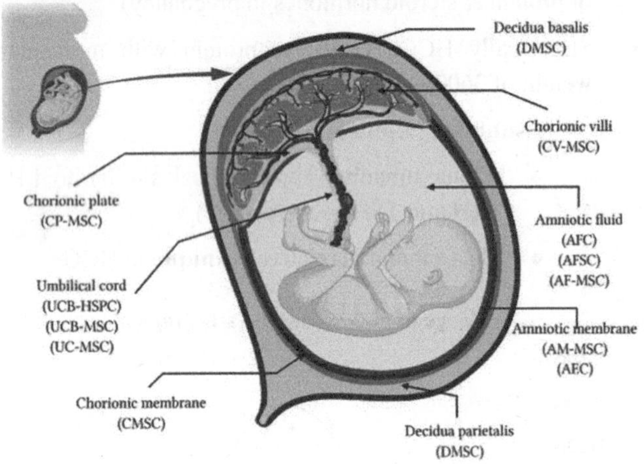

Amnion

- Innermost membrane
- Avascular

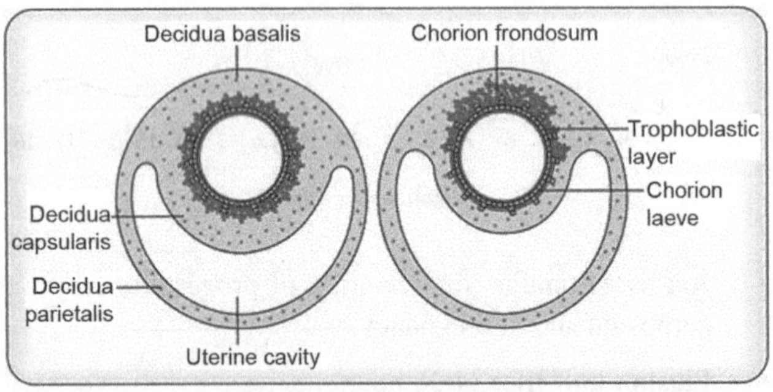

Chorion

- **Chorion laeve:**
  - o Gets merged with amnion
- **Chorion frondosum:**
  - o Form placental villi

UMBILICAL CORD

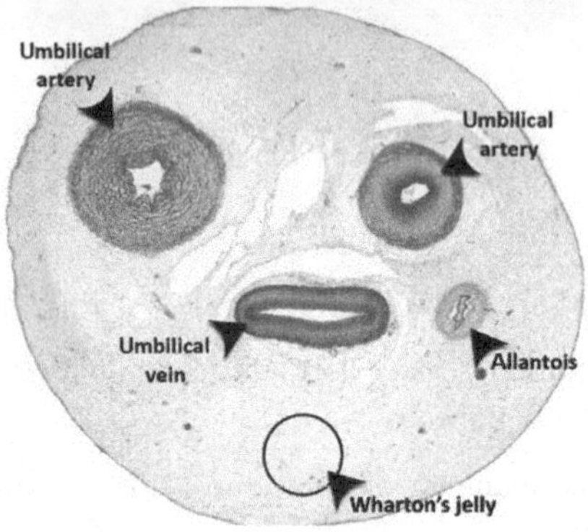

Umbilical cord

- Extends from the fetal surface of placenta/**chorionic plate** to the fetal umbilicus
- Attached to the placenta near the centre
- **Vessels in umbilical cord:**
  - o 2 arteries, 1 vein (initially there are 2 arteries and 2 veins, but later on right umbilical vein disappears)
- It is covered **only** by amnion (not by chorion)

Anomalies of umbilical cord

- **Battledore placenta/marginal placenta:**
  - o UC is attached to the **margin** of the placenta

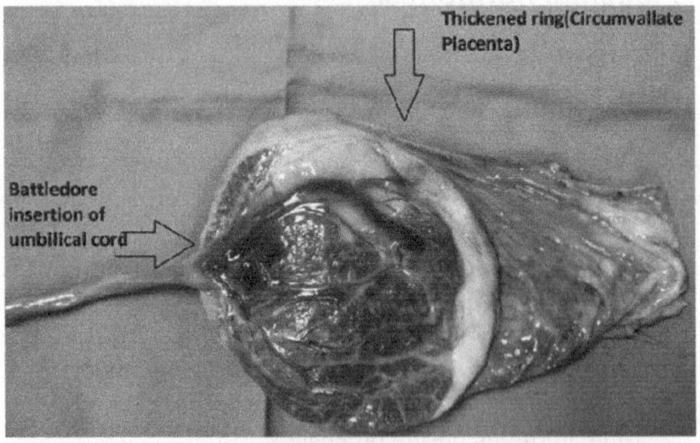

- **Velamentous insertion of UC:**
  - Here the UC is attached to the centre of placenta but the vessels split much before attaching to the placenta
  - Vessels attach to the **membrane** first and then they attach to the placenta
  - This can give rise to **vasa previa**

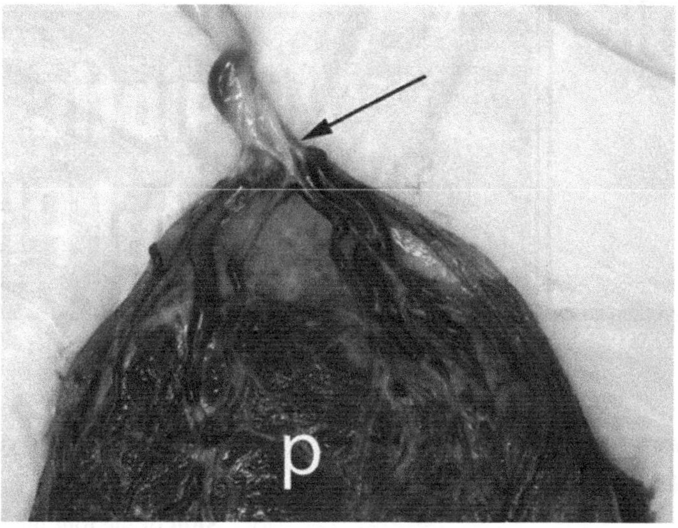

SECTION 3
OBSTETRICS

Chapter 3

Amniotic Fluid and Fetal Physiology

AMNIOTIC FLUID

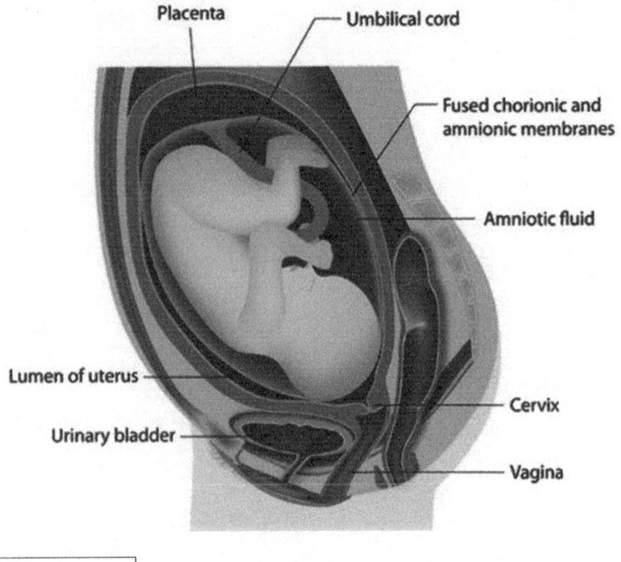

Features

- **Replaced every:** 3 hours
- Alkaline with specific gravity of 1.010
- **Contributor:**
  - o Fetal urine (**mainly**)
  - o Fetal lung
- Fetal amniotic fluid volume production is kept balanced by fetal swallowing (mainly)
- **Amniotic fluid index/AFI:**
  - o Abdomen is divided into **4** quadrants
  - o On USG, **largest vertical** pocket is measured in each quadrant
  - o **Sum** of the four measurements (in cms) is the AFI

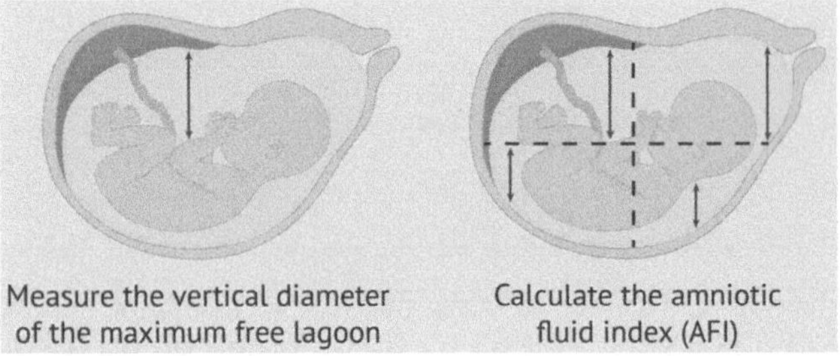

Amount

- **At 12 weeks:** 50 ml
- **At 20 weeks:** 400 ml
- **Maximum at:** 36-38 weeks (1000 ml)
- **Amount at term**: 600-800 ml
- There is reduction in volume in the pregnancies continued post-term (200 ml at 43 weeks)

Amniotic fluid appearance

- **Normal:**
  - o Pale straw colour (due to exfoliated lanugo and epidermal cells from fetal skin)
- **Golden yellow:**
  - o Rh incompatibility (due to increased bilirubin levels)

- **Green coloured (meconium stained) amniotic fluid indicates:**
  - o Fetal **distress** in presentations other than breech/ transverse (thick with presence of flakes suggest chronic fetal distress)

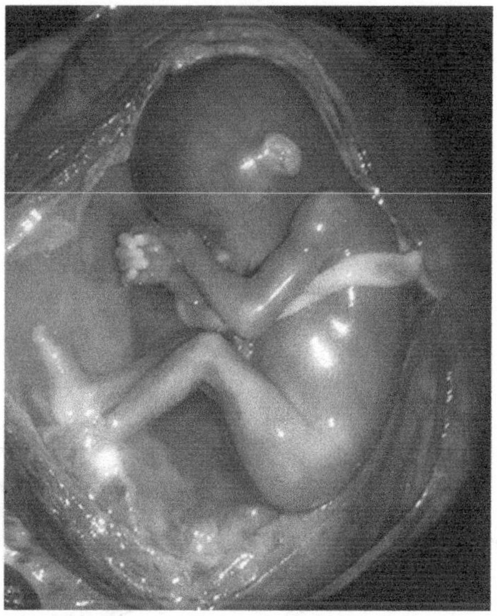

- **Greenish yellow/saffron:**
  - o Post-maturity
- **Dark maroon coloured:**
  - o Concealed accidental hemorrhage
- **Dark brown/tobacco juice/prune juice:**
  - o Intrauterine death (old HbA)

Functions

- To protect fetus (acts as a shock absorber)
- Maintains temperature
- No role in nutrition

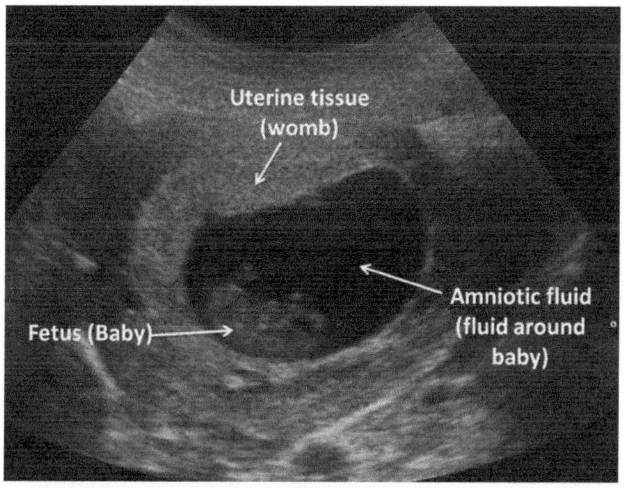

Oligohydramnios

- Liquor amnii is **less** than 200 ml at term
- AFI is **less** than 5 cm
- **Causes of oligohydramnios *(Mnemonic: Renal LIMP)***
  - o **Renal** anomalies of fetus resulting in decreased production of urine:
    - ♦ Renal agenesis
    - ♦ Urethral obstruction
    - ♦ Multicystic dysplastic kidneys (bilaterally)
- **L**eaking of fluid following procedures (amniocentesis/ Chorionic villous sampling)
- **I**UGR
- **M**aternal conditions (hypertension/pre-eclampsia)
- **P**remature rupture of membranes

Polyhydramnios

- Liquor amnii is > 2 litres
- AFI is $\geq$ to 25 cm
- **Polyhydramnios is seen in *(Mnemonic: MUPIS)***
  - o **M**ore **U**rine **P**roduction (fetus):
    - ♦ Twin/multifetal pregnancy
    - ♦ Maternal hyperglycemia/Diabetes
  - o **I**mpaired **S**wallowing (fetus):
    - ♦ Esophageal atresia/stenosis
    - ♦ Duodenal atresia/stenosis
    - ♦ Cleft lip and cleft palate
    - ♦ Bowel obstruction
    - ♦ Anencephaly

FETAL PHYSIOLOGY

Important terms

- **Embryo:**
  - o 3rd week to 8th week after fertilization (5th to 10th week of gestational age/GA)
  - o Period of organogenesis
  - o Most teratogenic period
- **Fetus:**
  - o **9th** week after fertilization till end of pregnancy (11th week of GA till end of pregnancy)

- **Last menstrual period:**
  - o Useful for calculating period of gestation
  - o **If a lady misses her period:**
    - ♦ It means fertilization has occurred
    - ♦ Around 2 weeks has passed since fertilization, considering fertilization occurred on 14th day of cycle (at the time of ovulation)
    - ♦ 28 days has passed since the first day of last menstrual period
  - o In pregnancy, all events are calculated from the first day of LMP and not from the day of fertilization, so if a lady misses her period, the pregnancy is 4 weeks old (and not 2 weeks old)

Fetal hemopoiesis

- **Age and site of RBC production** ***(Mnemonic: YoLiBo)***
  - o **Yo**lk sac: First site
  - o **Li**ver: 6th week onward
  - o **Bo**ne Marrow: 24th week onward

Fetal physiology

- **Source of oxygenated blood: Placenta** (not the fetal lungs)
- **Remember** umbilical vein carries oxygenated blood (being a vein, carries oxygenated blood) and umbilical artery carries deoxygenated blood (being an artery, carries deoxygenated blood)
- Oxygenated blood from placenta → through **umbilical vein/UV** → greater portion passes directly to **inferior vena cava/IVC** through **ductus venosus/DV** → oxygen rich blood reaches right atrium → most of the blood passes from right atrium to left atrium through **foramen ovale/FO** → remaining blood mixes with the blood coming from superior vena cava and passes to right ventricle → from right ventricle, blood enters pulmonary trunk → greater part of this blood is short circuited to aorta through **ductus arteriosus/DA** → blood from the aorta is carried by the **umbilical arteries** to the placenta

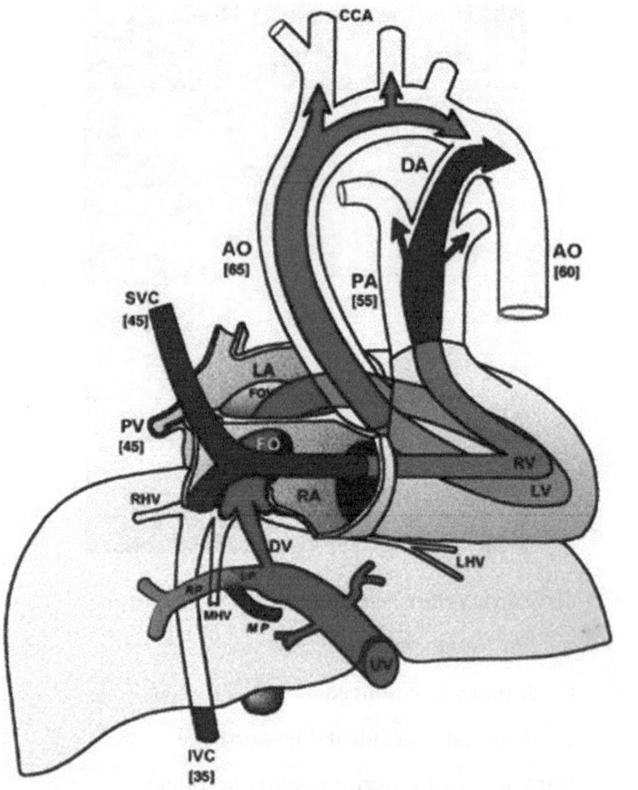

Structures occluded after birth

- Umbilical arteries contracts and their lumen is occluded
- Lumen of umbilical vein and ductus venosus is also occluded
- Ductus arteriosus is also occluded

SECTION 3

OBSTETRICS

Chapter 4

Pregnancy

PREGNANCY

Important points

- **Gravida:**
  - o Denotes pregnant state (**both** present and past), **irrespective** of the period of gestation
  - o Term is used in a lady, who is pregnant at present
  - o **Primigravida:**
    - ♦ Lady becoming pregnant for the **first** time
  - o **Elderly primigravida:**
    - ♦ Lady having first pregnancy at the age of **30** years or more
- **Parity:**
  - o Denotes only those previous pregnancies, which have **crossed** the period of viability
  - o **Period of viability:**
    - ♦ Physical ability of a fetus to lead a separate existence after birth apart from its mother
    - ♦ A child is viable after **210** days of intrauterine life
  - o **Grand multipara:**
    - ♦ Pregnant woman with past history of four births or more
- **Examples to understand gravida and parity:**
  - o **Lady with 12 weeks pregnancy and child of 3 years: G_2P_1** (G_2, because this is her second pregnancy and P_1, as previously, she had a pregnancy which crosses the period of viability)
  - o **Lady with 9 weeks pregnancy but previously 2 abortions at 18 weeks: G_3P_0** (G_3, as this is her third pregnancy and P_0, as previously none of her pregnancy crossed the period of viability mark)
- **Menstrual/Gestation age:**
  - o 10 lunar months/9 calendar months + 7 days/280 days/40 weeks, calculated from first day of last menstrual period
- **Calculation of expected date of delivery/EDD:**
  - o **Done by Naegele's formula:**
    - ♦ Forward counting: To the first day of LMP, add 7 days and 9 months
    - ♦ Backward counting: To the first day of LMP, add 7 days and subtract 3 months
  - o Only 4-6% of the females deliver on their exact date of EDD

Requirement during pregnancy

- **Calcium:** 1200 mg/day
- **Iodine:** 250 microgram/day
- **Folic acid:** 400 microgram/day
- **Iron:** 1000 mg/day
- **Extra calorie:** +350 Kcal/day (extra-calorie in lactation is +600 Kcal/day)

SIGNS OF PREGNANCY

First trimester

- Local vascular congestion of pelvis causing dusky/purplish hue of anterior vaginal wall & vestibule:
  - o Chadwick sign/Jacquemier's sign
  - o 8 weeks

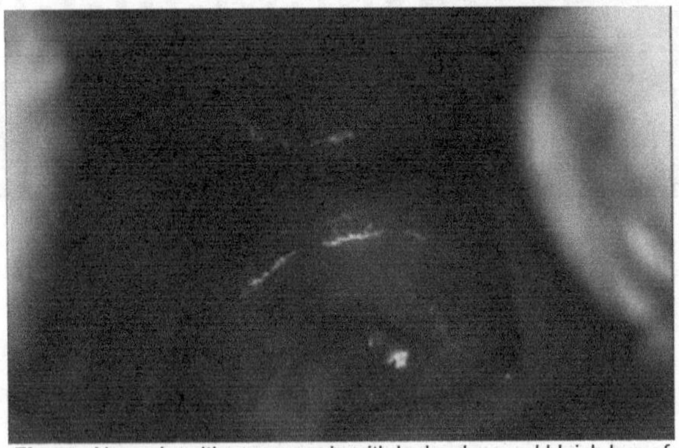

Figure: Normal multiparous cervix with leukorrhea and bluish hue of "Chadwick's sign"

- **Cyanosis & softening of cervix because of increased vascularity:**
  - o Goodell's sign
  - o 6 weeks
  - o Pregnant cervix feels like the **lips** of the mouth, while in the non-pregnant state, cervix feels like the of tip of the **nose**
- **Compressibility of isthmus on bimanual examination:**
  - o Hegar's sign
  - o 6-10 weeks

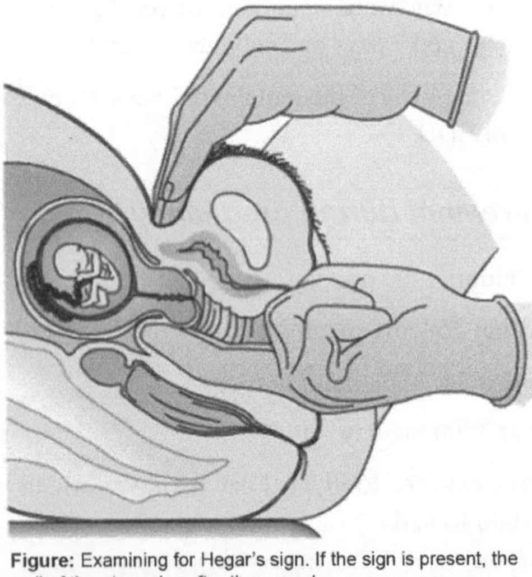

Figure: Examining for Hegar's sign. If the sign is present, the wall of the uterus is softer than usual

  - o Upper part of the body of uterus is enlarged by growing fetus
  - o Lower part of the body is empty & **isthmus** is extremely soft
  - o Cervix is comparatively firm
- **One half of the uterus is firmer than the other half in lateral implantation:**
  - o Piskacek's sign
  - o **Asymmetrical** enlargement of uterus in lateral implantation
- **Increased pulsations felt through lateral vaginal fornix:**
  - o Osiander's sign
  - o 8 weeks
- **Regular & rhythmic contractions of uterus, elicited by bimanual examination:**
  - o Palmer's sign
  - o 4-8 weeks
  - o **Valuable** sign when elicited

Second trimester

- **Quickening:**
  - o Perception of active fetal **movements** felt by 18 weeks of pregnancy in primipara and 16 weeks in multipara
- **Chloasma:**
  - o **Pigmentation** over forehead and cheeks

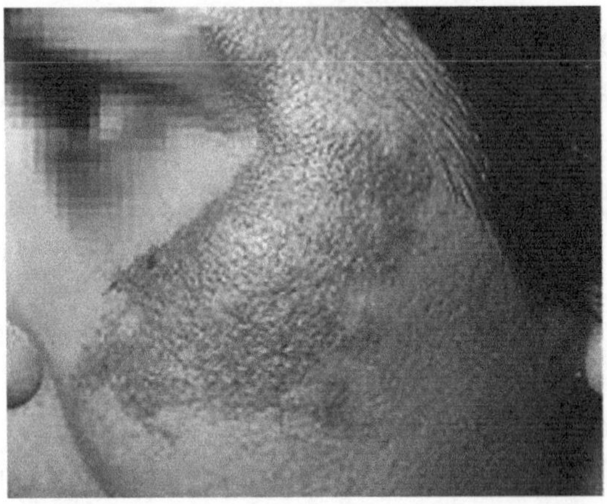

- **Lightening:**
  - o After 36 weeks, specially in primigravida, a sense of **relief** of the pressure symptoms is felt due to engagement of the presenting part

- **Braxton-Hick's contractions:**
  - o Irregular, infrequent spasmodic and painless contractions
- **External Ballottement of uterus:**
  - o On bimanual examination
  - o Gives the impression of **floating** object inside the uterus

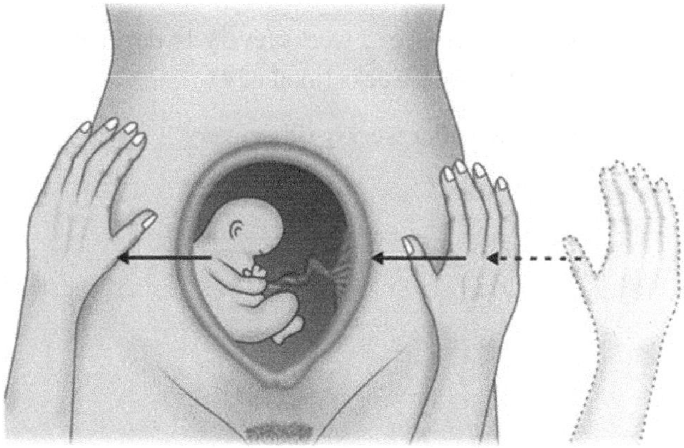

MATERNAL CHANGES IN PREGNANCY

Weight gain

- **Net weight gained during pregnancy:** 6 kg
- **Total weight gained during pregnancy: 11-12** kg

Hematological system

- **Parameters which increase:**
  - o **Blood volume** (by 40%; maximum increase occurs at 34 weeks)
  - o **Plasma volume** (by 40-50%)
  - o RBC volume (by 20-30%)
  - o Hemoglobin mass (hence oxygen carrying capacity also increases)
  - o WBC count
  - o Plasma protein mass
  - o Clotting factors (hence pregnancy is a **hyper-coagulable** state)
- **Parameters which decrease:**
  - o Hematocrit
  - o Blood viscosity
  - o Packed cell volume
  - o Platelet count
  - o Fibrinolytic activity

Cardiovascular system

- **Parameters which increase:**
  - o Heart rate (by 20%)
  - o **Cardiac output** (by 40%; peak at 28-32 weeks)
- **Parameters which decrease:**
  - o Blood pressure
  - o Arteriovenous oxygen gradient

Renal system

- **Parameters which increase:**
  - o Renal blood flow
  - o Glomerular filtration rate
  - o Creatinine clearance
- **Parameters which decrease:**
  - o Serum creatinine
  - o Serum urea

Genital system

- **Vagina:**
  - o **Jacquemier/Chadwick sign:** More oedematous and vascular vagina with a bluish hue
  - o Vaginal **pH** decreases (3.5 to 6) as there is an increase in Doderlein bacilli which converts glycogen to lactic acid, causing a fall in pH of vagina
- **Uterus:**
  - o Weight of non-pregnant is 70 grams but in pregnancy it is 1000 grams
  - o There is increase in uteroplacental blood flow
  - o **Braxton-Hick's contraction:** These are non-rhythmic, sporadic, painless contractions
  - o Isthmus forms the lower uterine segment. At term lower uterine segment is formed by isthmus and cervix. Taking up of cervix in the lower uterine segment is known as **effacement**
- **Cervix:**
  - o Marked softening of cervix is seen (Goodell's sign)
  - o Mucus forms a thick plug sealing the cervical canal

- At the time of true labor, dilatation of the cervix releases this mucus plus mixed with blood. This is known as **show**

ANTENATAL VISITS

Visits, timings and frequency

- **Minimum number of antenatal visits (as per WHO):**
  - **4** visits
    - 1st around 16th week
    - 2nd between 24-28 weeks
    - 3rd at 32 weeks
    - 4th at 36 weeks
- **Ideal number of antenatal visits:**
  - **12-14** visits
    - At an interval of 4 weeks (every month), up to 28 weeks (total of 7)
    - At interval of 2 weeks (every 14 days), between 28 and 36 weeks (total of 4)
    - Thereafter weekly till delivery

SECTION 3
OBSTETRICS

Chapter 5

Prenatal Diagnosis and Fetal Monitoring

PRENATAL DIAGNOSTIC TECHNIQUES

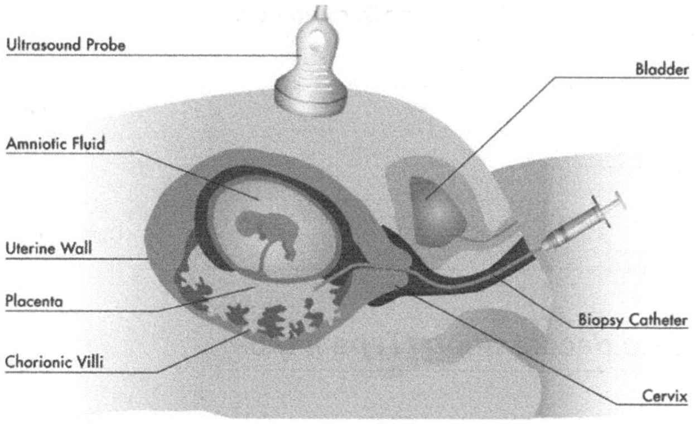

Chorionic villous sampling

- Prenatal diagnosis of genetic disorders
- **Material for study:** Trophoblast cells (from chorionic villi)
- A few villi are collected from the chorion frondosum under USG
- Accurate; may need amniocentesis
- MTP is **safe** (1st trimester), if needed as per report
- Anti-D (50 mcg IM) should be administered to Rh **negative** woman
- **CVS is preferably done at:**
  - o Done between 10 and 13 weeks
  - o 10-12 weeks (transcervically)
  - o **Transabdominally:** 10 weeks to term
- **Risks:**
  - o Chances of fetal loss/abortion
  - o **Fetal loss:** 0.5-1%
- **CVS if done before 10 weeks results in:** Oromandibular limb hypogenesis & Limb reduction defects/LRD

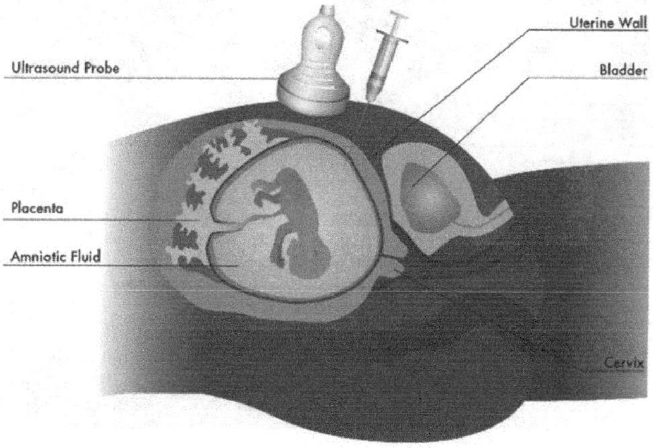

Amniocentesis

- Puncturing of amniotic sac (per abdomen) to diagnose aneuploidy and other genetic conditions
- Can be done any time between **15 and 20** weeks
- It can be diagnostic or therapeutic
- **Diagnostic use:**
  - o Antenatal diagnosis of chromosomal and genetic disorders

- Fetal lung maturity
- **Therapeutic use:**
  - Induction of abortion
  - Decompression of uterus in acute polyhydramnios
- **Complications:**
  - Hemorrhage
  - Abortion

SCREENING FOR DOWN SYNDROME

First trimester

- USG to detect nuchal thickness
- **Double screening:**
  - Increased maternal serum beta HCG
  - Decreased PAPP-A

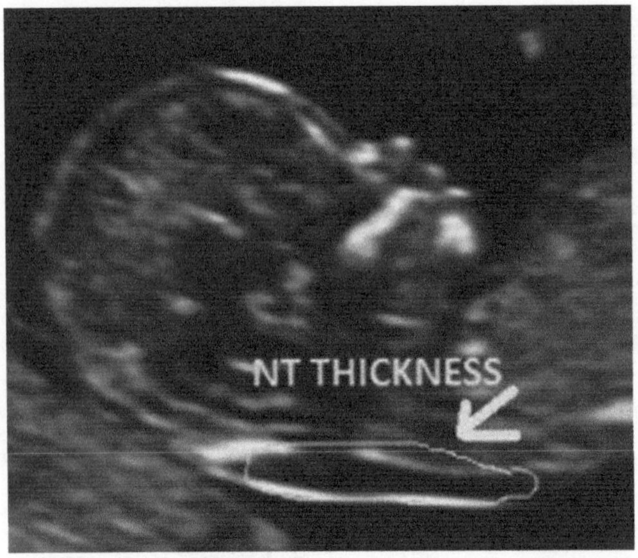

Second trimester

- **Triple test:**
  - Decreased alpha fetoprotein & serum estriol
  - Increased beta-HCG
- **Quadruple test:**
  - Decreased alpha fetoprotein & serum estriol
  - Increased beta-HCG & **Inhibin-A**

FETAL HEART RATE/FHR DECELERATIONS

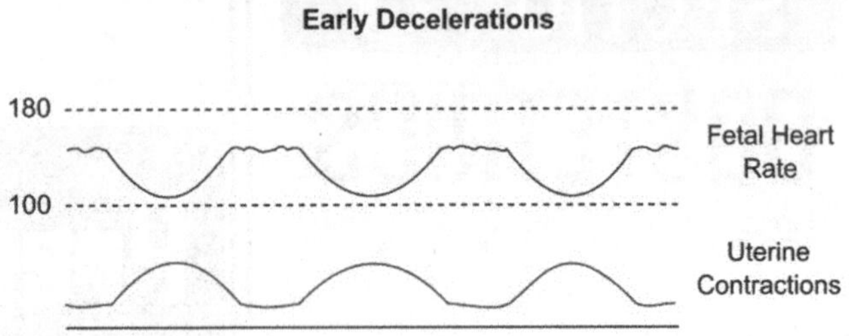

Early deceleration (Type I dips)

- **Head** compression (vagal nerve activation)
- Type I dips are uniform, repetitive periodic slowing of FHR
- Onset and recovery of deceleration coincides with the beginning, peak & ending of uterine contractions

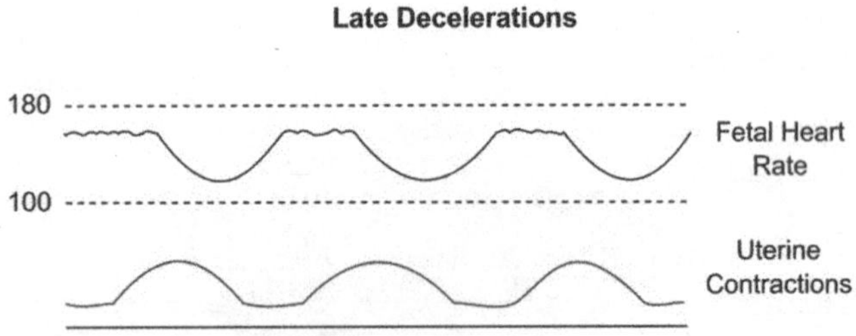

Late deceleration (Type II dips)

- Uteroplacental **insufficiency** & fetal hypoxia (5%)
- Type II dips are uniform, repetitive periodic slowing of FHR with onset mid to end of uterine contraction and nadir >20 seconds after the peak of the contraction and FHR return to normal after the contraction is over

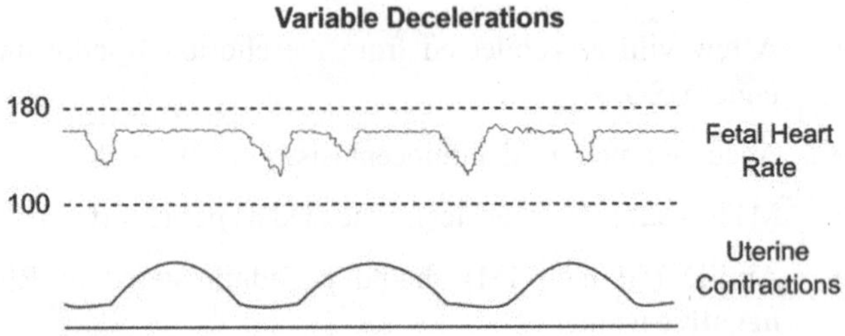

Variable deceleration

- Due to umbilical **cord** compression

BIOPHYSICAL SCORE/MANNING SCORE

Biophysical profile score

- Used to assess the status of fetal **well being** antenatally
- Highest score possible on a normal fetus is 10

5 Parameters in biophysical profile score

- NST (Non-stress test)
- Fetal breathing
- Gross body movements of fetus
- Fetal muscle tone
- Amniotic fluid volume

USG IN PREGNANCY

Important points

- **Earliest detection of pregnancy by USG is by demonstrating:**
  - o Intradecidual **Gestation sac**/GS
  - o GS can be identified as early as 29 – 35 days of gestation
- **Pregnancy is confirmed by:**
  - o Fetal heart rate
  - o Fetal movements
  - o Gestational sac on USG

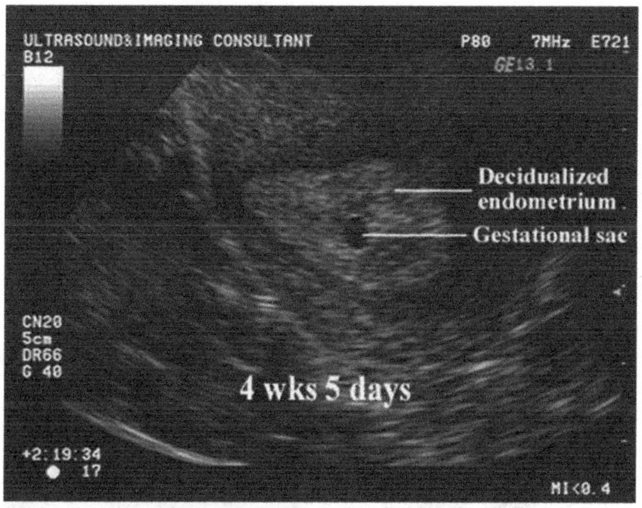

Fetal viability on transvaginal USG

- **Gestational sac & yolk sac:** 5th week
- **Fetal pole & cardiac activity:** 6th week
- **Embryonic movements:** 7th week

Use of USG in different trimesters

- **First trimester:**
  - o **For diagnosing pregnancy:**
    - ♦ By demonstrating gestational sac and fetal cardiac activity
    - ♦ Gestation sac is the **first** sign of pregnancy on USG
    - ♦ Yolk sac is the **first** anatomic structure to be seen within gestational sac

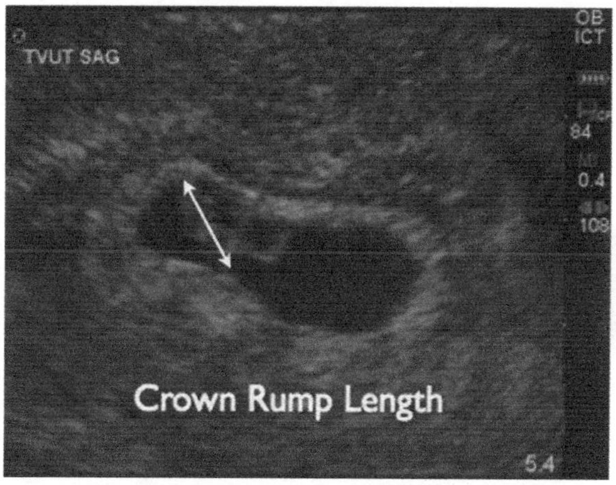

  - o **Determination of gestational age:**
    - ♦ Crown-Rump length is the **most** accurate method to establish or confirm gestational age
    - ♦ **Ideal** time to measure CRL is 7-10 weeks

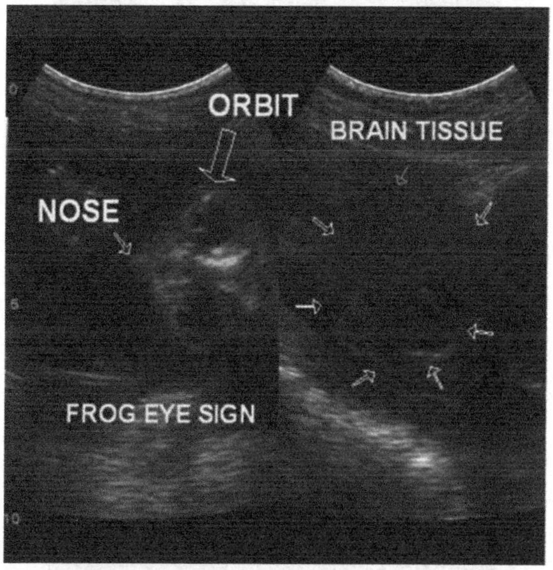

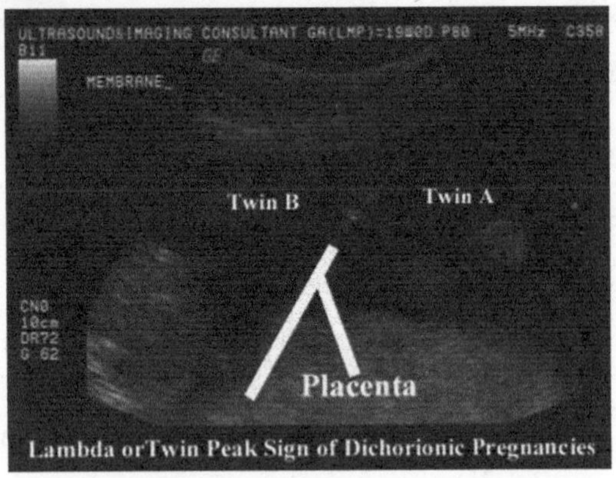

Lambda or Twin Peak Sign of Dichorionic Pregnancies

- o **Diagnosis of fetal anomalies:**
  - ♦ Anencephaly:
    - □ It is the **earliest** anomaly to be detected on USG
    - □ Can be detected earlier by 10th week
    - □ Face shows Mickey mouse sign
    - □ Eyes of the fetus are big (**Frog** eye sign)
  - ♦ Cystic hygroma/lymphangiectasia
  - ♦ Omphalocele
  - ♦ Gastroschisis
- o **Twin pregnancy:**
  - ♦ Twin **peak** sign is seen in dichorionic twins

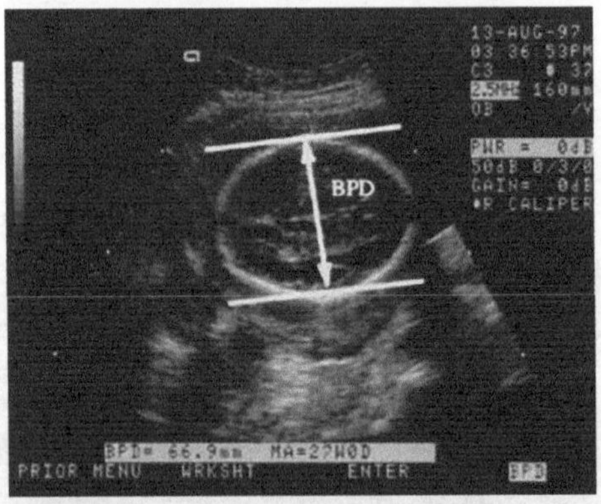

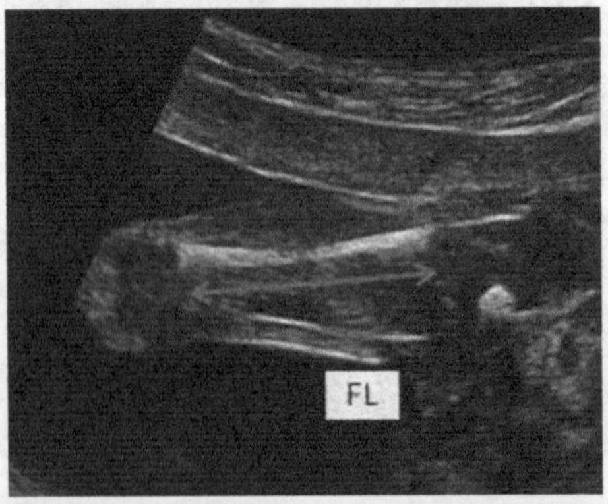

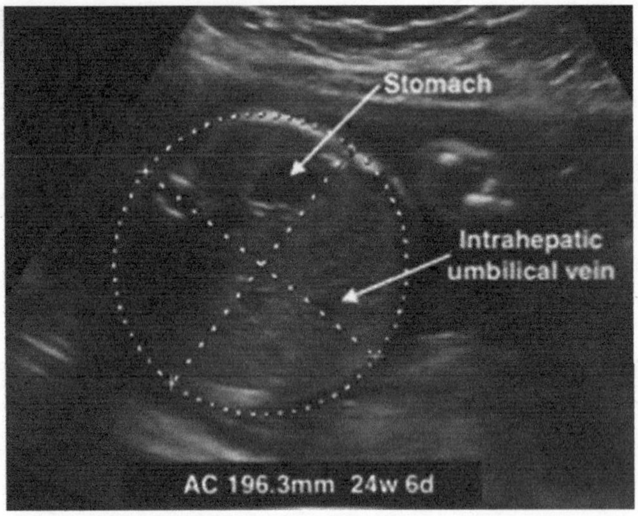

- **Second trimester:**
  - o **Biparietal diameter/BPD:**
    - ♦ **Best** parameter for fetal age after 14 weeks and until 20 weeks
  - o **Femur length/FL:**
    - ♦ **Best** parameter for fetal age in 3rd trimester
  - o **Abdominal circumference/AC:**
    - ♦ Single **best** parameter for fetal growth
    - ♦ AC ≥35 cms means macrosomia
  - o **Detection of congenital anomalies:**
    - ♦ Spina bifida:
      - □ Lemon sign (red arrow)
      - □ Banana sign (yellow arrow)

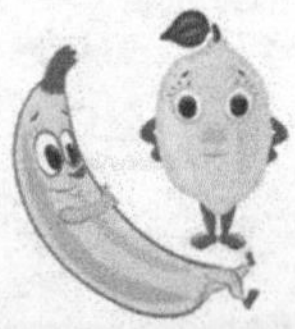

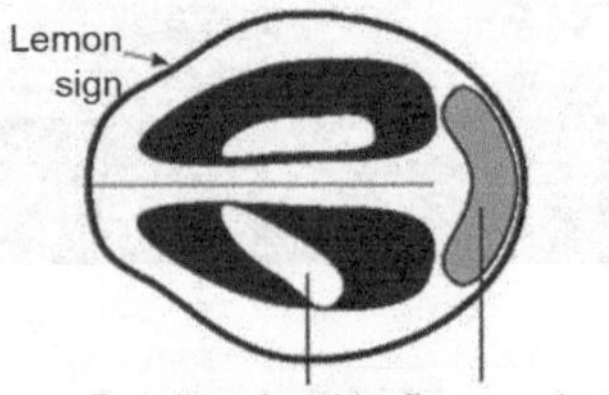

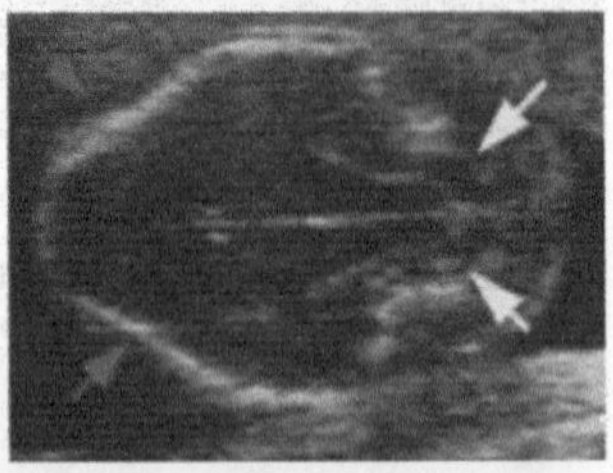

SECTION 3 OBSTETRICS

Chapter 6

Osteology in Relation to Obstetrics

MATERNAL PELVIS

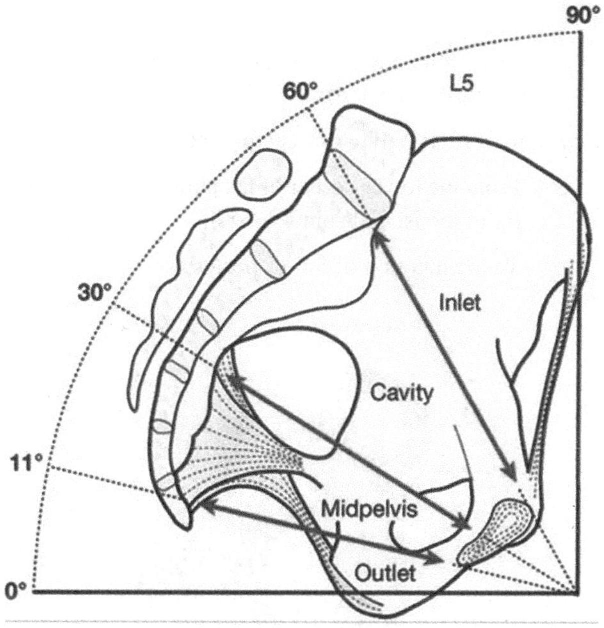

Landmarks

- **Pelvic Inlet:**
  - o Plane of inlet makes an angle of about **55** degrees with the horizontal
- **Pelvic Cavity:**
  - o Bounded above by plane of inlet & below by plane of least pelvic dimension
- **Midpelvis**
- **Anatomical outlet:**
  - o Bony outlet of pelvis

Pelvic inlet

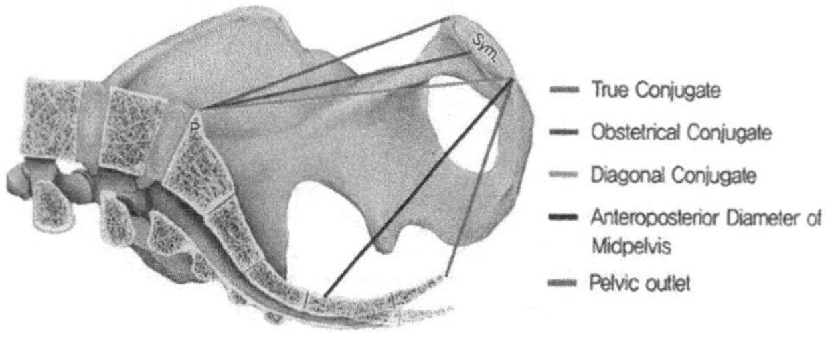

- **AP diameters** ***(Mnemonic: Anatomy Of Diagonal conjugate):***
  - o **True conjugate/Anatomical conjugate (11 cm):**
    - ♦ Measured from the midpoint of sacral promontory to the upper border of pubic symphysis
  - o **Obstetric conjugate (10 cm)**
    - ♦ Distance between the midpoint of the sacral promontory to prominent bony projection in the midline of the inner surface of the symphysis pubis
    - ♦ It **cannot** be measured clinically but is inferred from diagonal conjugate/DC by subtracting 3/4 inch from it (DC – 1.5 to 2 cm)
    - ♦ For a normal delivery, OC **must** measure 10 cm or more

- **Diagonal conjugate (12 cm):**
  - Measured from the midpoint of sacral promontory to the lower border of pubic symphysis
  - **Only** DC can be measured clinically

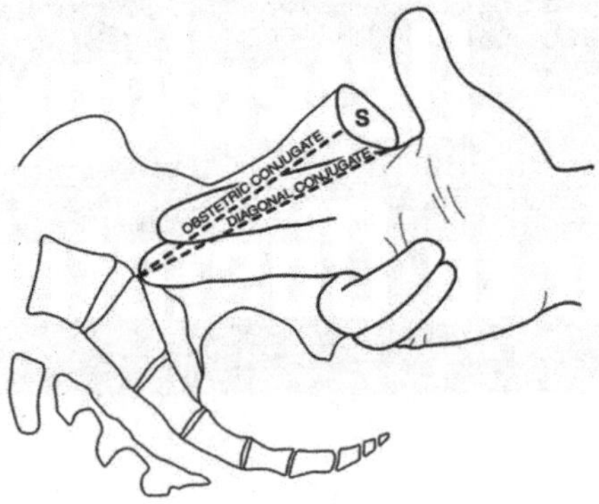

- **Transverse diameters:**
  - Distance between the farthest two points on iliopectineal line
- **Oblique diameters:**
  - There are two oblique diameters – right and left

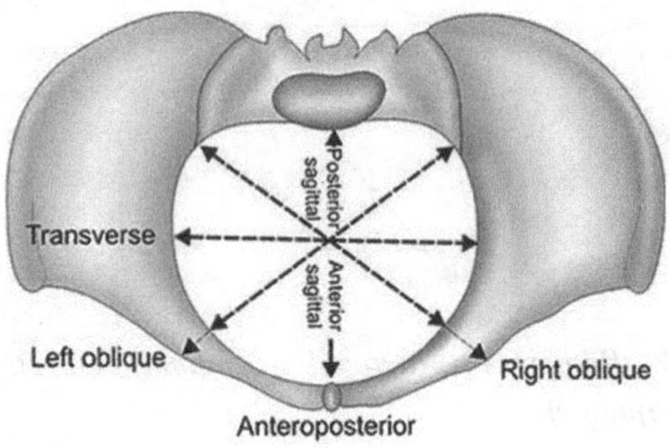

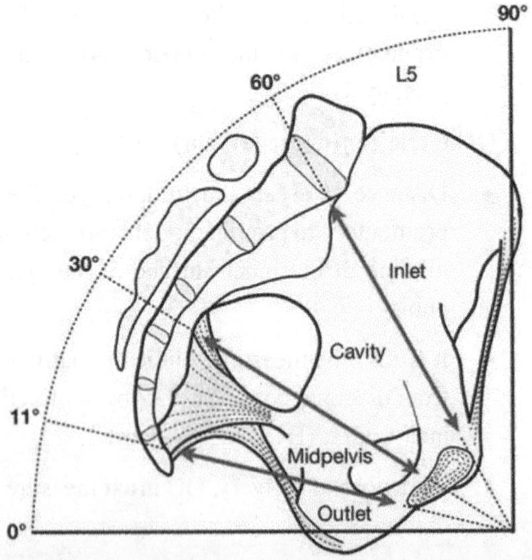

Pelvic cavity

- Round in shape
- **Boundaries:**
  - **Above:** Pelvic brim/inlet
  - **Below:** Plane of least pelvic dimension/midpelvis
  - **Anteriorly:** Symphysis pubis
  - **Posteriorly:** Sacrum

Midpelvis

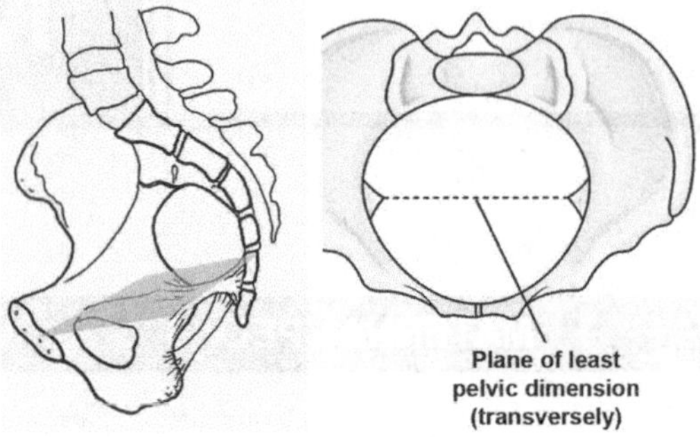

- Measured at the level of ischial **spine** (midplane/plane of least pelvic dimension)
- **Plane of least pelvic dimension extends**
  - From the lower border of the pubic symphysis to the tip of the ischial spines laterally
  - To the junction of S4-S5 posteriorly

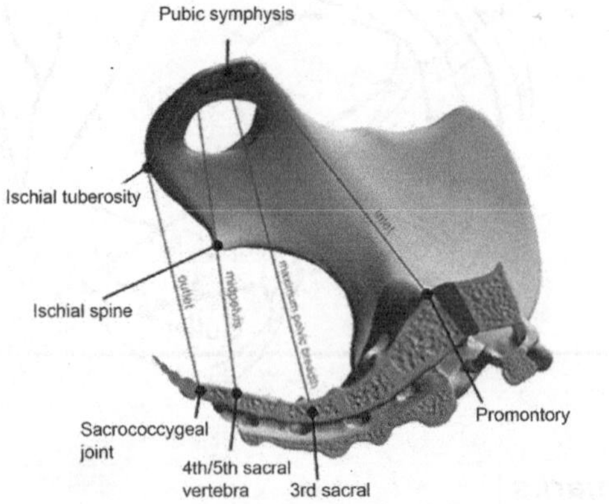

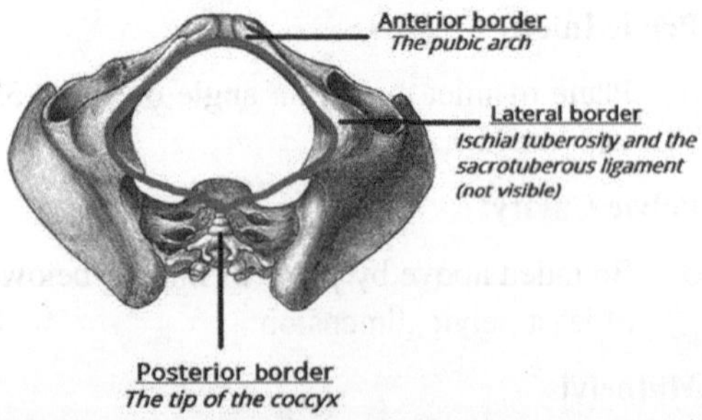

- **AP diameter of midpelvis:** 11.5-12 cm
- **Transverse/diameter/bispinous/interspinous diameter:** 10 cm

Pelvic outlet

- Lies at the level of ischial tuberosity
- **Anatomical pelvic outlet:**
  - o Rhombus shaped cavity
  - o **Bounded by:** Symphysis pubis, pubic arch, ischial tuberosity, sacrotuberous ligament, sacrospinous ligament and tip of coccyx on either side
- **Diameters:**
  - o **AP:** 11.5 to 13.5 cm
  - o **Transverse/intertuberous:** 11 cm
  - o **Posterior sagittal:** 7 cm

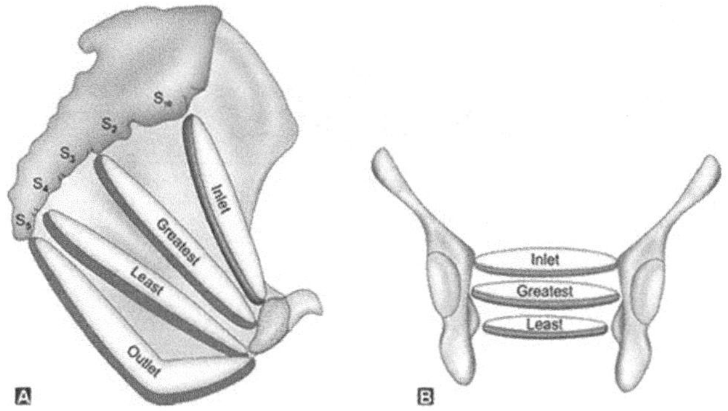

TYPES OF PELVISES

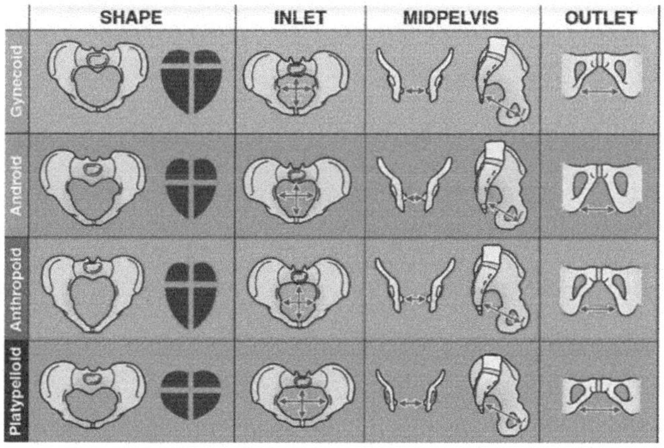

Gynecoid

- Female type
- **MC** type
- Transverse diameter of inlet is slightly bigger than AP diameter
- **Obstetrical importance:**
  - o Normal pelvis
  - o No difficulty in engagement
  - o **Normal** delivery
  - o **MC** position is LOA (Left Occipito Anterior)

Android

- **Male** type
- Ischial spine prominent
- Transverse diameter is more than AP diameter
- **Obstetrical importance:**
  - o Engagement is delayed
  - o Deep transverse arrest/**DTA** & Persistent occipito posterior/POP position is common
  - o **Difficult** instrumental delivery

Anthropoid

- **Ape** like pelvis
- Only pelvis with AP diameter more than transverse diameter
- **Obstetrical importance:**
  - o Diameter of engagement is AP diameter
  - o Direct occipito posterior position is **MC**
  - o Non-rotation is common
  - o Face to pubis delivery is **common**

Platypelloid

- **Flat** pelvis
- Transverse diameter is much more than AP diameter
- **Least** common type of pelvis
- **Obstetrical importance:**
  - o Diameter of engagement is transverse diameter, with **marked** asynclitism

FETAL SKULL

Important diameters

- **Shortest diameter of fetal skull:**

- Bimastoid (**7.5 cm**)
  - Distance between the tips of the mastoid processes
- **Largest diameter of fetal skull:**
  - Mentovertical (**14 cm**)
  - Extends from the mid-point of the chin to the highest point of sagittal suture

AP Diameters

- **Suboccipitobregmatic:** 9.5 cm
- **Mentovertical:** 14 cm
- **Submentobregmatic:** 9.5 cm
- **Submentovertical:** 11.5 cm

Transverse Diameters

- **Biparietal:** 9.5 cm
- **Bitemporal:** 8 cm
- **Bimastoid:** 7.5 cm

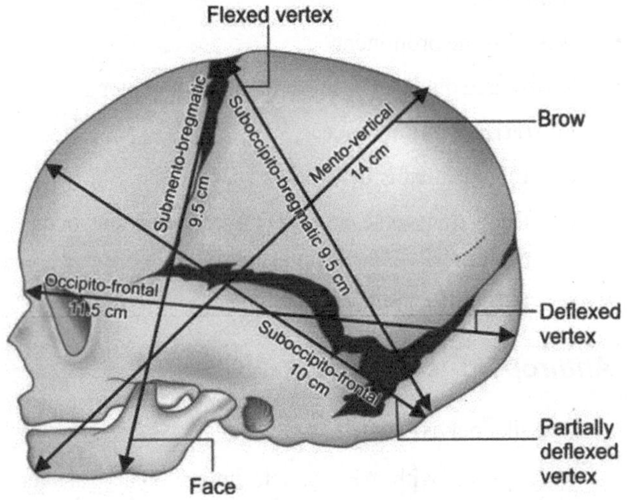

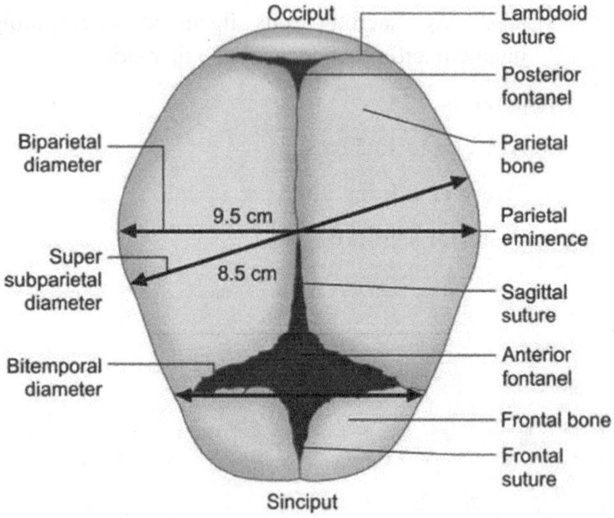

SECTION 3
OBSTETRICS

Chapter 7

Fetus in Utero

TERMINOLOGY

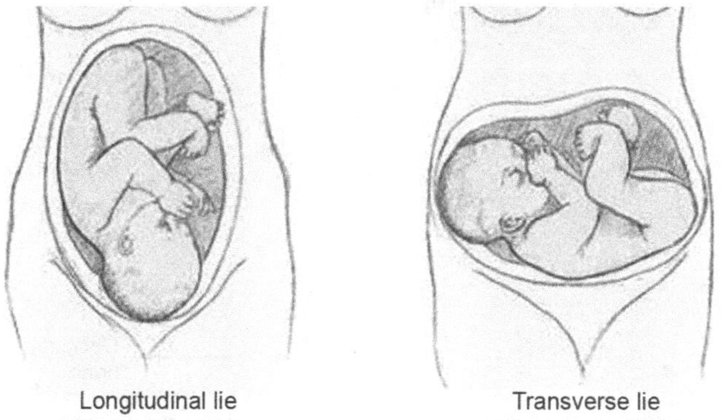

Lie

- It is the relationship of the long axis of the baby with respect to the long axis of maternal spine
- It can be longitudinal, transverse or oblique

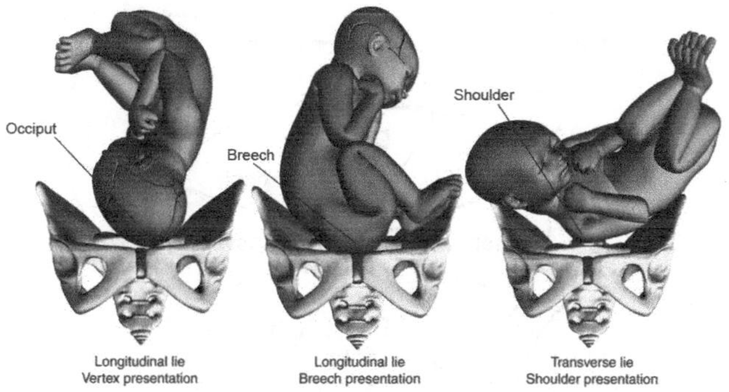

- Lie is longitudinal in **99.5%** cases

Presentation

- Defined as fetal part which occupies the lower pole of the uterus (lies over the pelvic inlet)
- **Types of presentation in longitudinal lie:**
  - **Cephalic (96.5%):** Head is in the lower pole of the uterus
  - **Podalic (3%):** Buttocks are in the lower pole of uterus
- **Types of presentation in transverse lie:**
  - Shoulder (0.5%)
- **Compound presentation:**
  - When more than one fetal part is present in the lower pole of the uterus
  - For example, Head with hand

Presenting part

- Most dependent part of the presentation which overlies the internal os & is felt by the examining finger through the cervical opening
- In cephalic presentation, the presenting part may be vertex (**MC**), brow or face (depending on the degree of flexion of head)

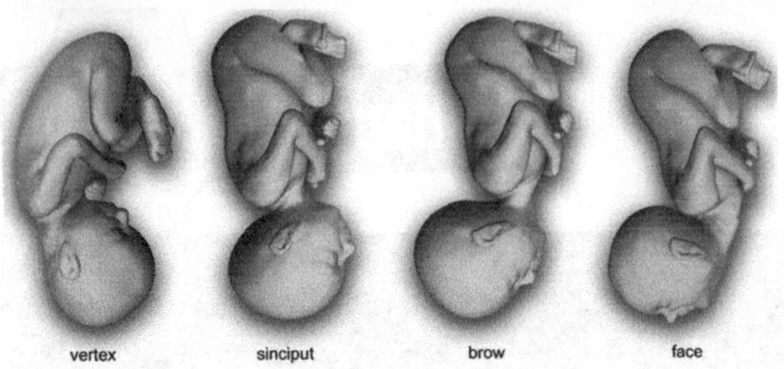

Engaging diameter & presenting part, in cephalic presentation

- **Suboccipitobregmatic:** Vertex
- **Mentovertical:** Brow
- **Submentovertical & Submentobregmatic diameter:** Face

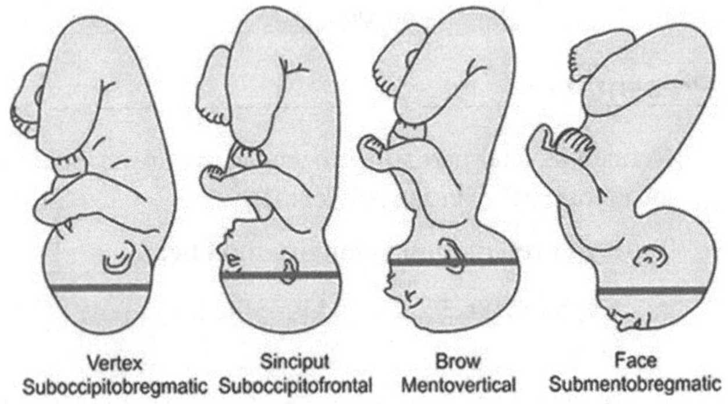

Extent of diameters

- **Submentovertical/SMV:** Extends from the junction of floor of mouth & neck to the highest point on the sagittal suture

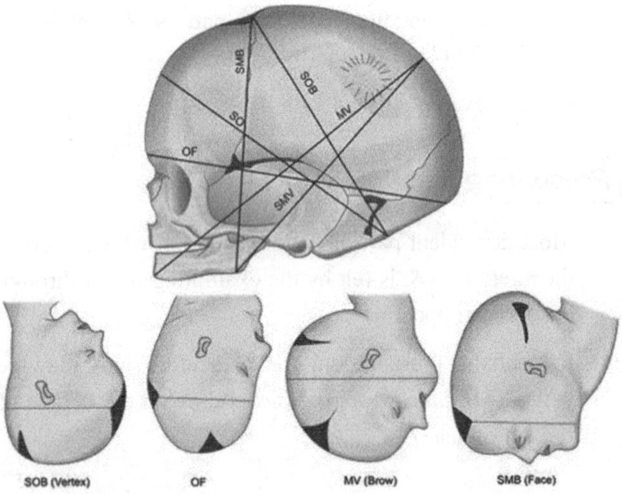

- **Submentobregmatic diameter/SMB:** Extends from the junction of the floor of the mouth & neck to the centre of bregma
- **Suboccipitobregmatic/SOB:** Extends from the nape of neck to the centre of bregma
- **Occipitofrontal diameter/OF:** Extends from the occipital eminence to the root of the nose

Definition of landmarks

- **Face:** Area bounded on one side by the root of the nose and supraorbital ridges and on the other, by the junction of the floor of the mouth with the neck
- **Vertex:** Quadrangular area bounded anteriorly by the bregma and coronal sutures, behind by lambda and laterally by lines passing through the parietal eminences

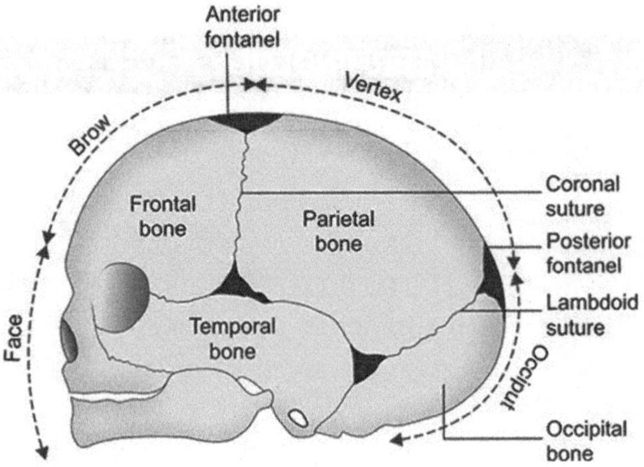

Denominator

- An arbitrary bony point on the presenting part of the fetus
- **If the presenting part is:**
    - o Vertex, the denominator is occiput

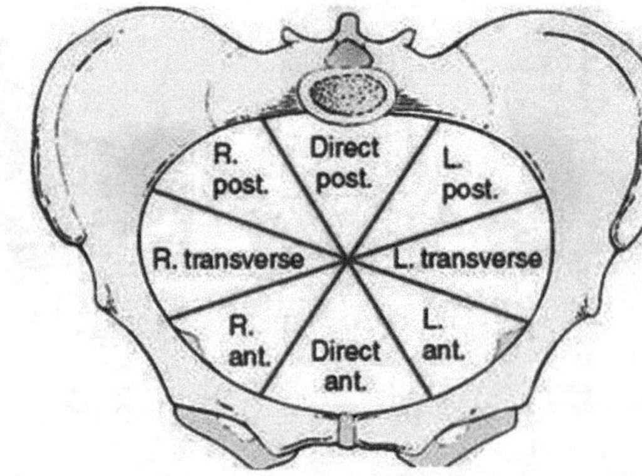

- o Face, the denominator is chin (mentum)
- o Breech, the denominator is sacrum
- It comes in relation with the various quadrants of the maternal pelvis and determines the position

Position

- Maternal pelvis is divided into 8 segments, 45 degrees apart
- Position of fetus is defined as the relationship of the denominator to the different quadrants of the maternal pelvis
- So, 8 positions are possible
- Occiput is the denominator in the vertex (**MC** presenting part), so 8 positions are possible
- MC position of fetus is **LOT** (Left Occipito-Transverse) > LOA (Left Occipito-Anterior)

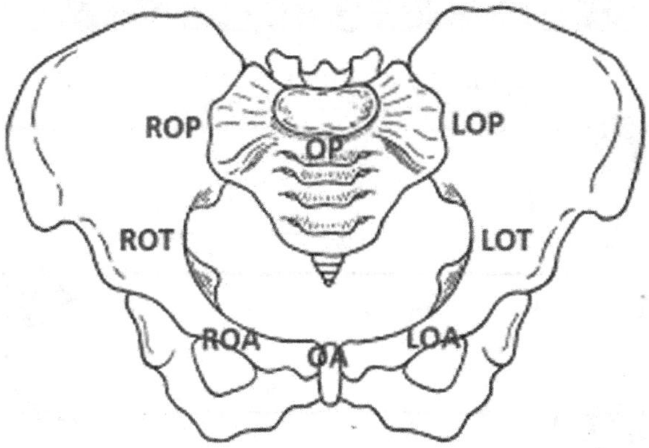

Attitude

- Relationship of different fetal parts to each other
- Normal attitude is of **universal** general flexion (all joints flexed)

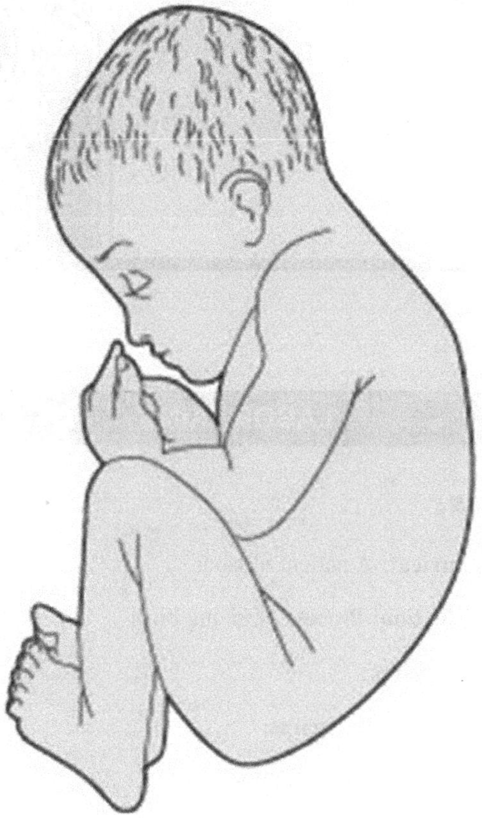

SECTION 3
OBSTETRICS

Chapter 8

Normal Labor

LABOR PAINS

Basics

- **Parturient:** A patient in labor
- **Parturition:** Process of giving birth
- **Labor pains:**
  - o **False labor pains:**
    - ♦ Dull & continuous
    - ♦ Confined to groin & lower abdomen
    - ♦ Dilatation and effacement of cervix is absent
    - ♦ There is **no** bag of water formation
  - o **True labor pains:**
    - ♦ **Painful** uterine contractions at regular intervals
    - ♦ Duration & intensity of contractions increases gradually
    - ♦ There is **progressive** uterine dilatation & effacement of the cervix
    - ♦ Descent of the presenting part
    - ♦ Formation of **bag** of waters
    - ♦ Per vaginum blood mixed with mucus (**show**)

STAGES OF LABOR

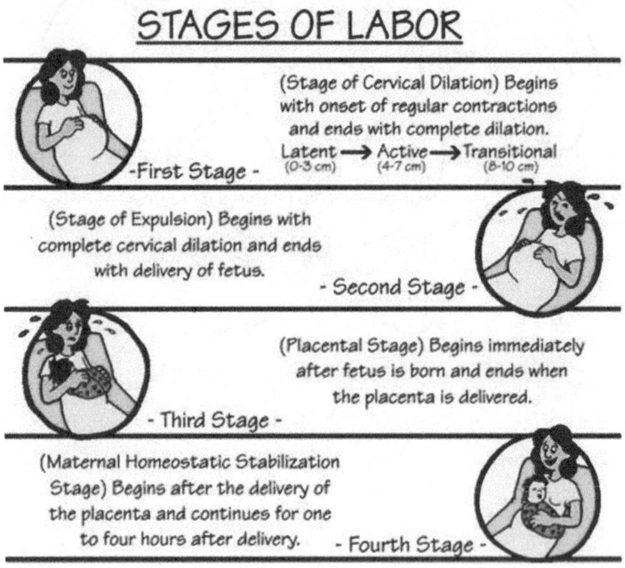

1st stage

- **Extends** from onset of true labor pains to full dilatation of cervix
- 1st stage is concerned with **preparation** of the birth canal so as to facilitate expulsion of the fetus in second stage
- **Average duration:**
  - o About 12 hours in primigravidae
  - o 6 hours in multipara

- 1st stage is clinically manifested by progressive uterine contraction, dilatation & effacement of cervix and ultimate rupture of membranes
- **Main events in 1st stage:**
    - o Dilatation & effacement of the cervix
    - o Full formation of lower uterine segment

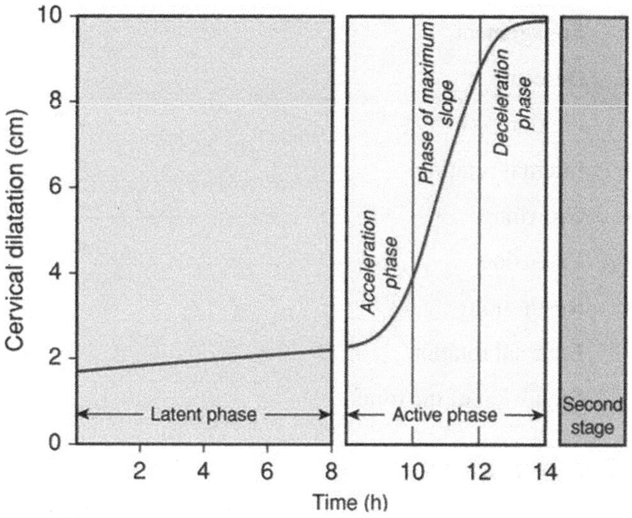

- **Phases:**
    - o **Latent phase:**
        - ♦ Up to 3 cm of cervical dilatation
        - ♦ Mainly concerned with cervical effacement and dilatation
    - o **Active phase:**
        - ♦ Begins with cervical dilatation of up to 10 cm of cervical dilatation
        - ♦ Minimum rate of dilatation should be 1 cm/ hour
        - ♦ Mainly concerned with cervical dilatation and **descent** of fetal head

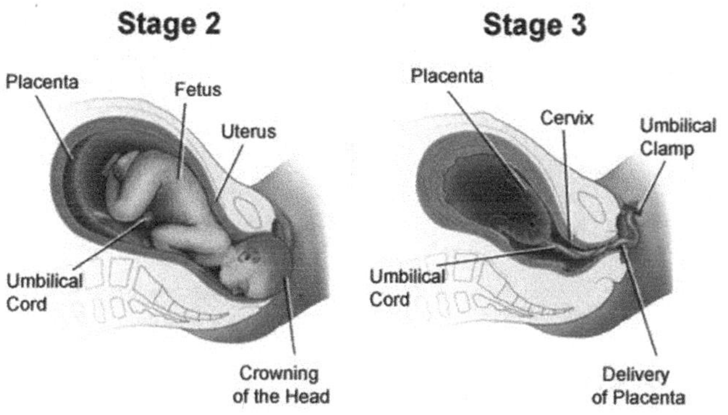

2nd stage

- **Extends** from full dilatation of cervix to complete birth of baby
- 2nd stage is **concerned** with the descent & delivery of the fetus through the birth canal
- 2nd stage is clinically manifested by increased frequency and intensity of uterine contractions with appearance of "**bearing** down" efforts which result in expulsion of fetus
- In the second stage, the expulsive efforts by a woman play more important role than uterine contractions
- **Average duration:**
    - o 2 hours in primigravidae
    - o 30 minutes in multipara
- **Immediate** care of newborn includes clearing the air passages & eyes, clamping and ligaturing of the umbilical cord & APGAR scoring
- **Phases of 2nd stage:**
    - o **Propulsive:** From full dilatation until head touches the pelvic floor
    - o **Expulsive (bear down):** Until the baby is delivered

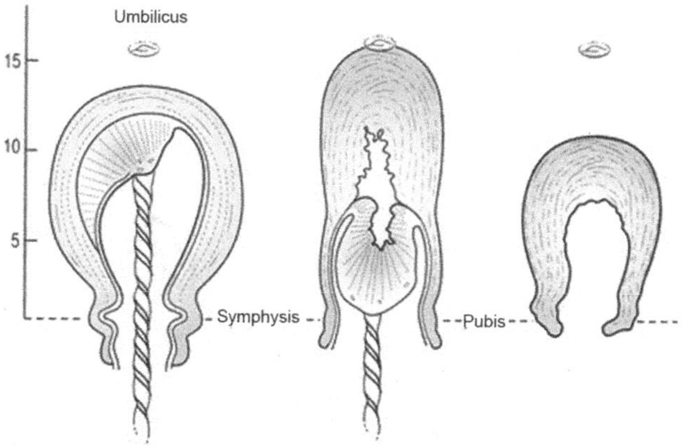

(A) Beginning of the third stage (B) Placenta in the lower segment (C) End of the third stage

3rd stage

- **Extends** from birth of infant to complete delivery of placenta and membranes and contraction and retraction of uterus
- 3rd stage comprises the phase of placental **separation**; its descent to the lower segment and finally its expulsion with the membranes

- Average duration of 3rd stage is 15-20 minutes
- The separation of placenta is achieved by marked reduction in the uterine surface area of the placental site following delivery due to retraction
- The placenta being inelastic shears off its attachment through the deep spongy decidual layer
- The bleeding is controlled by effective myometrial contraction & retraction (living ligature) and by thrombosis
- **Active management of third stage of labor:**
    - o **Oxytocin** slow I/V or I/M or Ergometrine I/V is administered within one minute following the delivery of the baby (to prevent postpartum hemorrhage)
    - o **Delayed cord clamping:**
        - ♦ Clamping of the cord between 1 and 3 minutes
        - ♦ This allows additional 80 ml of **blood** to go into fetal circulation and helps in preventing neonatal anemia
    - o Delivery of placenta by Controlled Cord **Traction**/ Modified Brandt-Andrew's technique)

Controlled cord traction

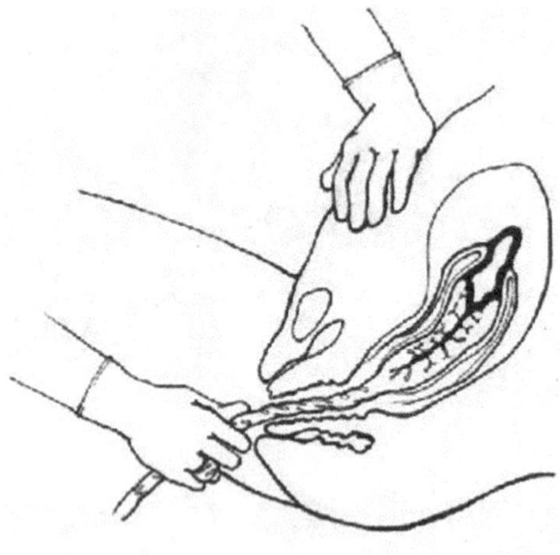

4th stage

- 1 hour observation period after the delivery of the placenta

MECHANISM OF NORMAL LABOR

Features

- **MC** position is LOT/LOA
- Engaging anteroposterior diameter of the head is either suboccipitobregmatic (9.5 cm) or suboccipitofrontal (10 cm)
- Engaging transverse diameter is **biparietal** (9.5 cm)

Principal movements (Mnemonic: Every Drunkard Favors ICE REE)

- Engagement
- Descent
- Flexion
- Internal rotation
- Crowning
- Extension
- Restitution
- External rotation
- Expulsion of the trunk

Different steps

- **Engagement:**
    - o When the greatest horizontal plane/greatest transverse diameter (**biparietal** in cephalic presentation), has passed the plane of the pelvic brim, the head is said to be engaged
    - o **Types:**
        - ♦ **Synclitic:** Sagittal suture of the fetus lies in the transverse diameter of the pelvic inlet
        - ♦ **Asynclitic:**
            - □ **Anterior:** Sagittal suture is **deflected** towards sacral promontory
            - □ **Posterior:** Sagittal suture is deflected towards pubis symphysis

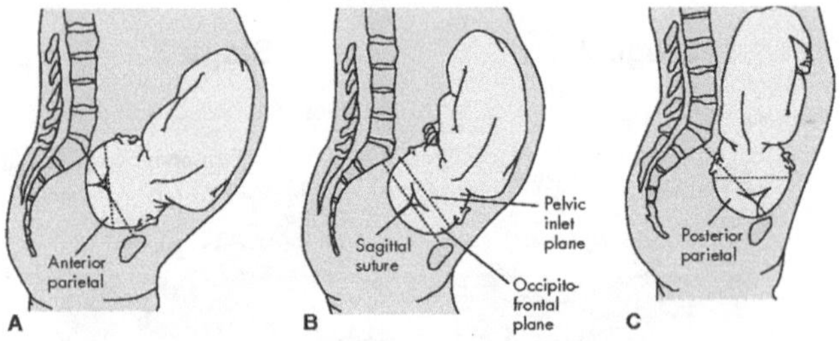

Figure: Synclitism and asynclitism. **A,** Anterior asynclitism. **B,** Normal synclitism. **C,** Posterior asynclitism

- **Descent:**
    - o It is because of uterine **contraction** & retraction, bearing down efforts and straightening of fetus

- **Flexion:**
  - Full flexion of fetal head occurs as the head meets **resistance** of the birth canal during descent
- **Internal rotation:**
  - This is of **great** importance without which there will be no further descent
  - Occiput comes to lie behind the symphysis pubis, rotating **1/8th** of a circle

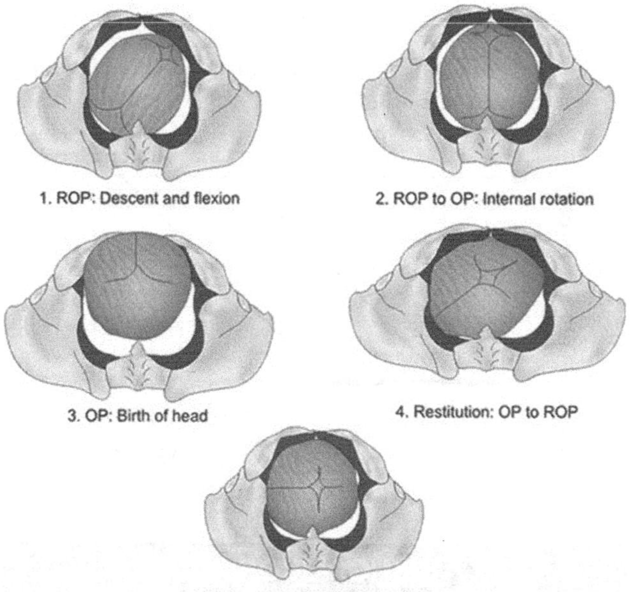

- **Crowning:**
  - After internal rotation of the head, further descent occurs until the suboccipu lies underneath the pubic arch
  - At this stage, the maximum diameter of the head (biparietal diameter) stretches the vulval outlet without any recession of the head even after contraction is over – called "**crowning** of the head"

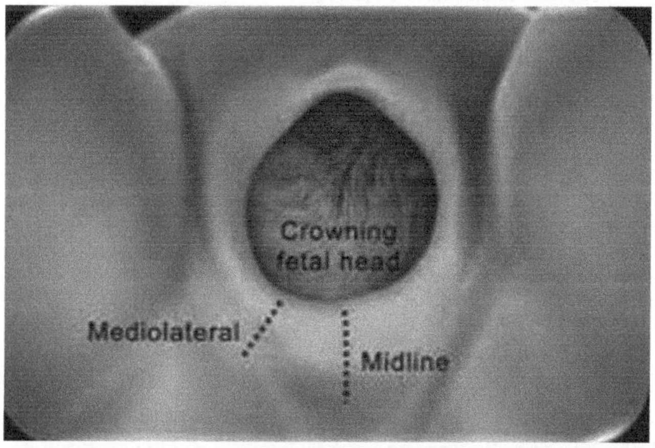

- **Extension:**
  - Delivery of the **head** takes place by extension
  - The successive parts of the fetal head to be born through the stretched vulval outlet are vertex, brow and face
- **Restitution:**
  - It is the visible passive movement of the head due to **untwisting** of the neck sustained during internal rotation
  - Movement of restitution occurs rotating the head through 1/8th of a circle in the direction **opposite** to that of internal rotation
  - The occiput thus points to the maternal thigh of the corresponding side to which it **originally** lay
- **External rotation:**
  - It is the movement of **rotation** of the head visible externally due to internal rotation of the shoulders
  - As the anterior shoulder rotates towards the symphysis pubis from the oblique diameter, it carries the head in a movement of external rotation through 1/8th of a circle in the **same** direction as restitution
  - The shoulders now **lie** in the anteroposterior plane
- **Expulsion of shoulders & trunk:**
  - After the shoulders are positioned in anteroposterior diameter of the outlet, further descent takes place until the **anterior** shoulder escapes below the pubis symphysis first
  - By the movement of lateral flexion of the spine, the **posterior** shoulder sweeps over perineum
  - The rest of the trunk is then expelled out by lateral flexion

PARTOGRAM

Uses

- Graphical representation of stages of labor
- **It includes:**
  - Cervical dilatation
  - Descent of head
  - Rotation of head
- **Assessment** of labor

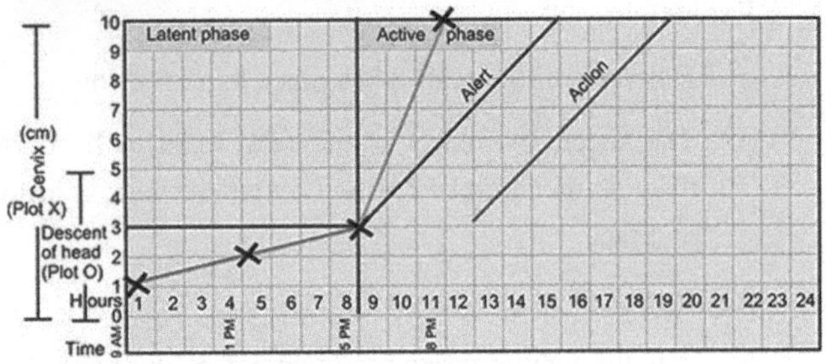

WHO partograph

- Main purpose is to **avoid** prolonged labor and intervene timely
- **X-axis:** Time in hours is plotted
- **Y-axis:** Cervical dilatation and descent of head is plotted
- Labor is expected to progress at the rate of **at least** 1 cm dilatation per hour, which corresponds to **alert** line
- **Action** line is drawn 4 hours to the right of the alert line
- Labor is considered normal if the progress of cervical dilatation is to the **left** of the alert line
- Prolonged labor is diagnosed once the alert line is **crossed**
- **Components:**
  - **Time:** Recorded every 30 minutes
  - **Fetal heart rate:** Recorded every 30 minutes
  - **State of membranes:**
    - I for intact membranes
    - In case of ruptured membranes:
      - Color of liquor is noted
      - C (clear liquor)
      - M (**meconium**-stained liquor)
      - B (blood-stained amniotic fluid)
  - **Moulding:** Degree of **moulding** is noted
  - Cervical dilatation
  - **Descent of head:**
    - Recorded as the number of **fifths** of head above the pelvic brim
  - **Uterine contractions:**
    - Can be assessed with electronic monitoring/ manually every 30 minutes
  - Drugs (Oxytocin) & fluids
  - **Maternal vitals:**
    - BP recorded every 2 hours
    - Pulse recorded every 30 minutes
    - Temperature

CERVICOGRAPH

Features

- Graph showing relationship between cervical dilatation & labor
- **Alert line:** Starts at 3 cm & ends at 10 cm dilatation (1 cm/hr)
- **Action line:** 3-4 hours to the right of alert line & parallel to it
- In a **normal** labor, the cervical dilatation should be either on the alert line or **left** to it

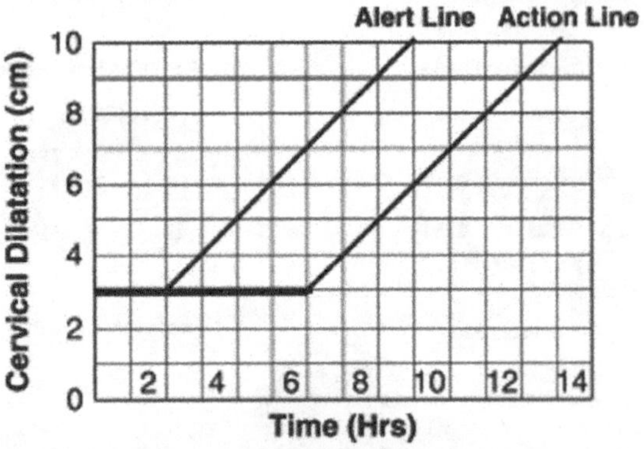

BISHOP SCORING

Used for

- Labor (It is a **pre-induction** cervical scoring system)
- Bishop score is a quantitative method for prediction of **successful** induction of labor

Induction of labor

- It means, stimulation of uterine contractions before the spontaneous onset of labor

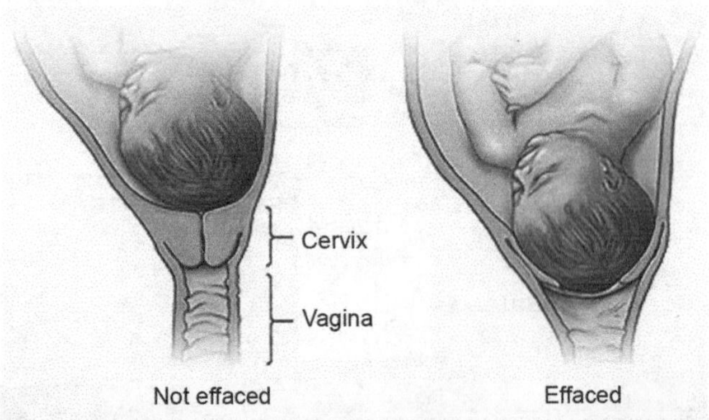

Includes (Mnemonic: Chandigarh Enforcement Directorate Police Station)

- Consistency of cervix
- Effacement of cervix
- Dilatation of cervix
- Position of cervix
- Station of fetal head
- **Modification** (1991) replaces effacement (%) with cervical length (in cm)

Score

- **Total score:** 13
- **Favorable score:** 6-13
- **Unfavorable score:** 0-5

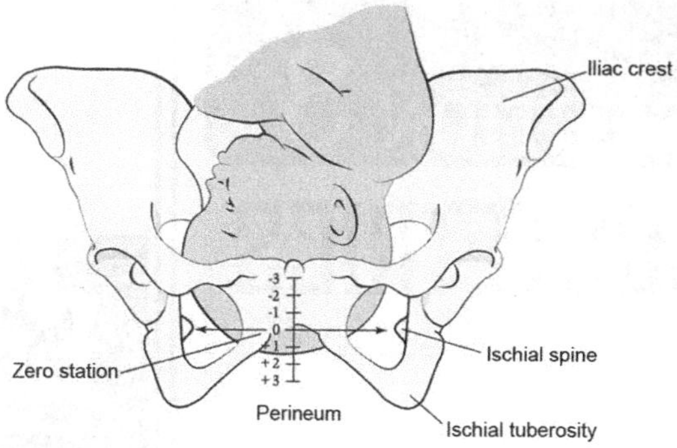

Methods for induction

- **Medical:**
  - o PGE$_1$ (Misoprostol)
  - o Oxytocin
  - o Mifepristone
- **Surgical:**
  - o Artificial rupture of membranes
  - o Stripping of membranes

SECTION 3

OBSTETRICS

Chapter 9

Complications of Third Stage of Labor

COMPLICATIONS OF 3rd STAGE OF LABOR

Complications

- Postpartum hemorrhage (**MC**)
- Retention of placenta
- Uterine inversion (**rare**)
- Pulmonary embolism (amniotic fluid/air)
- Shock (hemorrhagic & non-hemorrhagic)

POSTPARTUM HEMORRHAGE

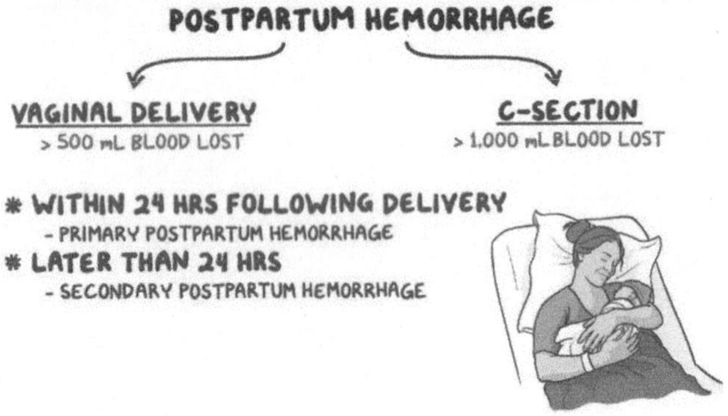

Types of PPH

- **Primary:**
  - Hemorrhage occurring **within** 24 hours following delivery
  - **MC** due to atonic uterus
- **Secondary:**
  - Hemorrhage occurring after 24 hours and up to 12 weeks postpartum
  - **MC** cause is retained placenta

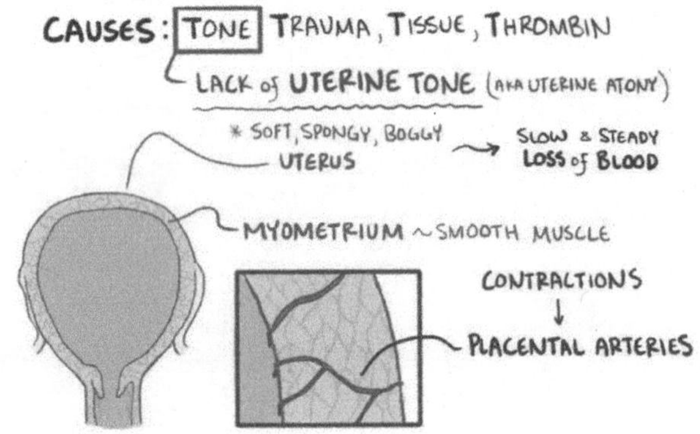

MC cause of PPH

- Atonic uterus (**80%**)
- With the separation of the placenta, the uterine sinuses are torn, which cannot be compressed effectively due to imperfect contraction and retraction of the uterine musculature and bleeding continues

PPH is said to occur if

- Blood loss is **more** than 500 cc, from the genital tract, following vaginal delivery (or **more** than 1000 ml following caesarean section)
- The average normal blood loss following vaginal delivery, caesarean delivery & caesarean hysterectomy is 500 ml, 1000 ml & 1500 ml respectively

Risk factors for PPH

- **Atonic uterus:**
  - o Grand multipara
  - o Anemia
  - o Ante partum hemorrhage
- **Traumatic PPH:**
  - o Instrumental delivery
  - o Precipitate labor
- **Blood coagulopathy:**
  - o Abruption
  - o Intrauterine death

Drugs used for PPH/Uterotonic drugs

- Misoprostol (PGE_1)
- Carboprost ($PGF_{2\ alpha}$)
- Ergometrine
- Oxytocin
- Carbotectin
- Dinoprostone (PGE_2)

Management of atonic uterus causing PPH

- **Step I:**
  - o **Massage** the uterus to make it hard
  - o I/V oxytocin infusion

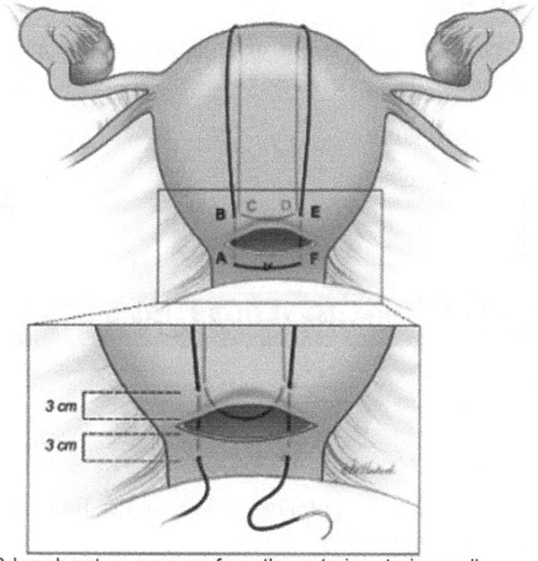

B-Lynch suture as seen from the anterior uterine wall

Figure: B-Lynch suture

  - o Inj. Methergin I/V
  - o Examine expelled placenta
- **Step II:** Explore uterus under GA
- **Step III:** Uterine massage & bimanual compression
- **Step IV:** Tight intrauterine packing under GA (tamponade)
- **Step V:** Surgical method to control PPH
  - o Ligation of arteries
  - o **B-lynch** compression suture
  - o Arterial embolization
  - o Hysterectomy (for completed family)

RETAINED PLACENTA

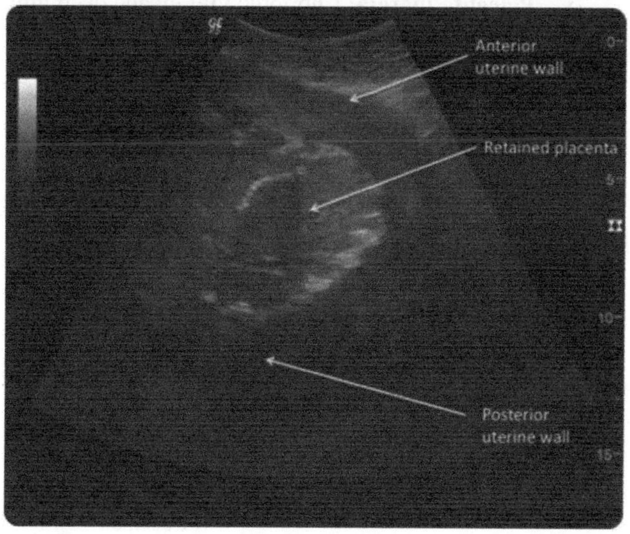

Types

- **Category I:** Separated **but** retained

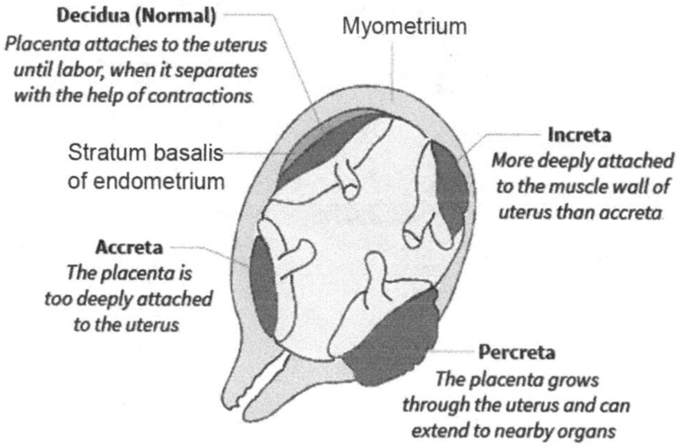

- **Placenta adherent to uterus:**
  - o **Category II: Simple** adherent placenta
  - o **Category III:** Morbidly adherent placenta
    - ♦ Placenta accreta
    - ♦ Placenta increta
    - ♦ Placenta percreta

Morbidly adherent placenta

- There is **defective** formation of decidua basalis and Nitabuch's layer
- Placenta is **firmly** adherent to the uterine wall
- **Types:**
  - o **Placenta percreta:** Chorionic villi penetrate the full thickness of myometrium and reach up to the serosa
  - o **Placenta increta:** Chorionic villi invade deep into the myometrium
  - o **Placenta accreta:** Chorionic villi are attached to the superficial myometrium
- One of the important risk factors is placenta previa in previous pregnancy

Management of retained placenta

- **Category I and II:**
  - o Use oxytocin
  - o Controlled cord traction for 30 minutes
  - o Otherwise, do **manual** removal of placenta, which is done in OT under general anesthesia

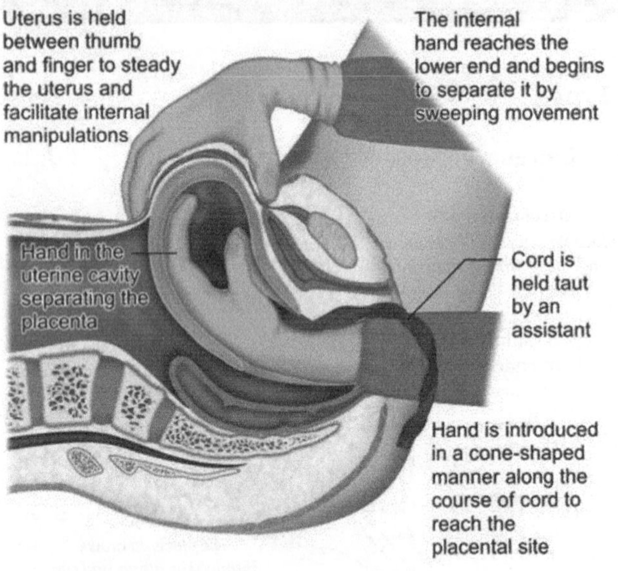

- **Category III:**
  - o ***Completed family size:*** Caesarean section delivery followed by hysterectomy

UTERINE INVERSION

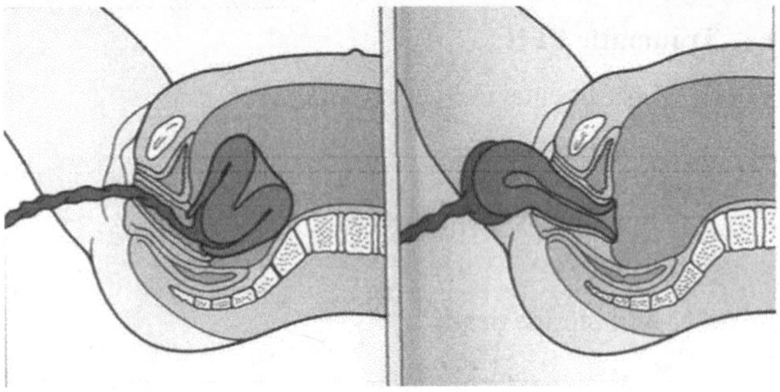

Features

- It is a condition in which there is **inside out** turning of the uterus
- **Causes:**
  - o Mismanaged 3rd stage of labor/faulty technique in manual removal of placenta is the **most** important cause
  - o Pulling the cord (cord traction) to deliver placenta that has **not** separated from the uterus, results in uterine inversion
  - o Spontaneous inversion with an atonic uterus (40%)
- Patient presents with features of shock **immediately** after delivery
- Degree of shock is **out of** proportion to the amount of bleeding during delivery
- **Management:**
  - o Resuscitation
  - o Replacement of uterus

AMNIOTIC FLUID EMBOLISM

Features

- Abrupt in onset
- Results due to **entering** of amniotic fluid into the maternal circulation

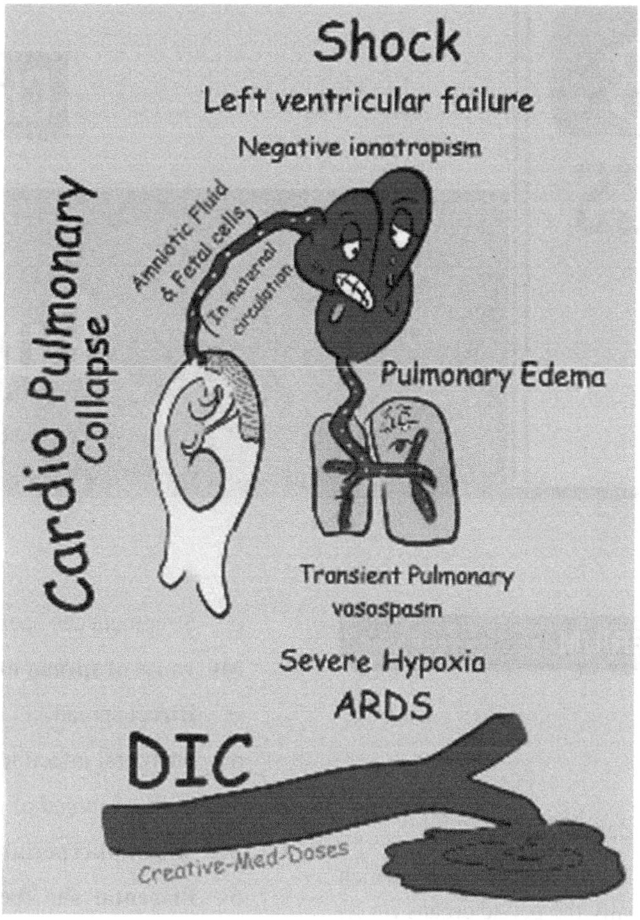

- **Manifest as:**
  - o Tachypnea
  - o Cyanosis
  - o Hypotension
  - o Altered mental status
  - o Disseminated intravascular coagulation/DIC

SECTION 3

OBSTETRICS

Chapter 10

Puerperium

PUERPERIUM

Events

- **Puerperium:**
  - o Lasts for **6** weeks after delivery
  - o It is the period following childbirth during which the body tissues, especially the pelvic organs revert back approximately to the **pre-pregnant** state both anatomically & physiologically
- **Uterus:**
  - o Uterus becomes a pelvic organ by **2** weeks of delivery
  - o There is a steady decrease in uterine height by **1.25** cm (half inch) per day
- **Involution of uterus is complete by:**
  - o **6** weeks
  - o **Immediately** following delivery, uterus weighs 1000 gm & measures 20 × 12 × 7.5 cm (length, breath & thickness)
  - o At the end of 6 weeks, it weighs **60** gm & measures 8 × 5 × 1.25 cm

Puerperal sepsis

- **MC cause of puerperial infection:**
  - o Streptococcus haemolyticus group A (***Mnemonic: GAS***; Group **A** Streptococci)
  - o Streptococcus haemolyticus group B (GBS)
- **MC route of spread of puerperial infection:**
  - o **Direct** spread
  - o Puerperal infection is essentially a wound infection
- MC route of spread of puerperial infection
- **MC site of puerperial infection:**
  - o **Placental** site (being a raw surface), lacerations of the genital tract (cervix, vagina, perineum) or caesarean section wounds may be infected

LOCHIA

Features

- It is the vaginal discharge for the first **fortnight** during puerperium
- **Duration:** The normal duration may extend up to 3 weeks
- **Clinical importance:** Character of the lochial discharge gives useful information about the abnormal puerperal state
- ***Mnemonic: RSA*** (**R**epublic of **S**outh **A**frica)

L. Rubra

- **Reddish** (1-4 days)
- Consists of blood, shreds of fetal membranes and decidua, vernix caseosa, lanugo & meconium

L. Serosa

- **Yellowish** (5-9 days)
- Consists of RBC but more leucocytes, wound exudates, mucus from the cervix and microorganisms (anaerobic streptococci & staphylococci)
- Presence of bacteria is not pathognomonic of infection

L. Alba

- Pale **white** (10-15 days)
- Contains plenty of decidual cells, leucocytes, mucus, cholestrin crystals, fatty and granular epithelial cells & microorganisms

SECTION 3
OBSTETRICS

Chapter 11

Malpositions and Malpresentations

OCCIPITO-POSTERIOR MALPOSITION

Malposition

- Refers to any position (of the vertex) **other** than occipito-anterior/OA or occipito-transverse/OT
- **MC** malposition is occipito-posterior

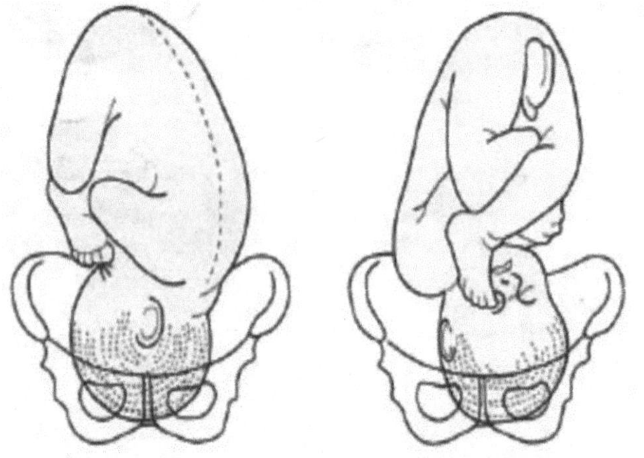

Normal Malposition (OP)

Occipito-posterior/OP position

- Occiput is placed posteriorly over the sacroiliac joint (right/left OP) or directly over the sacrum (direct OP position)
- **MC** cause is anthropoid or android pelvis
- OP position is the **MC** cause of non-engagement of fetal head at term in primigravidae

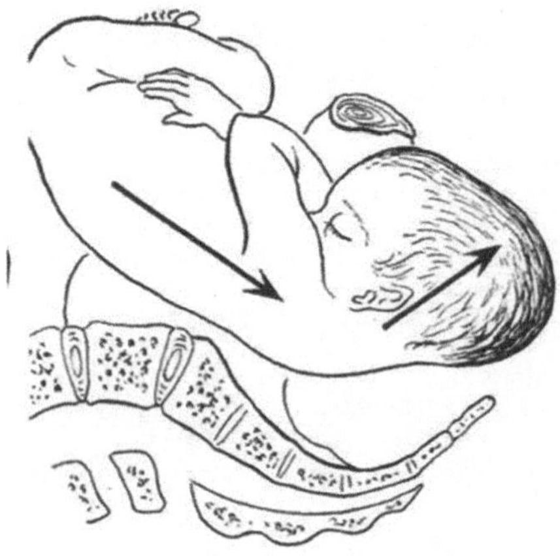

Figure: Occipito-posterior (OP)

- Engaging diameter in deflexed head is occipitofrontal diameter
- In **90%** of cases, normal delivery occurs as head moves through 3/8th of a circle
- So whenever, a diagnosis of OP position is made, labor is allowed to proceed in a manner **similar** to normal labor, in anticipation of normal vaginal delivery
- Hence the **best** management is Wait and watch
- **Deep transverse arrest/DTA:**
  - o In which the fetal head rotates **only** 1/8th of a circle (instead of $3/8^{th}$)
  - o Sagittal suture of the fetal head is placed in the transverse bispinous diameter of the pelvis and there is no further descent
  - o Caesarean section is the management of **choice** for DTA

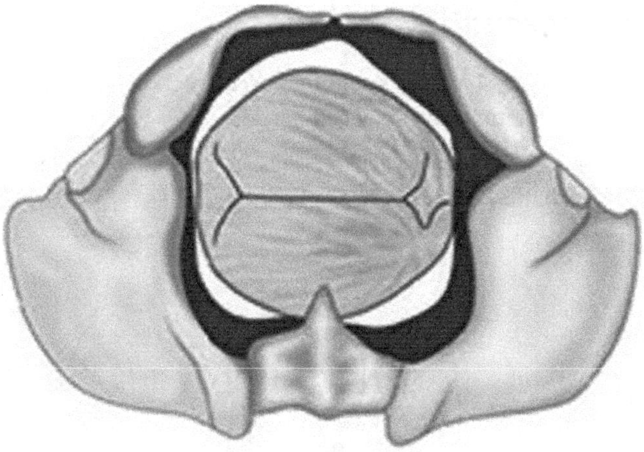

Deep transverse arrest

- **Malrotation:**
  - o Instead of rotating forward, the fetus turns backward and come to lie in direct OP position
  - o **MC** seen in anthropoid pelvis
  - o Then **Face** to pubis delivery occurs

BREECH

Malpresentation

- Refers to all presentations of the fetus **other** than the vertex
- **MC** malpresentation is breech
- **Breech:**
  - o In breech presentation, the lie is longitudinal and the podalic pole is present over the pelvic brim
  - o **MC** cause is prematurity

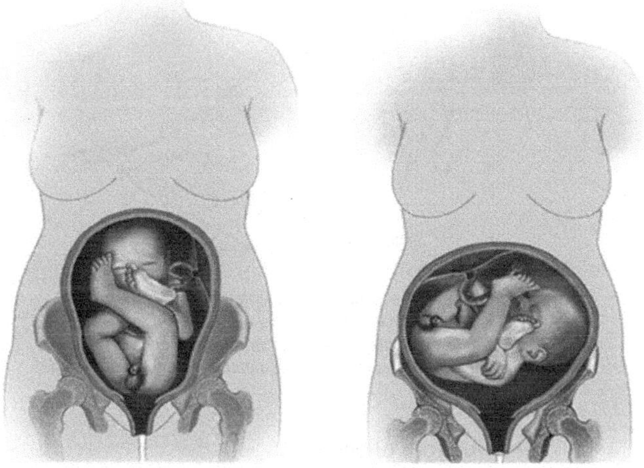

Longitudinal lie
Breech presentation

Transverse lie

Types of breech (Mnemonic: Frank extended his Completely flexed Foot)

- **Frank/extended** breech
- **Complete/flexed** breech
- **Foot**ling breech

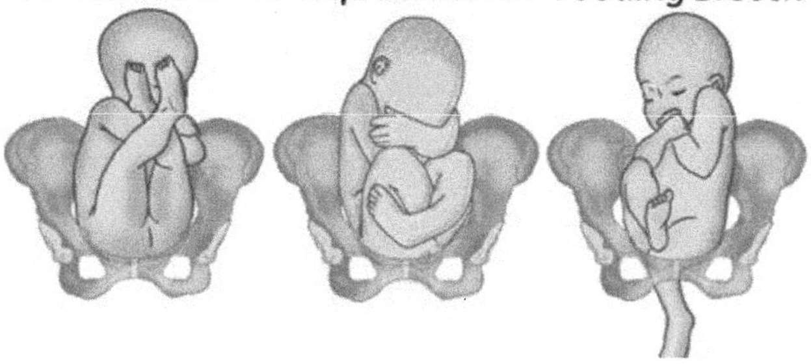

Frank breech/Breech with extended legs

- Hip is flexed
- Knee extended
- **Presenting** part consists of both the buttocks and external genitalia only
- Engagement occurs earliest
- Seen in primigravidae
- External cephalic version is **unsuccessful**
- **Least** chances of cord prolapse

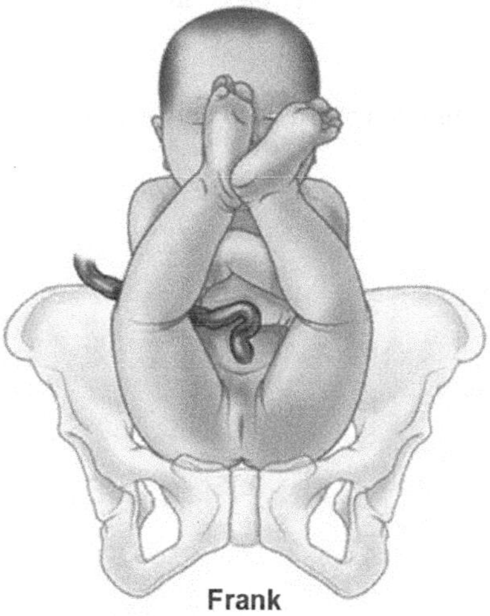

Frank

Complete breech/flexed breech

- **Normal** attitude of full flexion is maintained
- Knees & hip flexed
- **MC** type

- **Presenting** part consists of both the buttocks and external genitalia and two feet
- External cephalic version is **successful**
- Seen in multipara
- Intermediate chances of cord compression

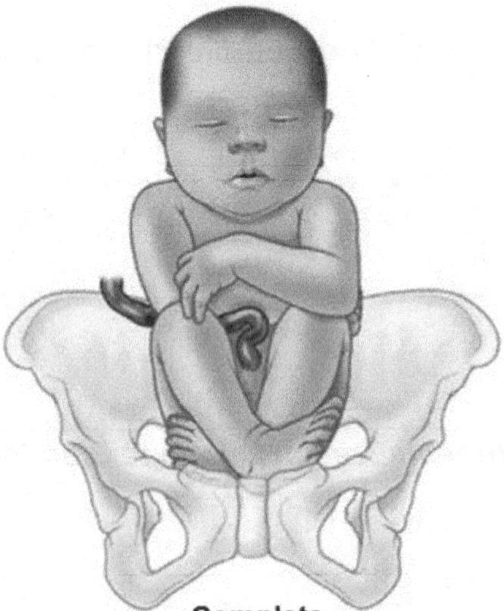

Complete

Footling breech

- Both the hips and the knee are **partially** extended so that **feet** become the presenting part
- Engagement is late
- Elective caesarean section is **indicated**
- **Worst** prognosis
- **Maximum** chances of cord compression

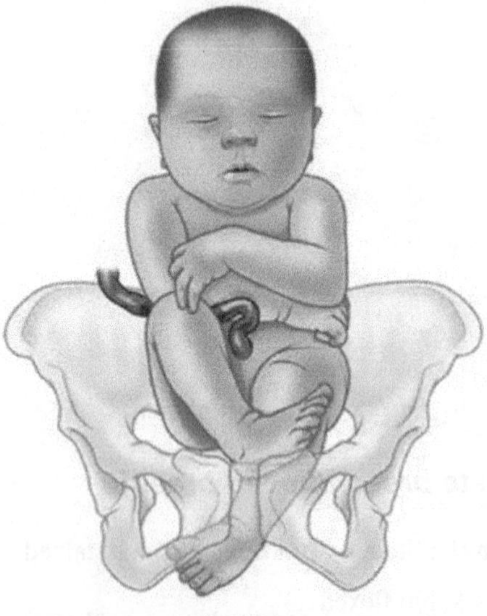

Footling

Management

- In 3 out 4 cases, **spontaneous** correction into vertex presentations by 34th week
- If patient with breech presents at >37 weeks, external cephalic version/**ECV** can be tried

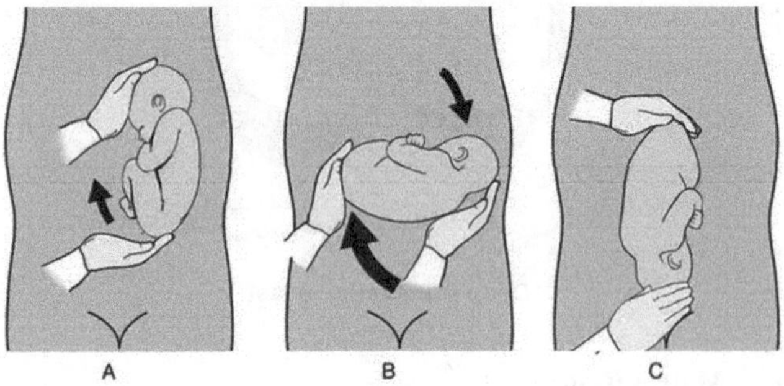

- 3 ways of delivery in breech, if ECV fails/contraindicated
  - o **Assisted breech delivery:**
    - ♦ Delivery of buttocks:
      - □ Groin traction
      - □ **Pinard** manoeuvre

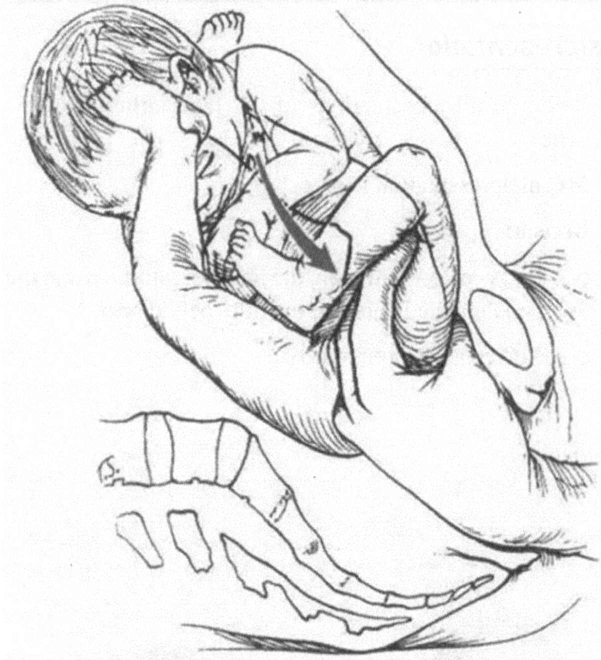

Figure: Frank breech decomposition using the Pinard maneuver. Two fingers are inserted along one extremity to the knee, which is the knee, which is then pushed away from the midline after spontaneous flexion traction is used to deliver a foot into the vagina

    - ♦ Delivery of shoulders:
      - □ **Lovset** manoeuvre

Lovset maneuver for delivery of arms

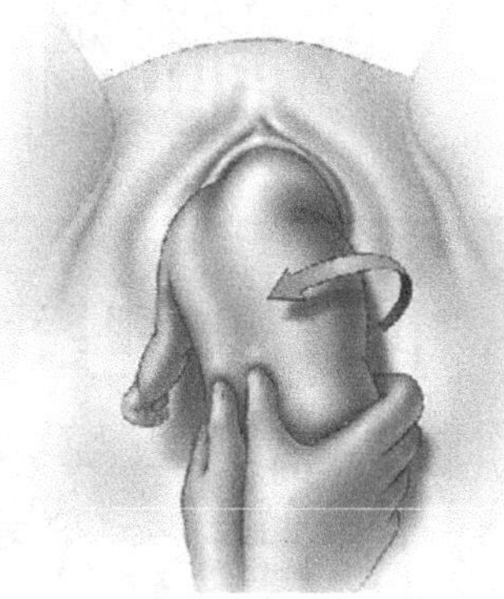

- Delivery of head in breech presentation:
  - □ **Burns-Marshall** technique
  - □ **Mauriceau**-Smellie-Veit method/Malar flexion and shoulder traction

The Burns–Marshall Maneuver

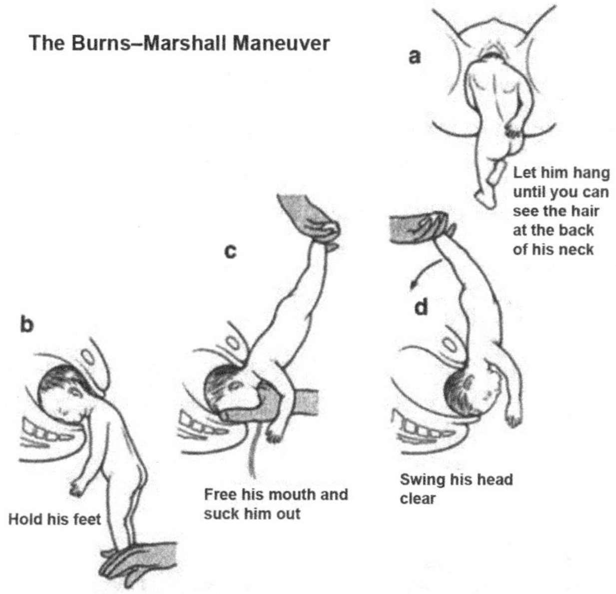

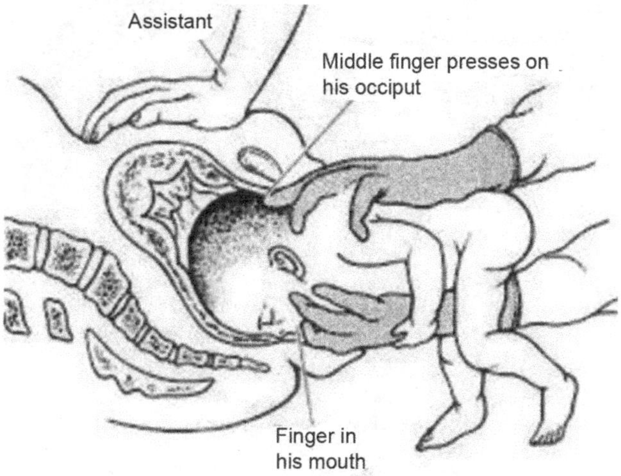

Mauriceau-Smellie-Veit maneuver

- o **Breech extraction:**
  - ♦ Part or the entire body of the fetus is extracted under general anesthesia
  - ♦ Rarely done
- o Cesarean section

TRANSVERSE LIE

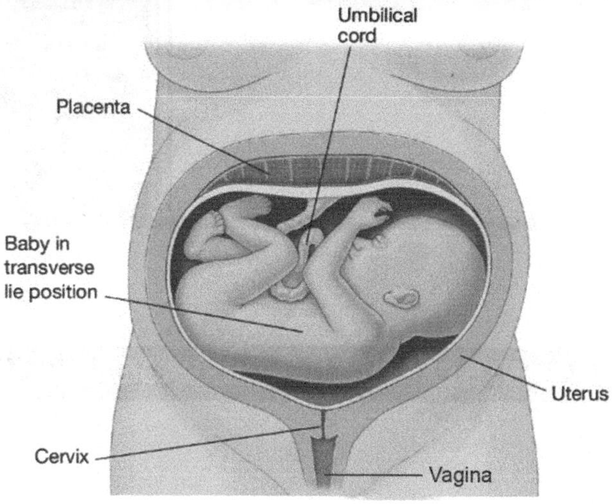

Features

- As the name suggest, lie is transverse
- Presentation is **shoulder**
- **MC** cause is prematurity
- **No** mechanism of labor
- Management is always caesarean section

CORD PROLAPSE

Features

- In this condition, umbilical cord **lies** below the presenting part after rupture of membranes
- **Maximum** chances of cord prolapse are seen in transverse lie

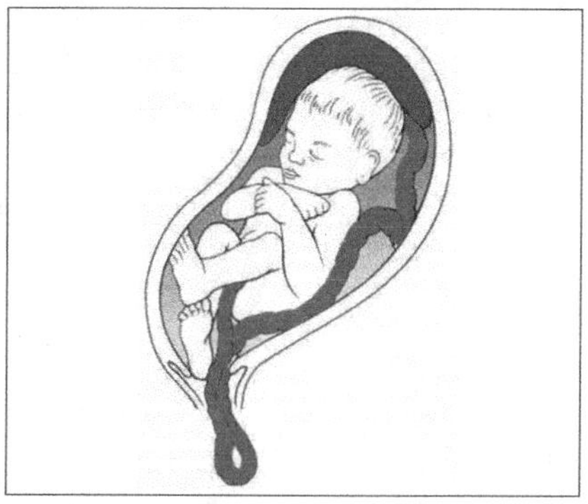

SECTION 3
OBSTETRICS

Chapter 12

Ante Partum Hemorrhage

ANTE PARTUM HEMORRHAGE/APH

APH

- Bleeding from or into genital tract after **28** weeks of pregnancy
- **Types:**
  - o **Placental bleeding:**
    - ♦ Abruptio placentae
    - ♦ Placenta praevia
  - o Unexplained/Intermediate
  - o **Extraplacental:**
    - ♦ Local trauma
    - ♦ Carcinoma of cervix
    - ♦ Cervical polyp

ABRUPTIO PLACENTAE

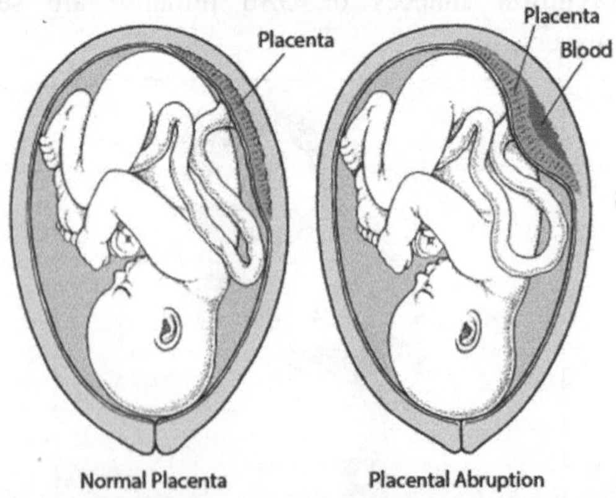

Features

- Also known as accidental hemorrhage
- It occurs due to premature **separation** of a normally situated placenta, resulting in hemorrhage
- Bleeding is always maternal in origin
- **Types:**
  - o **Concealed:**
    - ♦ Separation of placenta is in such a way that the blood collects behind the placenta and does not come out

Couvelaire Uterus

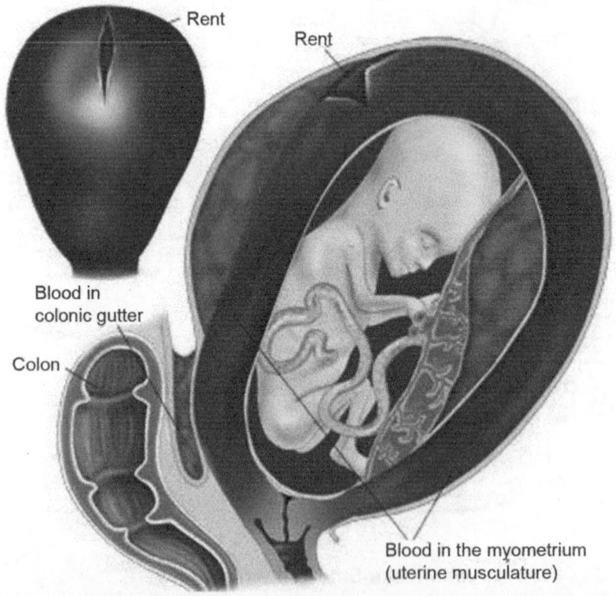

- ♦ **Couvelaire** uterus
  - o Revealed
  - o Mixed
- **Presentation:**
  - o Severe and constant abdominal **pain**
  - o Bleeding per vaginum (revealed)
  - o **Hypertension** may be present
  - o Fetal distress/absent fetal heart sounds

PLACENTA PREVIA

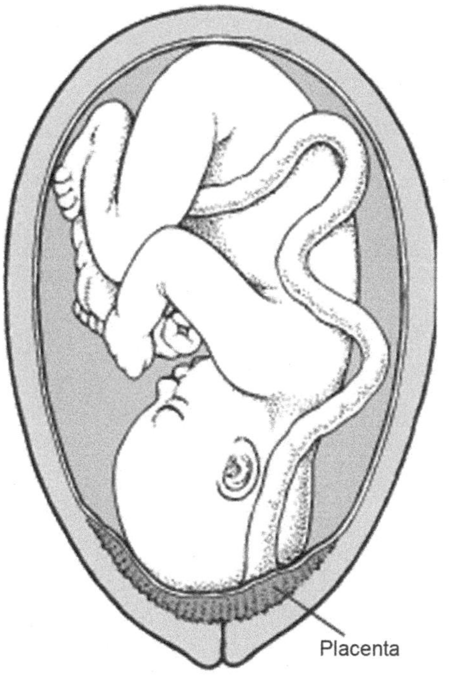

Placenta previa

Features

- Placenta is **implanted** partially or completely on to lower segment
- **Types:**
  - o **Type IV/Complete/Central:** Placenta covers the internal os completely
  - o **Type III/Partial:** Placenta covers the internal os partially
  - o **Type II/Marginal:** Lower edge of placenta touches the internal os but does not cover it
  - o **Type I/Low lying**

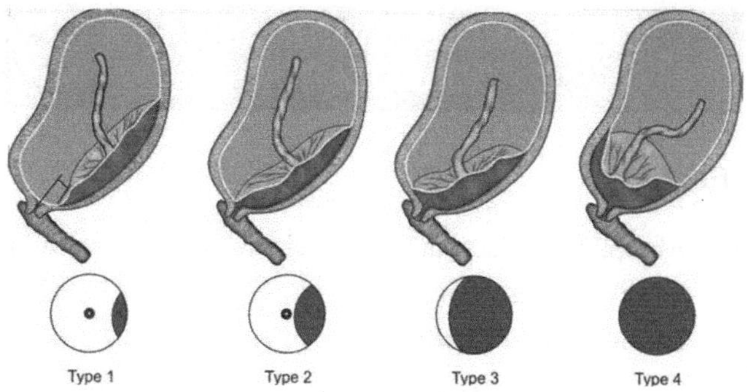

- **Clinical presentation:**
  - o **Bleeding** ***(Mnemonic: CPR)***
    - ♦ **C**auseless
    - ♦ **P**ainless
    - ♦ **R**ecurrent
  - o Fetal heart sounds are heard
- **Investigations:**
  - o Vaginal examination should be **avoided**
  - o Transvaginal USG is the investigation of **choice**
- **Management:**
  - o Caesarean section **preferred**

VASA PREVIA

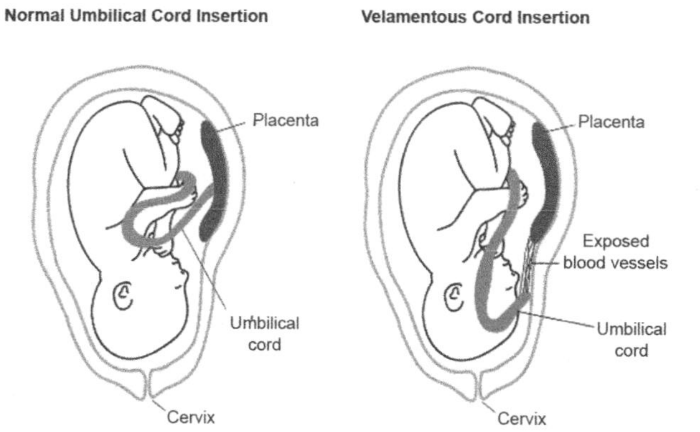

Features

- Occurs due to **velamentous** insertion of the umbilical cord (insertion of cord onto the fetal membranes)
- Rupture of membranes leads to **rupture** of the cord and hence bleeding
- Blood loss is of **fetal** origin so chances of fetal death are more
- **Emergency** caesarean section need to be done

DISSEMINATED INTRAVASCULAR COAGULATION

Features

- Abruption of placenta leads to release of thromboplastin, which leads to DIC
- **Other causes of DIC:**
  - o Intrauterine fetal death
  - o Amniotic fluid embolism
- **All clotting factors are consumed so:**
  - o Fibrinogen level **decreases**
  - o **PT, aPTT, FDP (fibrin degradation products) and D-dimer:** All **increases**
- **Management:**
  - o Fresh Frozen Plasma/**FFP**
  - o Cryoprecipitate

SECTION 3
OBSTETRICS

Chapter 13

Ectopic Pregnancy

ECTOPIC PREGNANCY/EP

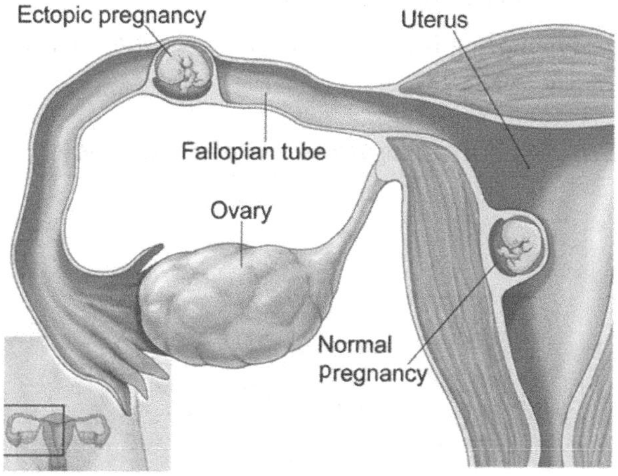

EP

- Defined as the **implantation** and development of the blastocyst at a site **other** than the endometrial lining of the uterus
- **MC** site is fallopian tube
- In fallopian tube, ampulla is the **MC** site (fertilization occurs in ampulla)
- **Causes/Risk factors:**
  - o Previous history of ectopic pregnancy
  - o Previous tubal surgical procedure
  - o Salpingitis/Pelvic inflammatory disease (**MC** cause) increases the risk of ectopic pregnancy by 6-10 folds. Chlamydia trachomatis infection is the **MC** risk factor
  - o Progestasert IUCD (**highest** rate of ectopic pregnancy among contraceptives)
  - o Tubal Endometriosis

Presentation

- Pain in the abdomen (**MC** and most consistent symptom)
- **Classic triad of symptoms of disturbed tubal pregnancy are *(Mnemonic: Ante Partum Bleed)*:**
  - o **A**menorrhoea (75%)
  - o Abdominal **pa**in (100%)
  - o Lastly, appearance of vaginal **bleed**ing (70%)
- **Expelled products in EP have origin from:** Decidua vera

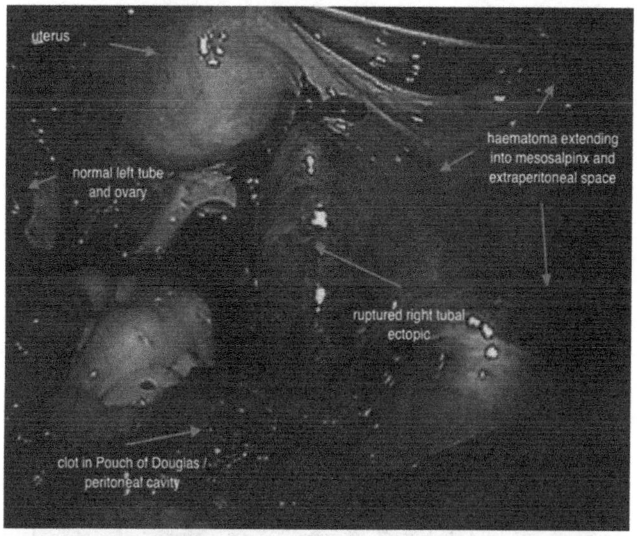

- **Fate of ectopic pregnancy:**
  - o Tubal abortion
  - o Rupture of the tube
- **Ruptured EP:**
  - o Patient will be in **shock** (hypotension and tachycardia)
  - o **Per abdomen examination:**
    - ♦ Tenderness
    - ♦ Guarding
    - ♦ Rigidity
- **MC type of EP which ruptures is:**
  - o Tubal rupture is **commoner** in isthmic & interstitial implantation
  - o As the isthmic portion is narrow and the wall is less distensible, the wall may be **easily** eroded by chorionic villi
  - o Isthmic rupture usually occurs at 6-8 weeks & interstitial one at 4 months

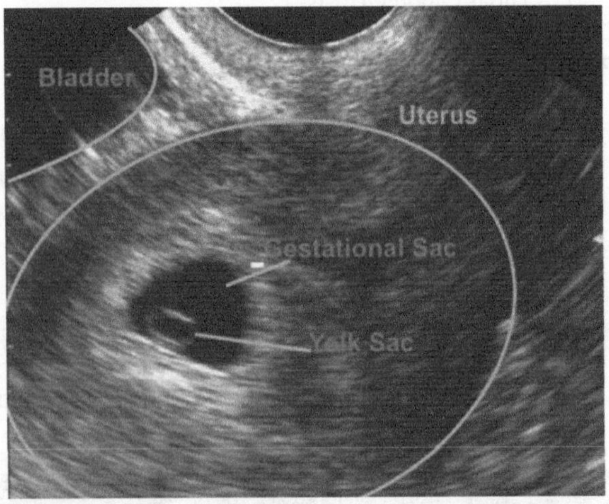

Diagnostic features of ectopic pregnancy on TVS

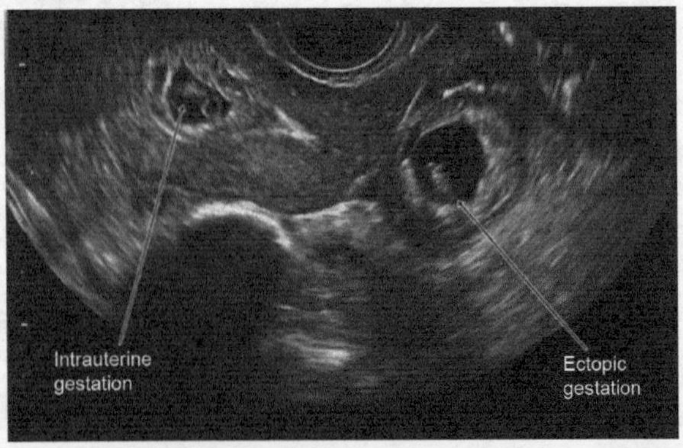

- **Absence** of intrauterine pregnancy with a **positive** pregnancy test
- Fluid (echogenic) in the pouch of Douglas
- Adnexal mass clearly separated from the ovary

Medical management of unruptured tubal EP

- **Salpingocentesis:**
  - o Methotrexate (drug of **choice**)
  - o Potassium chloride
  - o PGF2 alpha
  - o Hyperosmolar glucose
  - o Actinomycin-D etc.
- **Requirements for starting medical management:**
  - o Serum HCG level <3000 IU/L
  - o Tubal diameter <4 cm without any fetal cardiac activity
  - o No intra-abdominal hemorrhage
- **Monitoring** is done by measuring beta-HCG on Day 4 and Day 7

Surgery for unruptured tubal pregnancy

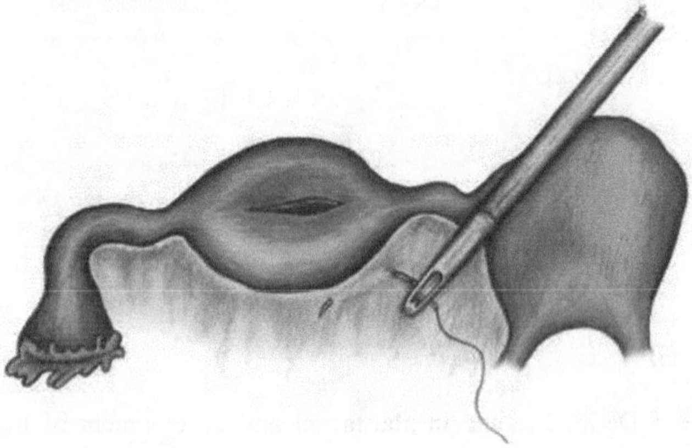

- **Linear Salpingostomy:**
  - o If the patient has **not** completed family size
  - o A longitudinal incision is made on the antimesenteric border directly over the site of ectopic pregnancy
  - o Remove the products
  - o The incision line is kept **open**, allowing it to heal by secondary intention
- **Salpingectomy:**
  - o Completed family size

Management of ruptured tubal pregnancy

- Management of shock
- Laparotomy and **salpingectomy**

Clinical presentation of EP

- A young lady with 6 weeks amenorrhea with lower abdominal mass (irregular & tender) & empty uterus on USG (unruptured)
- A young lady with 8 weeks amenorrhea & shock. The pulse is rapid & feeble, hypotension & cold clammy extremities (ruptured)
- A young lady with 6 weeks amenorrhea with abdominal pain & free **fluid** (echogenic) in pouch of Douglas (ruptured)

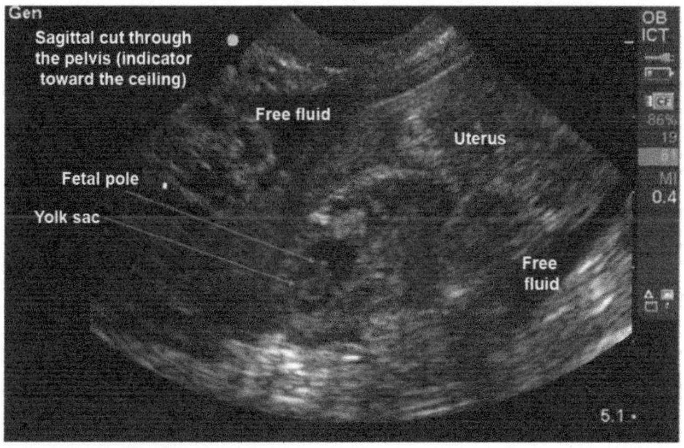

Other sites of EP

- **Abdominal:**
  - o Manifest as abdominal pain and bleeding
- **Ovarian:**
  - o **Spiegelberg** criteria
- **Cervical:**
  - o Painless vaginal bleeding

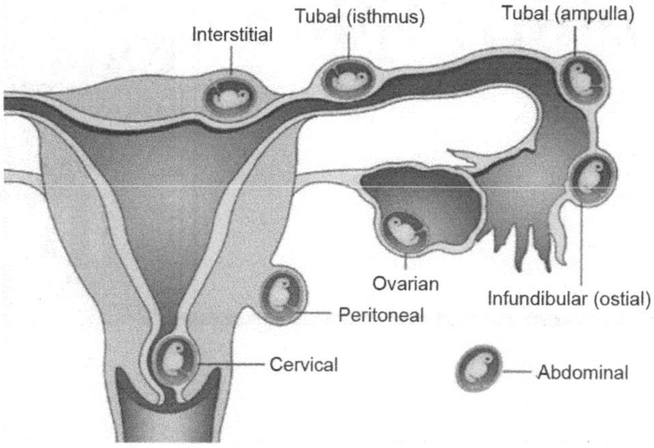

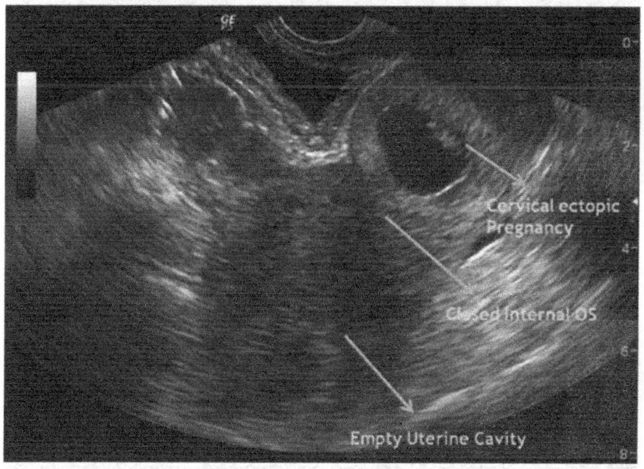

SECTION 3
OBSTETRICS

Chapter 14

Gestational Trophoblastic Disease

TROPHOBLASTIC DISEASES

Classification

- **Gestational trophoblastic disease/GTD:**
    - o Partial mole
    - o Complete mole
- **Gestational trophoblastic neoplasia/GTN:**
    - o Invasive mole
    - o Choriocarcinoma

HYDATIDIFORM MOLE/VESICULAR MOLE

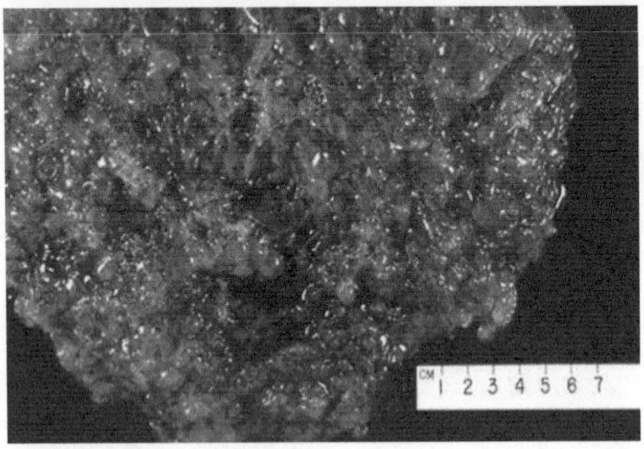

Pathology

- **MC** form of gestational trophoblastic disease
- Abnormal condition of the placenta where there are partly degenerative and partly proliferative changes in the young chorionic villi
- This results in formation of clusters of small **cysts** of varying sizes
- Because of its superficial **resemblance** to hydatid cyst, it is named as hydatidiform mole
- It is best regarded as benign neoplasia of the chorion with malignant **potential**

Complete mole is associated with

- PIH (hypertension, oedema and/or proteinuria)
- Thyrotoxicosis (tremors or tachycardia)
- Hyperemesis gravidarum (15%)

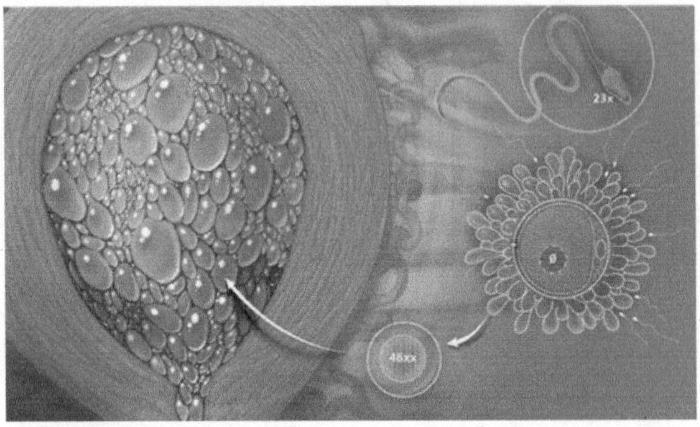

Symptoms

- **MC** presentation is vaginal bleeding (90%)
- Abdominal pain

- Expulsion of grape like vesicles per vaginum is **diagnostic** (in the absence of an intact fetus)
- **Molar pregnancy is usually diagnosed in:**
  - o 1st trimester
  - o Patient gives a history of amenorrhoea of 8-12 weeks with initial features suggestive of normal pregnancy

Per abdomen examination

- Size of uterus is **more** than the period of amenorrhoea (70%)
- Fetal parts **not** felt, nor any fetal movements
- **Absence** of fetal heart sounds

Per vaginal examination

- Unilateral/bilateral enlargement of the ovary (theca lutein **cyst**)
- Finding of vesicles in the vaginal discharge is **pathognomonic** of H. mole

Histological feature

- Hydropic degeneration (leads to marked thinning of stromal tissue)
- **Absence** of blood vessels in chorionic villi

Investigations

- **Quantitative estimation of HCG:**
  - o High **hCG** titer in urine (1 in 200 to 1 in 500) beyond 100 days of gestation
  - o Rapidly increasing serum HCG (>100,000 mIU/ml)

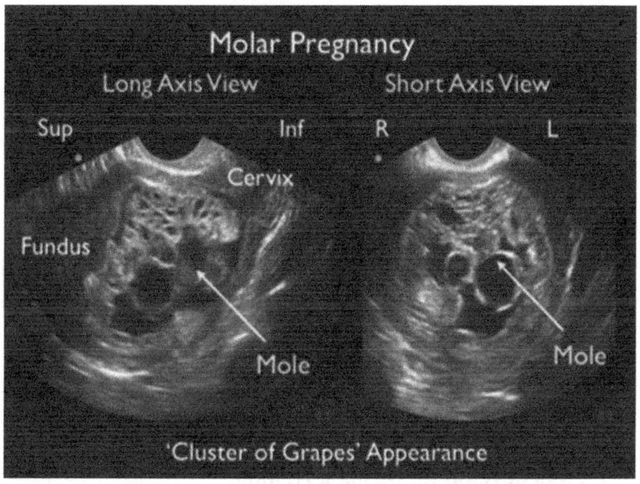

Imaging investigations

- Sonography
- Plain X-ray abdomen & chest (for pulmonary embolization)
- **Definitive** diagnosis is made by histological examination

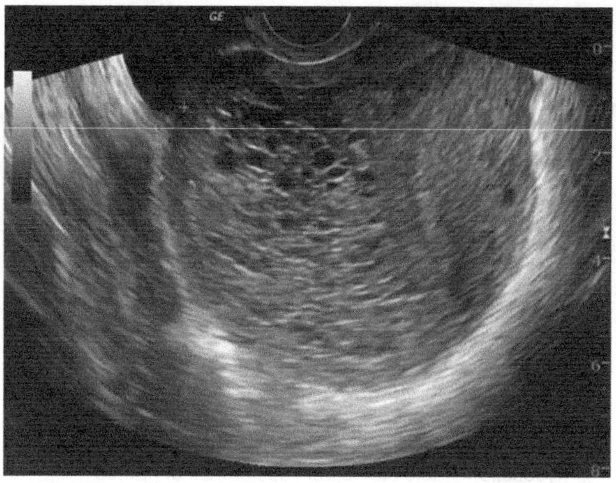

USG

- Investigation of **choice**
- Characteristic feature of molar pregnancy is **'snow storm'** appearance

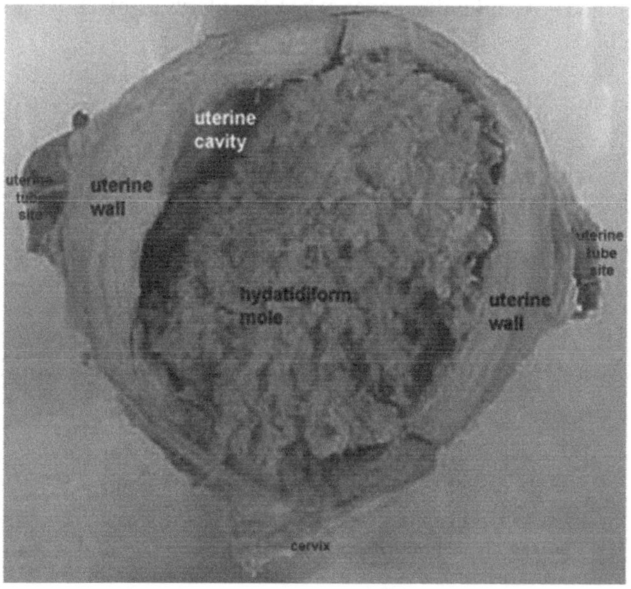

Complications (more in complete mole)

- Hemorrhage & shock

- Sepsis
- Perforation of the uterus
- Pre-eclampsia
- Coagulation failure
- **Choriocarcinoma** (2-10%)

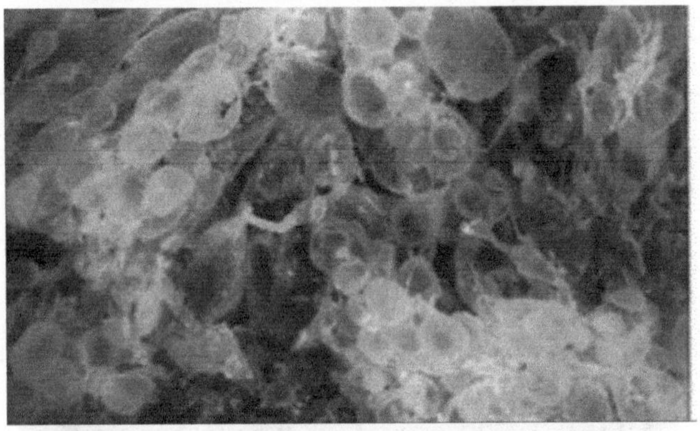

Complete hydatidiform mole: Macroscopically, these microscopic changes transform the chorionic villi into clusters of vesicles with variable dimensions the name hydatidiform mole stems from this "bunch of grapes"

Treatment of choice

- **Suction – evacuation**
    - o It is safe, rapid and **effective**
    - o Can be done even when the uterus is of 28 weeks gestation

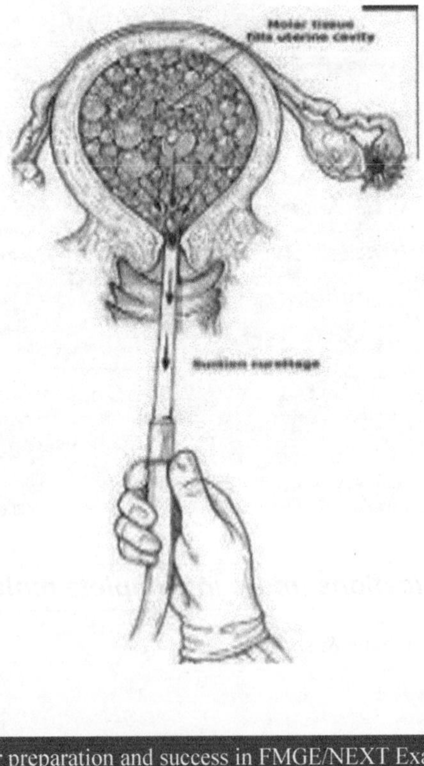

- **Hysterectomy:**
    - o Completed family size

Follow-up

- **Mandatory** for all cases for at least 1 year, as occurrence of choriocarcinoma is confined to this period
- HCG levels following evacuation should regress to normal within 3-month time
- For 4-8 weeks, check-up should be done once weekly
- After 56 days (when HCG is negative), for next 6 months, check-up is done every one month

Partial mole

- **Karyotype: Triploid** (69 XXY or 69 XXX)
- **Pathology:** Some villi, blood vessels and fetal tissue is present
- **Examination:** Height of uterus equal/less than the period of gestation
- **USG:** Confused with missed abortion
- **HCG levels:** Not markedly raised

Complete mole (Mnemonic: CD)

- **Karyotype: D**iploid (46 XX)
- **Pathology: No** villi formation, no blood vessels and no fetal tissue
- **Examination:**
    - o Passage of **grape** like vesicles common
    - o Height of uterus is **more** than the period of gestation
- **USG:** Typical **snow-storm** appearance
- **HCG levels: Markedly** raised

CHORIOCARCINOMA

Features

- **MC** malignant tumour of the uterus
- **50%** develop following a H. mole

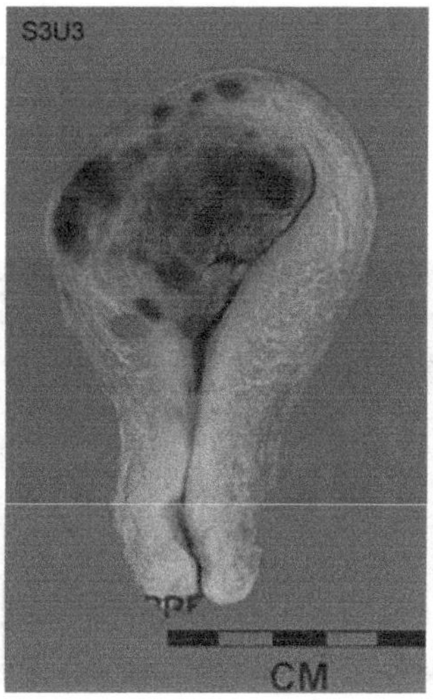

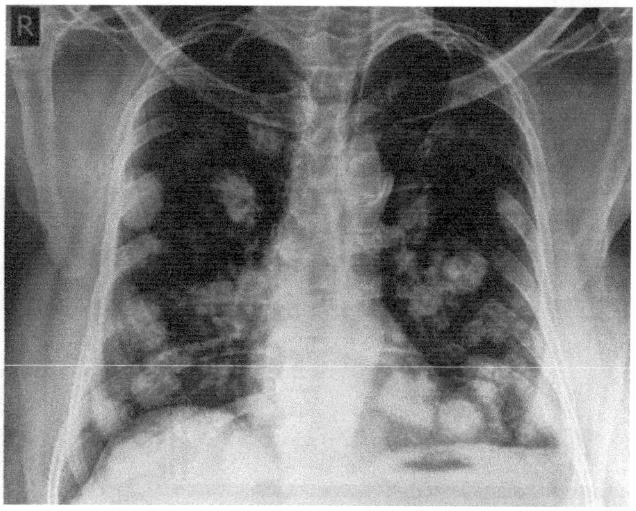

- **MC site of metastasis:**
  - o **Lung**
  - o **MC presentation of lung metastasis:** Discrete rounded densities (Canon-ball shadows)
- MC route of metastasis is hematogenous
- **Tumour marker:** Beta-HCG
- Chemotherapy with methotrexate is the treatment of **choice**

SECTION 3
OBSTETRICS

Chapter 15

Twin Pregnancy

TWIN PREGNANCY

Features

- **Zygosity:**
  - o Defines the type of conception
  - o Monozygotic or dizygotic
- **Chorionicity:**
  - o Defines the type of placentation
  - o Dizygotic twins have their own placenta, chorion and amnion
  - o In monozygotic twins, the timing of division of fertilized ovum decides whether the twins will have separate or common structures

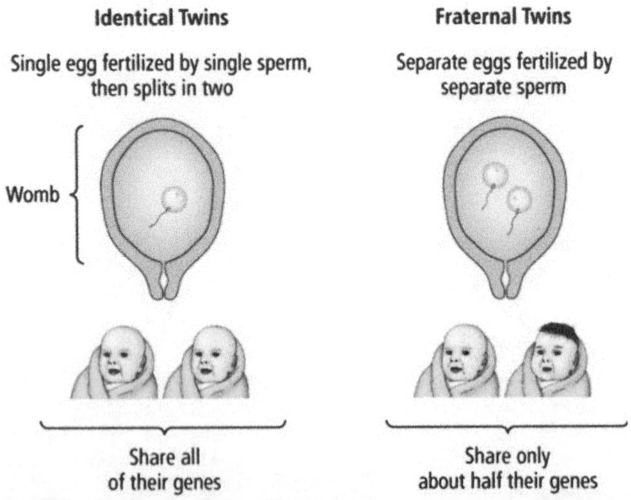

Types

- **Dizygotic/fraternal twins:**
  - o Most common (80%)
  - o Results from fertilization of two ova by 2 different spermatozoa's
  - o 2 zygotes are formed
- **Monozygotic/identical/uniovular:**
  - o 20%
  - o Results from fertilization of a single ovum
  - o There is splitting of a single fertilized ovum
  - o Babies have the same gender and look alike

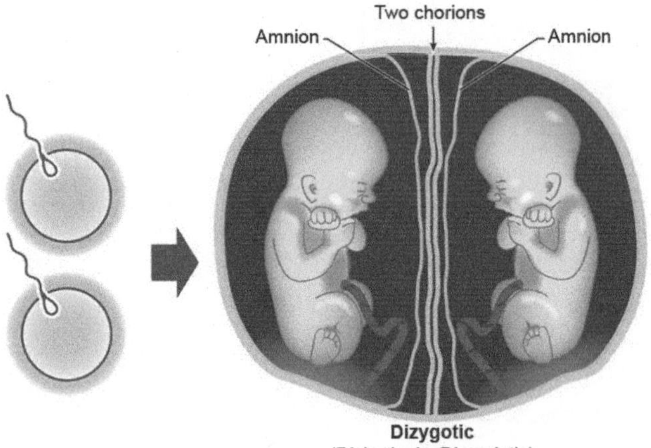

Dizygotic
(Dichorionic, Diamniotic)

Dizygotic twins

- **More** common variety

- Gender of the babies can be same or different
- Babies have different genetic features, same DNA imprints
- Dizygotic twins always have 2 chorions and 2 amnions (dichorionic and diamniotic)

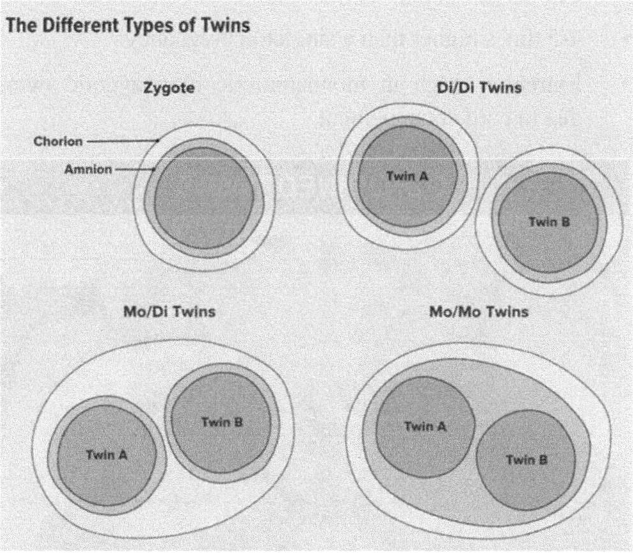

Monozygotic twins

- Gender of the babies is **always** same
- Babies have same genetic features, same DNA imprints
- The number of amnion and chorion depend at the time of differentiation
- The important timelines discussed are till 3rd day, 4th to 8th days and beyond 8th day

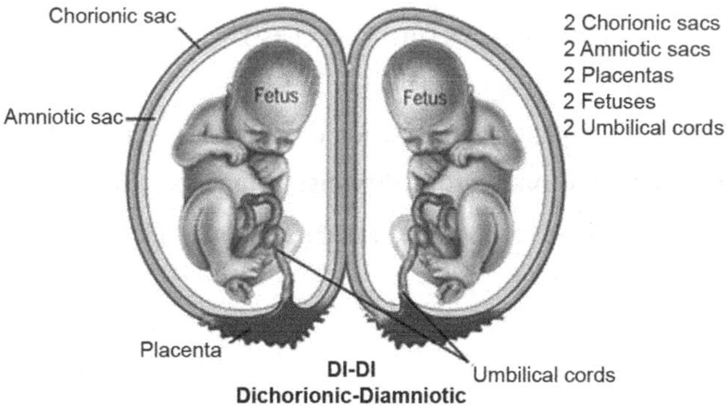

DI-DI
Dichorionic-Diamniotic

- **DADC (Diamniotic – dichorionic):**
  - o 30%
  - o Division takes place within 72 hours (3 days) after fertilization (prior to morula stage)
  - o The resulting embryos have 2 separate placenta, chorions and amnions
  - o There are 4 layers between the twins (2 amnions and 2 chorions)
  - o Twin peak sign seen on USG
- **DAMC (Diamniotic – monochorionic):**
  - o 60% (amongst monozygotic)
  - o Division takes place between the 4th and 8th day after formation of inner cell mass when chorion has already developed, so chorion will be common in both the twins
  - o There are 2 layers between the twins (2 amnions)
  - o **Bad** prognosis
  - o Twin to twin transfusion syndrome is seen

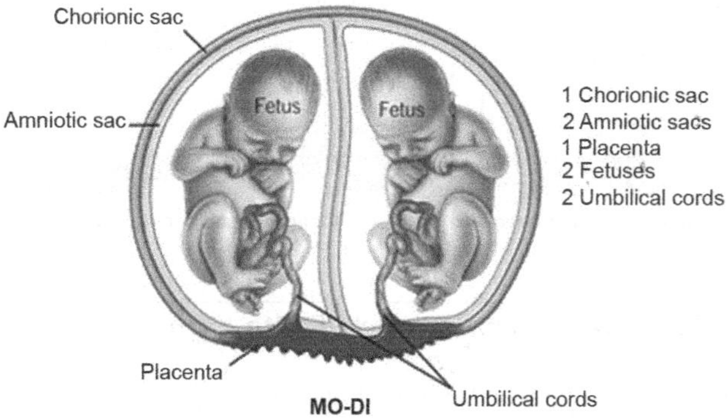

MO-DI
Monochorionic-Diamniotic

- **MAMC (Monoamniotic – monochorionic):**
  - o 3%
  - o Division occurs after 8th day of fertilization, when the amniotic cavity has already formed so amnion and chorion will be common
  - o **No** layers between the twins

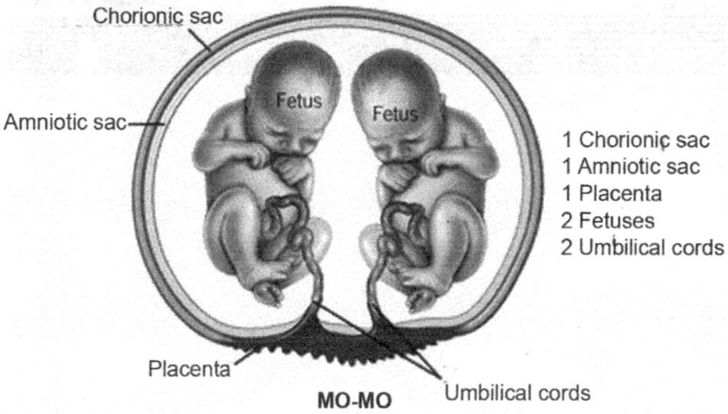

MO-MO
Monochorionic-Monoamniotic

Division <3 days	Division between 3 and 8 days	Division >8 days
Both membranes are separate for each fetus	Chorion is common/Single chorion (monochorionic) for both the fetus	Both membranes are common
Two chorions and two amnions	Amnion separate/Two amnions	Single chorion and single amnion for both fetus

Important points

- 2 sacs (before 10th week) indicates dichorionic pregnancy
- 2 placenta indicates dichorionic pregnancy
- 1 sac indicate monochorionic pregnancy
- Different genders of fetus indicate dichorionic, but same/concordant gender does **not** indicate monochorionic pregnancy

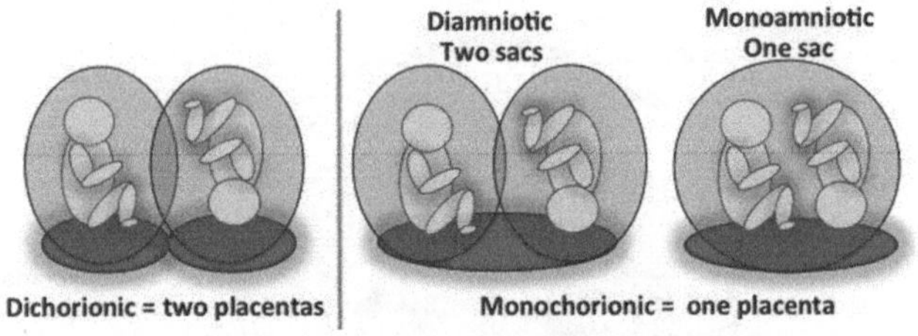

Twin peak sign/Lambda/Delta sign

- **Characteristic** finding of dichorionic pregnancies

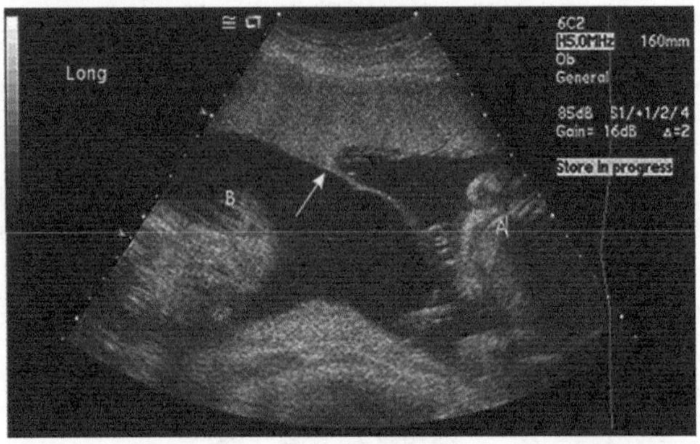

- Seen due to the presence of chorionic tissue between the two layers of the intertwin membrane at the placenta origin

Perinatal mortality in twins

- **MC cause:** Prematurity
- 4-5 times higher than a singleton pregnancy
- Extremely high in monoamniotic monozygotic twins due to cord entanglement

CONJOINED TWINS

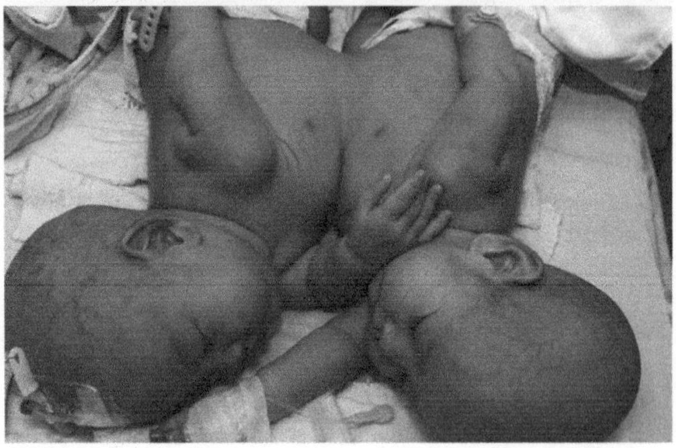

Features

- Also known as Siamese twins
- Division of single fertilized ovum occurs after 14th day of fertilization
- **Types:**
  - o Thoracopagus (fusion at chest)
  - o Craniopagus (Fusion of heads)
  - o Omphalopagus (Fusion of anterior abdominal wall)
- **MC type on conjoined twins:** Thoracopagus
- Conjoined twins are extremely **rare** (1:100,000 to 1:50,000)

SECTION 3
OBSTETRICS

Chapter 16

Pregnancy in Medical Disorders

DIABETES IN PREGNANCY

Important facts

- Pregnancy is a diabetogenic **state**
- There is hyperinsulinemia and insulin resistance
- **DM in pregnancy:**
  - o **Gestational DM:**
    - ♦ Previously **normoglycemic** females develop DM in pregnancy due to insulin resistance, which is maximum at 24-28 weeks of pregnancy
    - ♦ By 24th week of pregnancy, almost the organogenesis is over, so fetus does not develop any congenital malformations
  - o **Overt DM:**
    - ♦ Previously **hyperglycaemic** (known case of DM) female becomes pregnant
    - ♦ These females have high blood sugars from day 1, so high chances of having fetal malformations

Screening test for gestational diabetes

- **1st step/Glucose challenge test:**
  - o Performed between **24 and 28** weeks of gestation
  - o Patient is given **50** mg of glucose, irrespective of previous meals (no fasting required)
  - o Plasma glucose is measured after 1 hour
  - o Cut off value is **<140** mg% plasma glucose levels are between 140 and 180 mg/dl, screening test is considered positive and the 2nd step (confirmatory test) is carried out

Fetal complications of gestational diabetes

- Fetal hyperglycemia
- **Macrosomia** (birth weight of > 4 kilograms)
- Shoulder dystocia (difficulty in delivery of the shoulder following delivery of head)

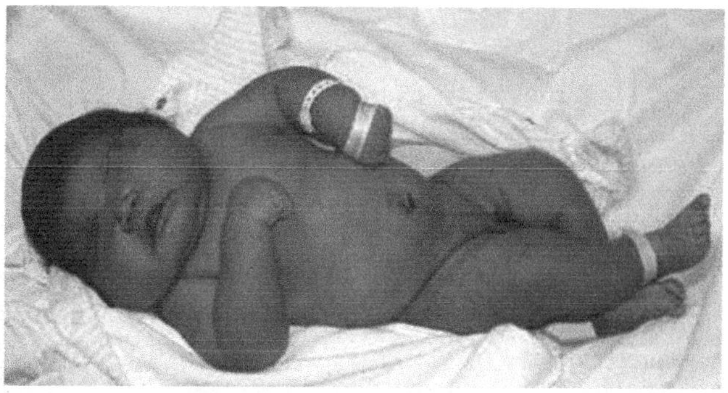

PREGNANCY IN RH NEGATIVE WOMEN

Important facts

- Alloimmunization/isoimmunization is defined as **production** of immune antibodies in an individual in response to foreign red cell antigen derived from another individual of the same species provided, the first one lacks antigen

- **Mother** is Rh –ve (D -ve)
- **Fetus**/husband is Rh +ve
- Fetal blood carrying Rh-antigen enters maternal circulation (mostly at the time of delivery) and stimulates production of antibodies in mother
- At least 0.1 ml of fetal blood must enter into maternal circulation to generate antibody response
- Detectable antibodies usually develop after 6 months after this fetomaternal leak
- It is the **IgG** antibodies that cross the placenta and causes damage the fetus
- Since IgG appears at a later period, therefore the first pregnancy is not affected
- IgM antibodies are larger molecules and cannot pass through placental barrier and hence is not harmful to the fetus
- Degree of affection of fetus depends upon the degree of destruction of the fetal RBC by the antibodies
- Alloimmunization is preventable by the anti-D Ig prophylaxis
- It should be given **within** 72 hours of delivery

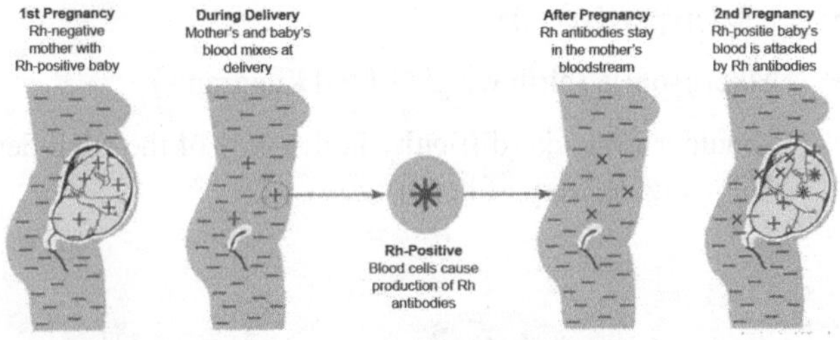

Fetal affection by maternal Rh-antibodies

- Maternal antibodies (IgG) formed in the previous pregnancy (mother RH +ve and fetus Rh -ve) crosses placental barrier and enters fetal circulation in second pregnancy
- If the fetus in second pregnancy is Rh -ve, nothing will happen
- If the fetus in second pregnancy is Rh +ve, these IgG antibodies attach to the antigen sites on fetal RBCs and destroy them
- **Various spectrum of fetal hemolytic disease** as per the degree of agglutination and destruction of fetal RBCs include:
  - o **Hydrops fetalis:**
    - ♦ **Most** serious form
    - ♦ Excessive destruction of fetal RBCs
    - ♦ **Severe** anemia
    - ♦ Generalized edema/hydrops fetalis
  - o Icterus gravidarum neonatorum
  - o **Congenital anemia of the newborn:**
    - ♦ **Mildest** form
    - ♦ Hemolysis is going on slowly

Antenatal investigations include

- **Indirect Coomb's test (Antibody detection):**
  - o Done on maternal blood
  - o **If +ve:** Indicates that Rh antibodies have formed in the mother
  - o **If -ve:** Rh antibodies have not formed
- Serial antibody measurement
- Serial USG
- Fetal blood sampling (cordocentesis)

USG

- Helpful in identifying an affected fetus & its severity
- Done at 1-3 weeks interval
- **Findings suggestive of fetal anemia:**
  - o Skin oedema, ascites, pleural/pericardial effusions/ increased placental thickness
- **Doppler blood flow in the middle cerebral artery can predict fetal anemia:**
  - o Peak velocity in the fetal MCA greater than 1.5 multiples of the median (MOMs) for the corresponding gestational age predicts moderate to severe fetal anemia

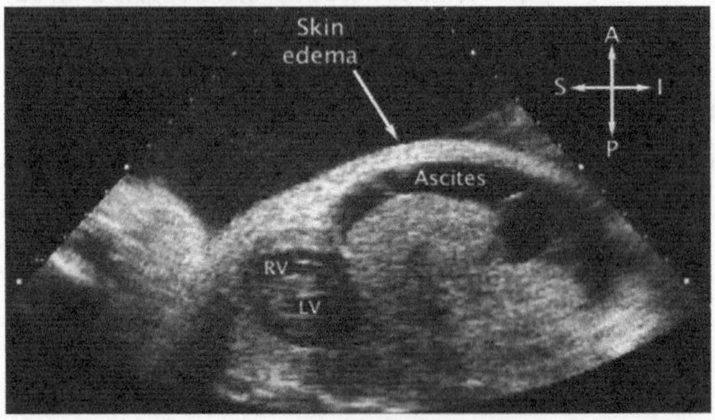

- **Earliest sign of IH on USG:**
  - **Skin edema**
  - Real time USG combined with pulse Doppler detects edema in the skin, scalp and pleural or pericardial effusion & echogenic bowel

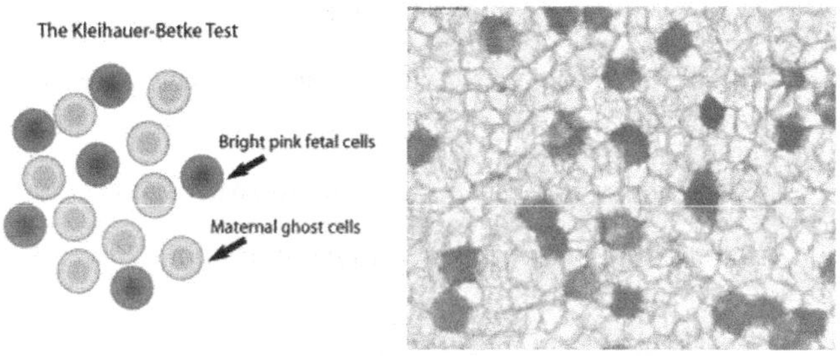

Fetomaternal transfusion is detected by

- **Kleihauer-Betke test**
  - Approximate volume of fetal blood cells entering into the maternal circulation is to be estimated by "Kleihauer-Betke" test using acid elution technique to note the number of fetal RBCs (dark, refractile bodies) per 50 low power fields
- If there are 80 fetal erythrocytes in 50 low power fields in maternal peripheral blood films, it represents a transplacental hemorrhage to the extent of 4 ml of fetal blood

Management is

- **Immediate** cord ligation (to minimize even minute amount of antibody to cross to the fetus from the mother)
- The cord should be kept long (15-20 cm) for exchange transfusion, if required
- Anti-D Ig (I/M) to mother (**within** 72 hours)
- To prevent active immunization of Rh -ve yet unimmunized, Rh anti-D Ig is administered I/M to the mother following child birth
- It should be given provided the baby born is Rh +ve & direct Coomb's test is -ve

Anti-D immunoprophylaxis in Rh (D) negative women is given after

- Miscarriage
- Ectopic pregnancy
- MTP
- Chorionic villous sampling
- Amniocentesis
- One dose of anti-D (300 mcg) Ig is given prophylactically at around 28 weeks and a second dose is given after delivery within 72 hours if the infant is Rh (D) positive

Dose of anti-D Ig

- **Following delivery:** 300 mcg
- **Induced/spontaneous abortion, ectopic/molar pregnancy or CVS in first trimester:** 50 mcg
- **Women with pregnancy >12 weeks:** 300 mcg (full dose)

HEART DISEASES/HD & PREGNANCY

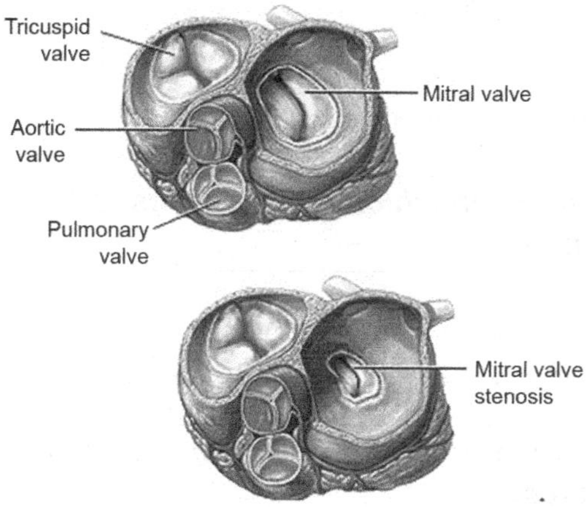

Mitral stenosis

- Mitral stenosis/MS is the **MC** heart disease associated with pregnancy
- Symptoms of MS appears when the stenosis narrows mitral valve area to less than 2.5 cm^2
- In symptomatic cases, mortality ranges between 5 and 15%
- **Best time of surgery:** 14-18 weeks

HD carrying worst prognosis in pregnancy

- Pulmonary hypertension
- Maternal mortality is 50%
- **Termination** of pregnancy is indicated
- Women with pulmonary HTN & right ventricular dysfunction are strongly discouraged to become pregnant

HD showing highest mortality

- Eisenmenger complex
- Patient have pulmonary HTN with shunt (right to left) through an open ductus, an atrial or ventricular septal defect
- **Maternal mortality:** 50%
- **Perinatal loss:** 50%
- **Termination** of pregnancy should be seriously considered

Anatomical & physiological changes during pregnancy that mimic cardiac disease

- Hyperdynamic circulation
- **Systolic** ejection murmur at left sternal border
- Dyspnoea, fatigue
- Tachycardia
- Continuous murmur at 2nd to 4th ICS

Conditions in which pregnancy is to be terminated

- Primary pulmonary HTN
- Eisenmenger syndrome etc.

Risk of maternal mortality (%) with heart diseases

- **Minimal risk (ASD, VSD, PDA, corrected TOF):** 0-1%
- **Moderate risk (MS, AS, uncorrected TOF):** 5-15%
- **Major risk (Pulmonary HTN, COA):** 25-50%

HIV & PREGNANCY

HIV & AIDS

- HIV is an incurable infection that finally leads to terminal disease called AIDS
- 25-30% are women
- 90% of them are 20-49 years of age

Virus

- HIV viruses (HIV-1 & HIV-2) are **RNA** retroviruses having the enzyme reverse transcriptase, which permits genomic RNA to be transcribed into double stranded DNA
- Virus attaches to T lymphocytes known as CD_4^+ cells (which combat viruses & bacteria)
- There is gradual depletion of **CD_4^+** cells
- This leads to progressive loss of host immune defense & development of AIDS
- CD_4^+ count <200 cells/mm^3 is **diagnostic** of AIDS
- Median time from infection to AIDS is about 10 years

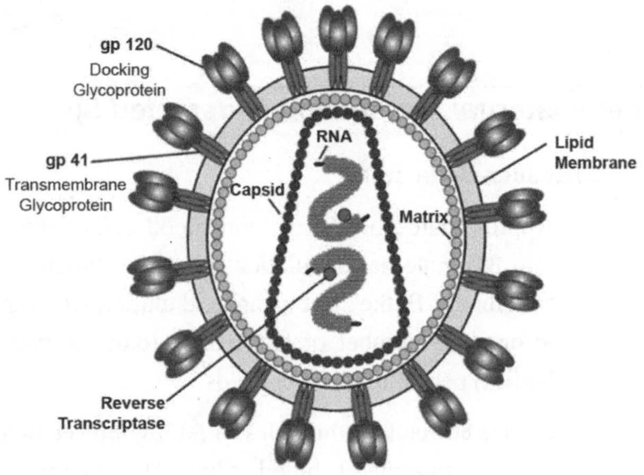

Perinatal transmission

- **Vertical transmission:**
  - **Total:** 14-25%
  - **HIV-1:** 15-40%
  - **HIV-2:** 1-4%
- Risk is **directly** proportional to maternal viral load (HIV-RNA) & inversely to maternal immune status (CD_4^+count)

Diagnosis

- **Screening:** ELISA (**sensitivity** 99.5%)
- PCR can be done
- **Confirmatory:** Western blot test/Immunofluorescence assay (IFA)
- Western blot/WB detects specific viral antigens (p24/capsid, GP41/envelope & GP120/160)
- **False positive WB test:** <1 in 10,000

Incidence of perinatal transmission of HIV can be reduced by

- **Antiretroviral prophylaxis:**
  - o HAART (Highly active antiretroviral therapy) to HIV-1 positive women reduces viral load (HIV RNA)
  - o **Triple** chemotherapy is preferred (2 drugs from NRTI + 1 from NNRTI/PI)
  - o Started between 14-28 weeks
  - o **In resource poor settings:** Zidovudine reduces perinatal transmission from 25% to 7%
- **LSCS at 38 weeks for women taking HAART:**
  - o Who have plasma viral load >50 copies/mL
  - o Elective CS reduces the risk of vertical transmission by 50%
- **Intrapartum nevirapine:**
  - o A single dose of Nevirapine at the onset of labor and a single dose of it to the newborn at age 48 hours is an effective alternative requirement for women who had no prior therapy
- **Avoid breastfeeding:**
  - o Breastfeeding **double** the risk of MTCT (from 14 to 28%) but where alternative forms of nutrition are not safe, the risk associated with breastfeeding may be accepted

IRON DEFICIENCY ANEMIA IN PREGNANCY

Important facts

- WHO defines anemia in pregnancy as Hb concentration of <**11** gm%
- Total amount of iron **requirement** during pregnancy is 1000 mg
- **Diagnosis:**
  - o **Earliest indicator:** Fall in serum ferritin levels
  - o **Most** sensitive index is MCHC

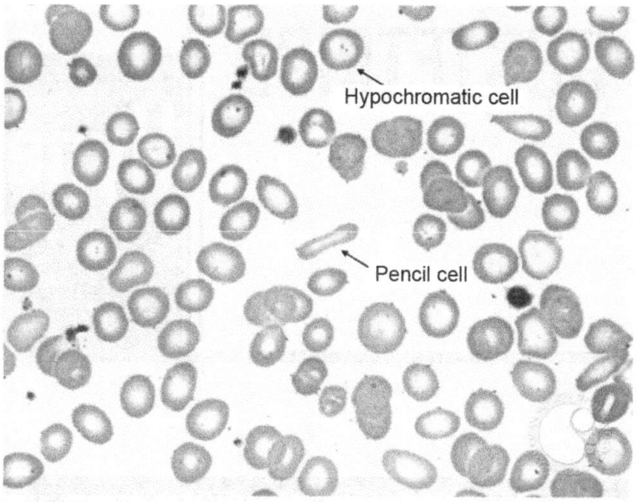

  - o Peripheral blood smear shows microcytic, hypochromic anemia
  - o All indices are **decreased**
  - o **TIBC** (Total Iron Binding Capacity) and Red Cell Distribution Width (RCDW) is increased
- **Treatment:**
  - o **Oral:**
    - ♦ Oral iron is given till blood parameters become normal and continued for **100** days after pregnancy for replenishing iron stores
  - o **Parenteral:**
    - ♦ To be used in patients with severe anemia
    - ♦ Parenteral iron therapy is **not** given for rapid rise in hemoglobin, as the rate of improvement in hemoglobin after oral and parenteral therapy is same

SECTION 3
OBSTETRICS

Chapter 17

Hypertensive Disorders in Pregnancy

PREGNANCY INDUCED HYPERTENSION/PIH

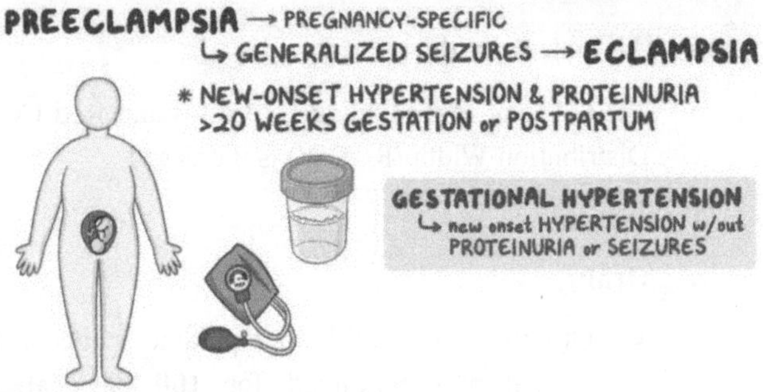

PIH includes

- **Gestational hypertension** (BP 140/90 mm HG for the **first** time in pregnancy after 20 weeks, **without** proteinuria)
- **Pre-eclampsia** (Gestational HTN with proteinuria)
- **Eclampsia** (Pre-eclampsia complicated **with** convulsions and/or coma)

Pathological organ changes

- **Blood:** Thrombocytopenia, coagulopathy
- **Uteroplacental bed:** Placental abruption, IUGR
- **Kidney:** Proteinuria, oliguria
- **Liver:** Necrosis, raised level of AST & ALT
- **CNS:** Seizures, posterior reversible encephalopathy, cortical blindness

Clinical manifestations & pathological changes

- Vasoconstriction → HTN
- Diminished organ perfusion → Oliguria
- Increased vascular permeability → Oedema & proteinuria
- Endothelial damage → Thrombocytopenia & HELLP syndrome

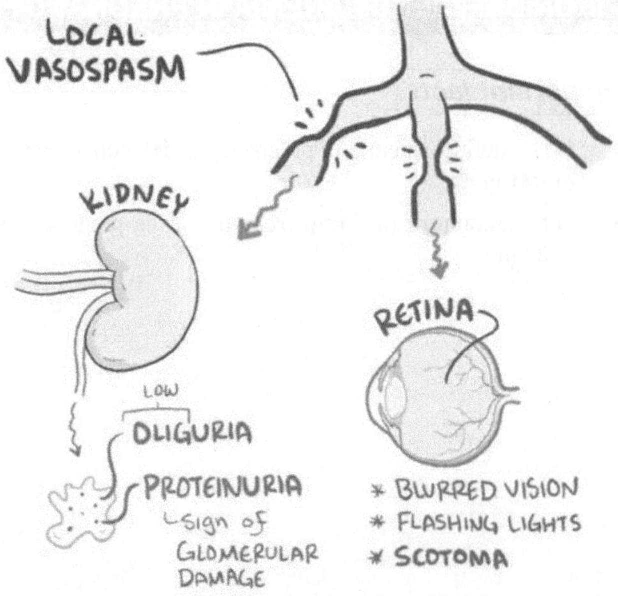

Management objectives

- **Control** BP
- Prevent complications like eclampsia
- Termination of the pregnancy is the only **definitive** treatment of pre-eclampsia

PRE-ECLAMPSIA

Features

- Syndrome of multiple organ dysfunction
- Manifest **first** time beyond the 20th week
- **Characterised** by the appearance of hypertension to the extent of 140/90 mm Hg or more and proteinuria with or without pathological edema
- **Basic** pathology is endothelial dysfunction & vasospasm

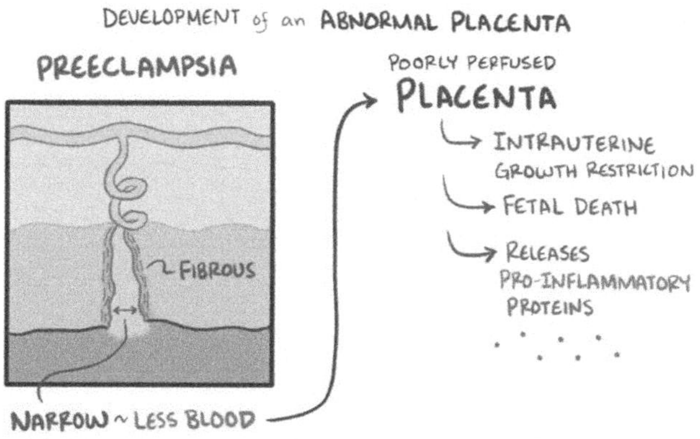

Earliest sign of pre-eclampsia

- Raised BP
- DBP usually tends to rise **first** followed by the SBP

Gant's rolling over test

- For **prediction** of pre-eclampsia
- Done between 28 and 32 weeks
- BP measured with patient on her side
- Patient is asked to roll on her back to check the BP once again
- Increase of 20 mm Hg of DBP from side to back position is **positive** test

Symptom of pre-eclampsia

- **Weight change:**
  - o Rapid gain in weight **(earliest)**
  - o A rapid gain in weight of more than 5 lb a month or more than 1 lb a week in later months of pregnancy is **significant**
- **Visual changes:**
  - o Blurring, scotomata, dimness of vision or at time complete blindness in PIH is due to retinal infarction and retinal detachment
  - o Vision is usually **regained** within 4-6 weeks following delivery
  - o Reattachment of the retina occurs following sub-sidence of oedema and normalization of BP after delivery
- **Complications of pre-eclampsia:**
  - o Eclampsia
  - o **HELLP syndrome:**
    - ♦ **H**emolysis
    - ♦ **E**levated **L**iver enzymes
    - ♦ **L**ow **P**latelet count (Thrombocytopenia)
  - o Accidental hemorrhage
  - o Dimness of vision/blindness
  - o Cerebral hemorrhage
  - o ARDS

Treatment

- **DOC** in severe pre-eclampsia (a persistent rise of SBP >160 mm HG or DBP >110 mm Hg, protein excretion >5 gm/day, Oliguria <400 ml/day, platelet count <1 lakh/mm^3, HELLP syndrome, cerebral/visual disturbances) is Methyldopa (central & peripheral anti-adrenergic action)

ECLAMPSIA

Features

- **Eclampsia is defined as:** HTN, proteinuria, edema & convulsions
- Pre-eclampsia when complicated by generalized tonic-clonic convulsions and/or coma is called eclampsia
- **MC eclampsia is:** Ante partum type (50%)

Cause of convulsion in eclampsia is

- Cerebral anoxia

- Spasm of vessels → increased vascular resistance → fall in oxygen consumption → anoxia → cerebral irritation → convulsions

Convulsions in eclampsia has got 4 stages

- **Premonitory:** Twitching of muscles
- **Tonic stage:** Tonic spasm
- **Clonic stage:** Alternate contraction & relaxation of voluntary muscles
- Stage of coma

Treatment for controlling convulsions in eclampsia

- Magnesium sulphate (**$MgSO_4$**)
- **Ideally** the patient should be delivered within a period of 6-8 hours even if the fits are controlled
- It acts as a membrane stabilizer and neuroprotector
- It has got **no** detrimental effects on the neonate within therapeutic levels
- It does **not** control hypertension

Toxicity of $MgSO_4$ is monitored by (Mnemonic: RUK)

- **R**espiratory rate
- **U**rinary output
- **K**nee jerk
- **Therapeutic level of $MgSO_4$:** 4-7 mEq/L
- **Repeat** injections are given only if the knee jerks are present, urine output is > 30 ml/hour and the respiration rate is >12 per minute

SECTION 3
OBSTETRICS

Chapter 18

Abortion

MISCARRIAGE/SPONTANEOUS ABORTION

Definition

- Expulsion/extraction from its mother, of an embryo/fetus weighing **500** gm or less when it is not capable of independent survival
- This 500 gm of fetal development is attained approximately at **22** weeks (154 days) of gestation

Types of abortions (Mnemonic: TIICM; The Indian Institute of Cash Management)

- Threatened:
  - o **Bleeding: Painless**
  - o **Cervix:** Closed
  - o Uterine size = Period of gestation
- Inevitable:
  - o **Bleeding:** Painful
  - o **Cervix:** Open
  - o Uterine size = Period of gestation
- Incomplete:
  - o POC (Product of Conception) coming out through internal os
  - o **Bleeding:** Painful
  - o **Cervix:** Open
  - o Uterine size < Period of gestation
- Complete:
  - o History of expulsion of fleshy mass (POC: Product of Conception) per vaginum
  - o **Bleeding:** Scanty
  - o **Cervix:** Closed
  - o Uterine size < Period of gestation
- Missed:
  - o Amenorrhoea continuing with subsidence of symptoms of pregnancy
  - o **Bleeding:** No (brown coloured vaginal discharge)
  - o **Cervix:** Closed
  - o Uterine size < Period of gestation

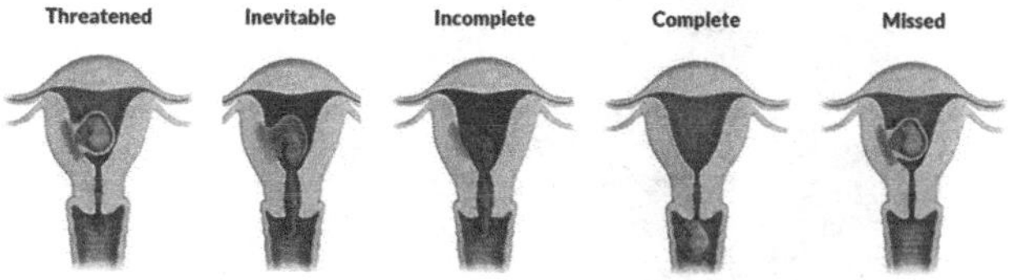

First trimester abortion

- **Causes:** Genetic factors (50%), endocrine disorders (luteal phase defects/LPD, thyroid abnormalities, DM), immunological disorders (autoimmune), infection
- **MC cause of 1st trimester abortion:** Autosomal trisomy (50%) (**MC** is trisomy 16 amongst all trisomies – 30%)

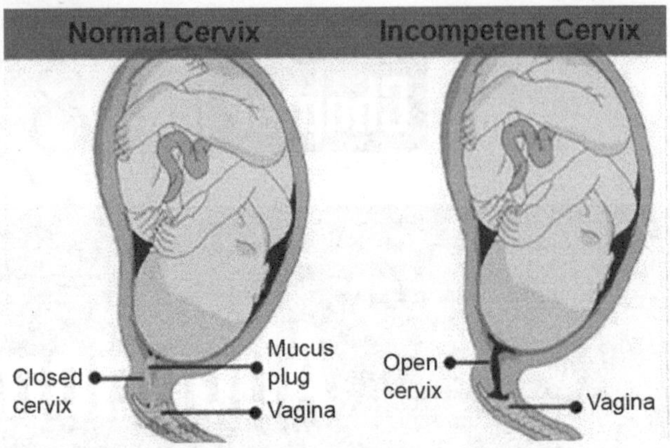

Second trimester abortion

- **MC cause of 2nd trimester abortion:** Cervical incompetence
- Cervical incompetence is characterized by painless, cervical dilatation in the second or early third trimester
- There is associated ballooning of the amniotic sac in to the vagina, followed by rupture of membranes and expulsion of the fetus

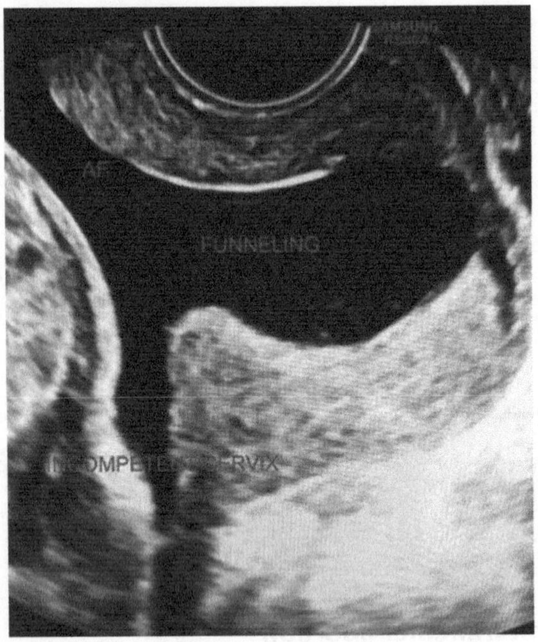

- Management of cervical incompetence, which causes second trimester abortion is by **Cerclage** operation:
  - o Shirodkar's procedure
  - o McDonald's procedure
- **Principle:** The procedure reinforces the weak cervix by a non-absorbable tape, placed around the cervix at the level of internal os
- **Time of operation:** Prophylactic cerclage should be done around **14** weeks of pregnancy or at least **2** weeks earlier than the lowest period of previous wastage, as early as 10th week

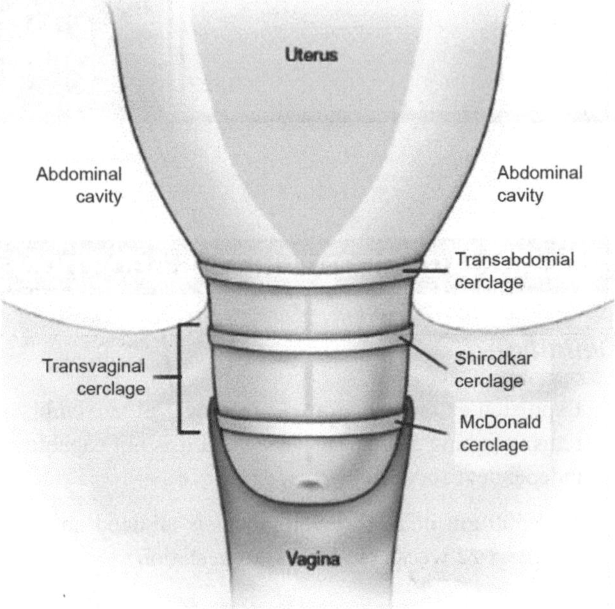

Figure: Suture placement in transvaginal and transabdominal cerclage procedures

Antiphospholipid antibody syndrome/APLA

- It is a treatable, autoimmune disorder associated with recurrent second trimester pregnancy loss
- Female with recurrent abortion & **raised** APTT
- APLA includes LAC (lupus anticoagulant) and aCL (anticardiolipin) **antibodies**
- Spiral artery and placental intervillous thrombosis, placental infarction and fetal hypoxia is the ultimate **pathology**

SECTION 3
OBSTETRICS

Chapter 19

Miscellaneous

POST-TERM PREGNANCY/ POST-MATURITY

Features

- Pregnancy continuing beyond **2** weeks of the EDD (>42 weeks or >294 days)
- **MC** cause is wrong dates calculation (if the patient gives wrong information about LMP)
- USG and amniocentesis are done to **confirm** fetal maturity and to detect any evidence of placental insufficiency
- Perinatal mortality and morbidity are much increased

SHOULDER DYSTOCIA

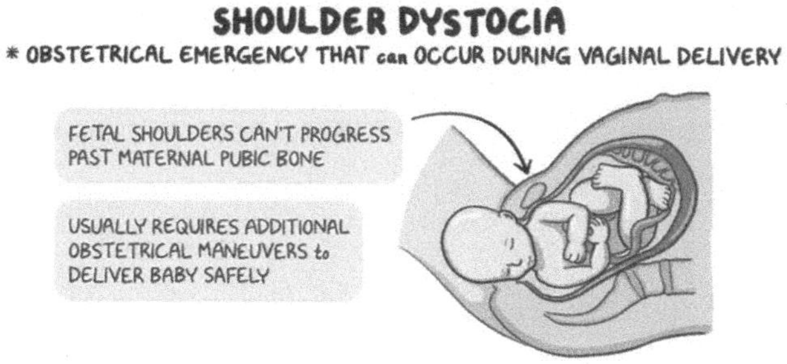

Shoulder dystocia

- The term shoulder dystocia is defined to describe a wide range of additional obstetric maneuvers to deliver the fetus, after the head has been born, and gentle traction has failed to deliver the shoulder
- Shoulder dystocia occurs when either the anterior or the posterior (rare) fetal shoulder impacts on the maternal symphysis or on the maternal sacral promontory respectively
- **Predisposing factors:**
  - Anencephaly
  - Fetal ascites
  - Fetal macrosomia
  - Obesity
  - Diabetes postmaturity
  - Associated with prolonged labor

Unilateral Shoulder Dystocia

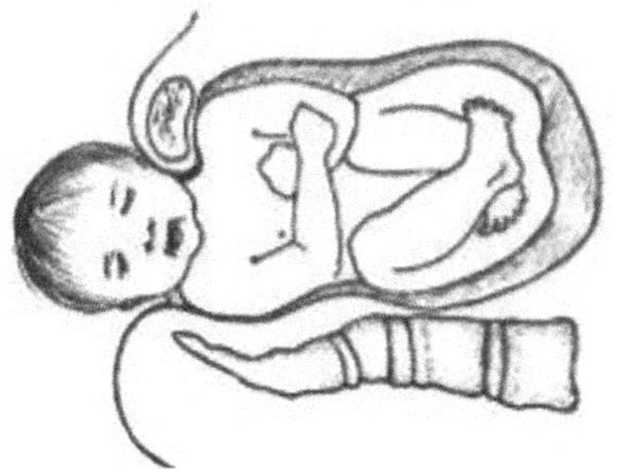

- **Fetal Complications:**
  - Brachial plexus injury
  - Fracture of clavicle/humerus
- **Maternal complications:**
  - Uterine rupture
  - Perineal tears
  - Hemorrhage

- **Management steps:**
  - o Apply **suprapubic** pressure (never apply fundal pressure as it causes further impaction of the shoulder and may cause orthopedic/neurological damage)
  - o McRobert's maneuver
  - o Wood's corkscrew maneuver
  - o Extraction of posterior arm
  - o Cleidotomy

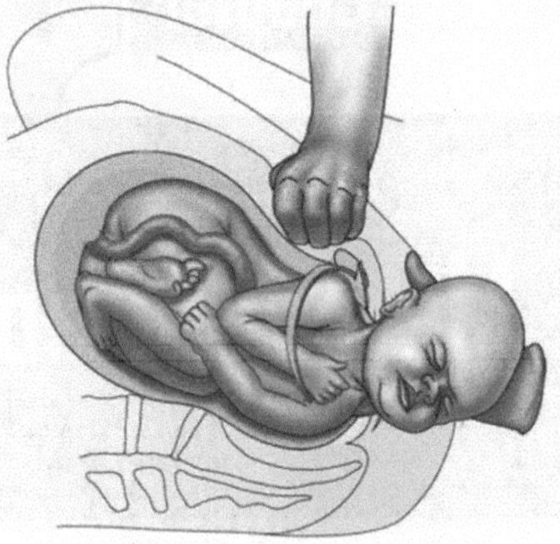

Shoulder Dystocia

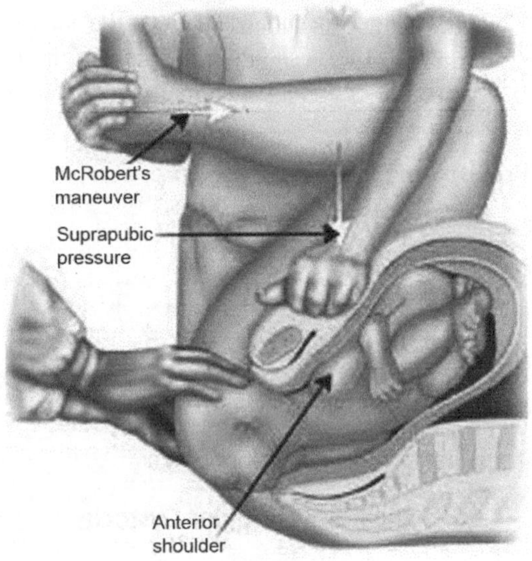

DRUGS IN PREGNANCY

Drugs indicated in pregnancy

- **Anti-thyroid:** Propylthiouracil
- **Anti-TB:** INH
- **Anti-coagulant:** Heparin
- **Anti-malarial:** Chloroquine

Contraindicated in pregnancy

- **Anti-TB:** Streptomycin
- **Anti-malarial:** Primaquine
- **Anti-convulsant:** Valproate (causes NTD)
- **Anti-folate:** Methotrexate
- **Anti-hypertensives:** ACE inhibitors
- All **live** vaccines are contraindicated
- **Yellow** fever vaccine, being a live vaccine can be given in special circumstances

SECTION 4 GYNECOLOGY

Chapter 1 Anatomy and Physiology

EMBRYOLOGY

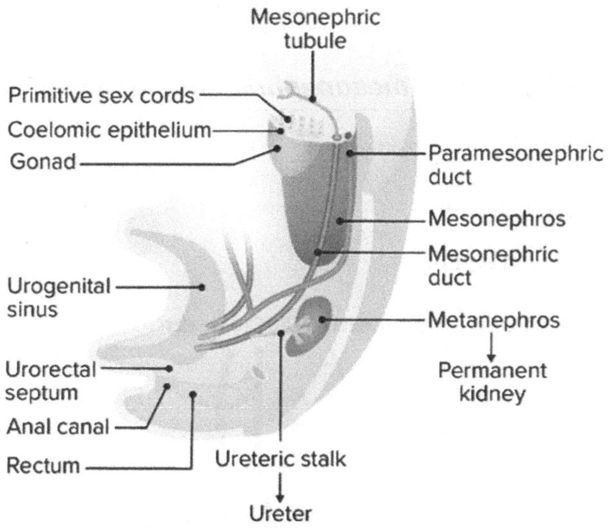

Development of genital organs

- **Bartholin's glands:** Caudal part of urogenital sinus
- **Vagina:**
  - **Upper 4/5th & hymen:**
    - Musculature develops from mesoderm of the **two** fused Mullerian duct
    - Mucus membrane is derived from the endoderm of the canalized sinovaginal bulbs
  - **Lower 1/5th below hymen: Endoderm** of urogenital sinus

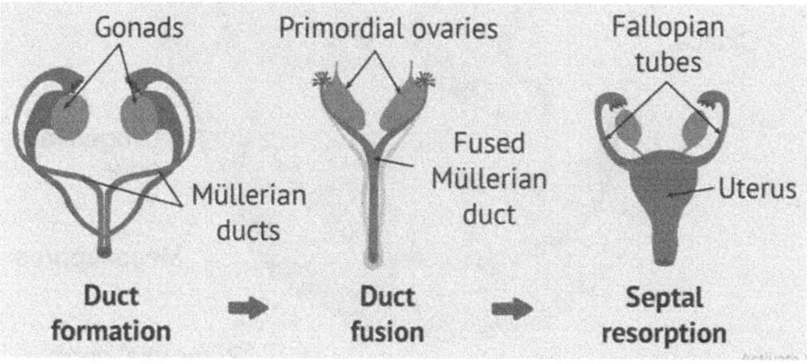

- **SRY** (sex-determining region of the Y chromosome) gene directly controls the testicular differentiation from the bipotential gonads
- SRY gene encodes the testicular determining factor (TDF), which induces the differentiation
- Testicular development is an active event whereas ovarian development is a default pathway due to **absent** SRY gene

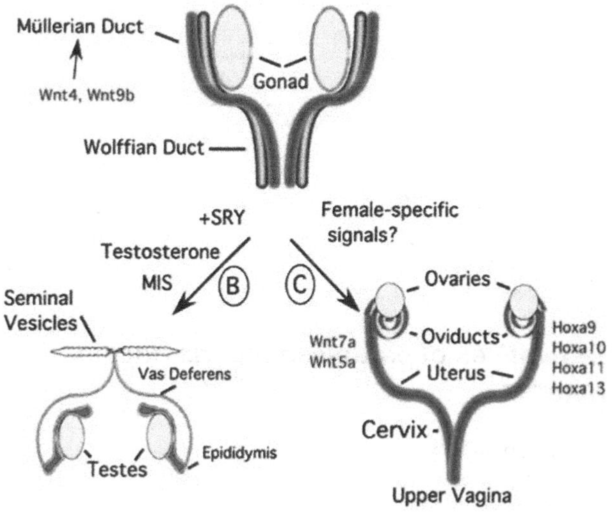

Development of ovary

- Develops from gonadal **ridge**
- **Cortex + covering epithelium:** Coelomic epithelium
- **Medulla:** Mesenchyme
- **Germ cells:** Endodermal in origin
- **Number of oogonia at 20th week:** 7 million
- **Estimated number of oogonia at birth:** 2 million

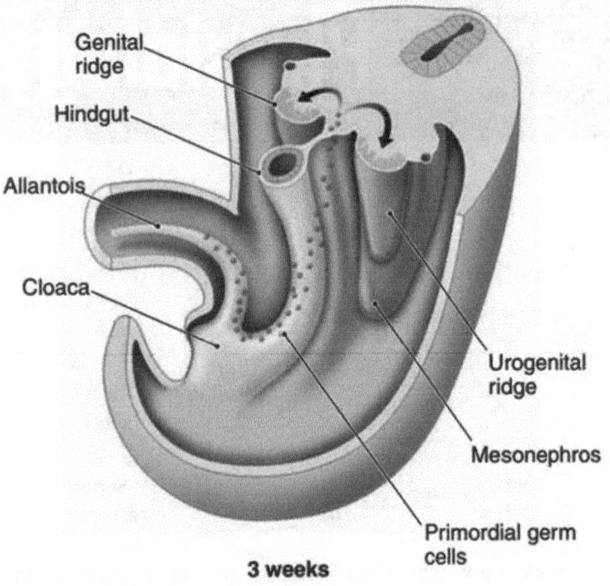

Genital ridge

- Cranial end forms infundibulopelvic ligament
- Middle part **forms** ovary
- Ovaries descend during 7th to 9th months and at birth they are situated at the pelvic brim

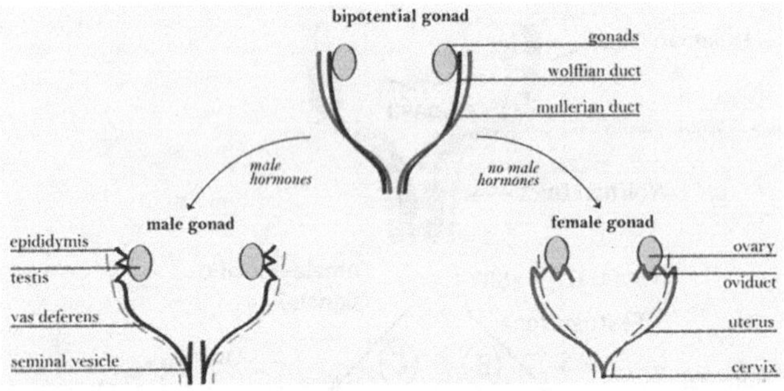

Derivatives of paramesonephric duct in females

- Fallopian tubes
- Uterus
- Cervix
- **Upper** 2/3rd of vagina

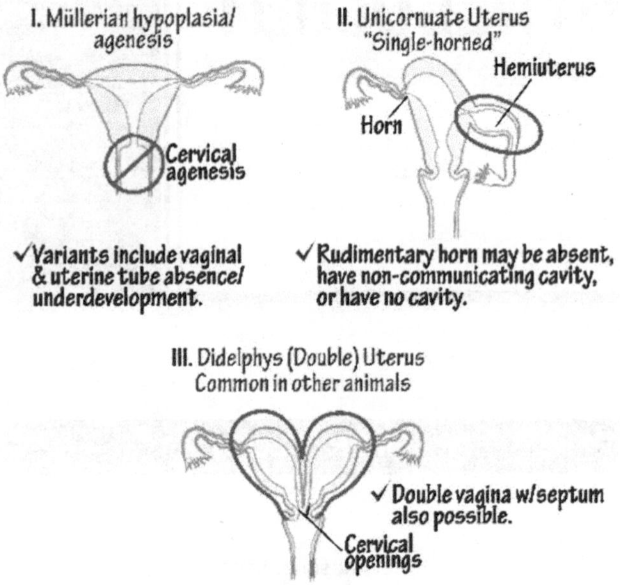

Derivatives of mesonephric duct in males

- Epididymis
- Vas deferens
- Seminal vesicles

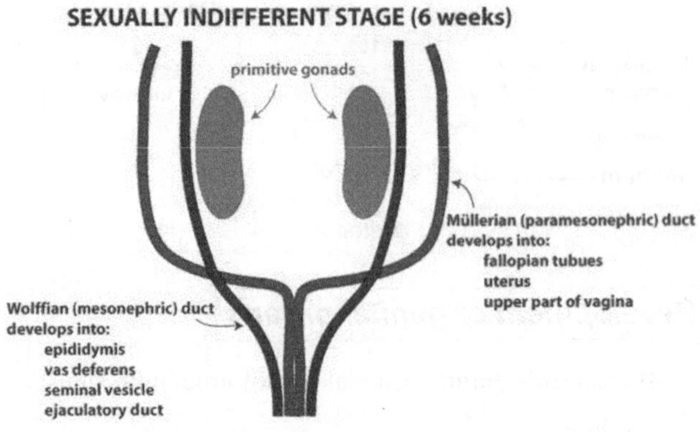

Derivatives of urogenital sinus

- **Vagina:** From sinovaginal bulbs, which grows from the posterior aspect of the urogenital **sinus**
- **Urinary bladder (except trigone):** From the upper vesicourethral part

FEMALE REPRODUCTIVE TRACT DEVELOPMENT

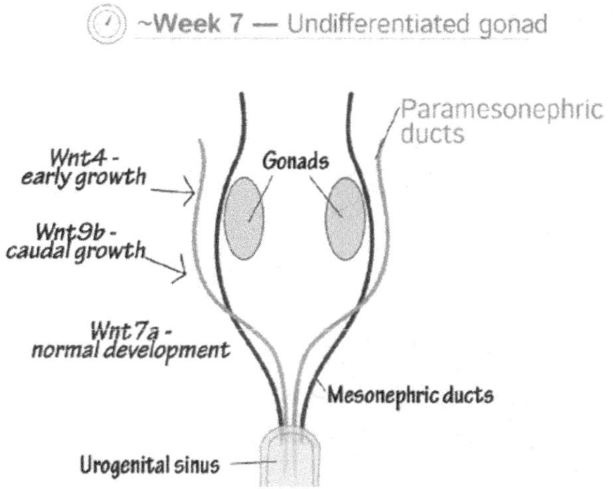

PELVIC ORGANS

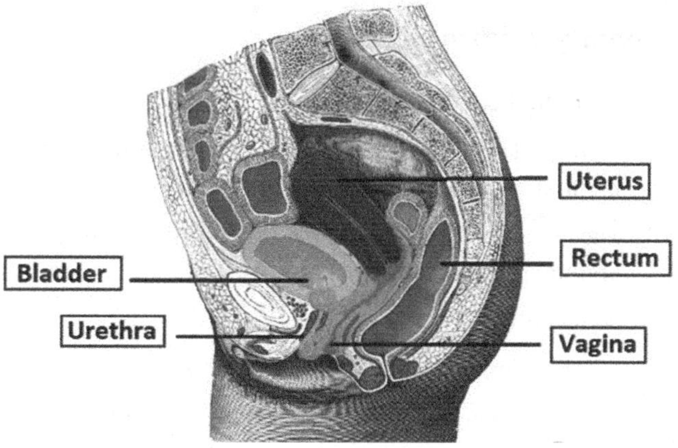

Uterus

- **Position:** 90 degrees forward with long axis of vagina
- **Parts:**
  - o Corpus/body
  - o Isthmus
  - o Cervix

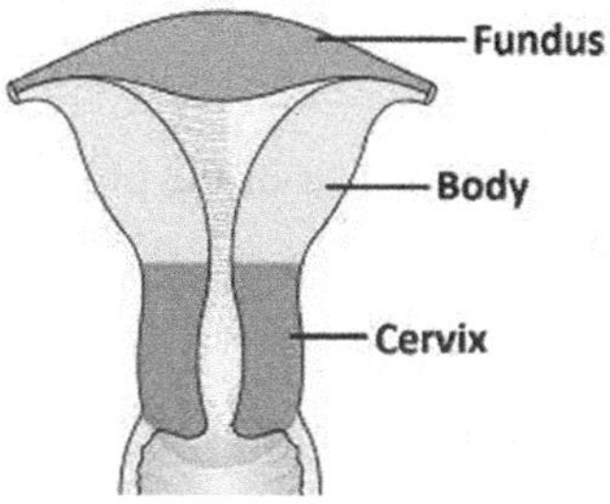

- Measures 8 cm & weighs 50-80 grams
- Isthmus is bounded **above** by the anatomical internal os & **below** by the histological internal os
- Epithelium/endometrium is ciliated columnar type

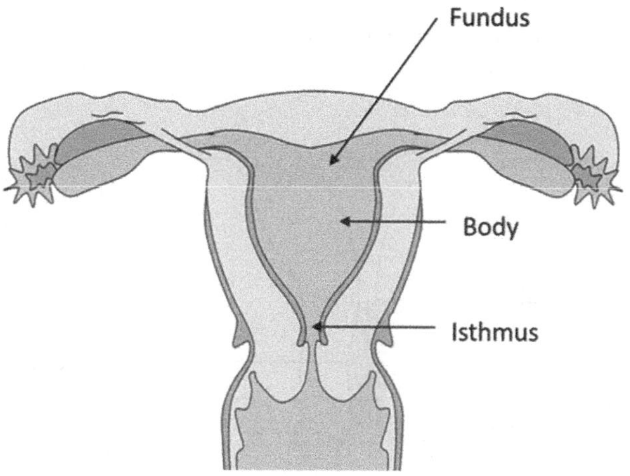

- Cervical canal is lined by tall columnar epithelium
- Squamocolumnar junction of the cervix is situated at the external os
- **Blood supply:** Uterine artery which is a branch of anterior division of internal iliac artery
- **Lymphatic drainage:**
  - o **Fundus & upper part of body:** Pre-aortic & lateral aortic group LN (lymph nodes)
  - o **Cornua:** Superficial inguinal LN
  - o **Lower part of body:** External iliac LN
  - o **Cervix:** External iliac LN, internal iliac LN, obturator LN & sacral group

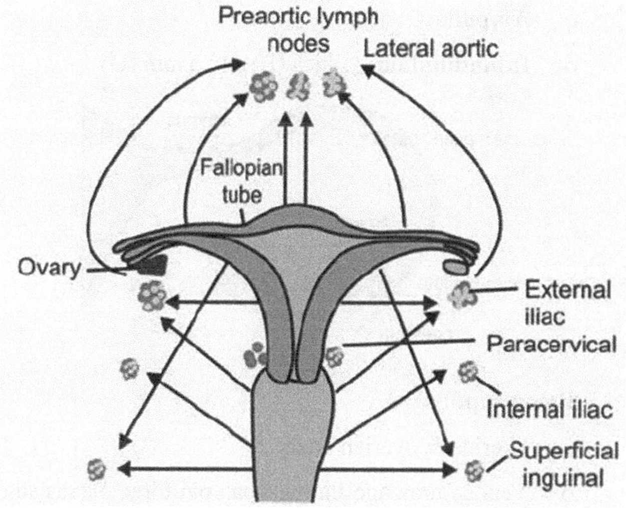

Cervix

- **Size:** 2.5 cm
- **Lining:**
  - **Ectocervix:** Non-keratinized stratified squamous
  - **Endocervix:** Simple columnar

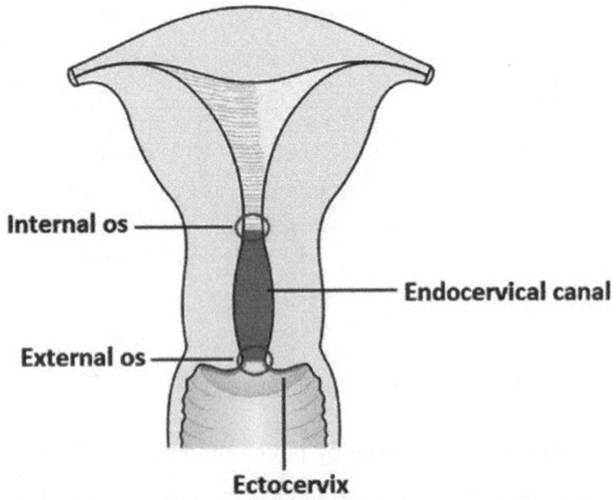

Fallopian tube

- Situated in the medial 3/4th of the upper free margin of the broad ligaments
- **2 openings:** Uterine (1 mm in diameter) & pelvic/ abdominal ostium (2 mm in diameter)
- **4 parts:**
  - **Intramural/interstitial:** ½ inch in length (L) and 1 mm in diameter (D)
  - **Isthmus:** 1 inch (L) and 2.5 mm (D)
  - **Ampulla:** 2 inch (L)
  - **Infundibulum:** ½ inch (L) and 6 mm (D)

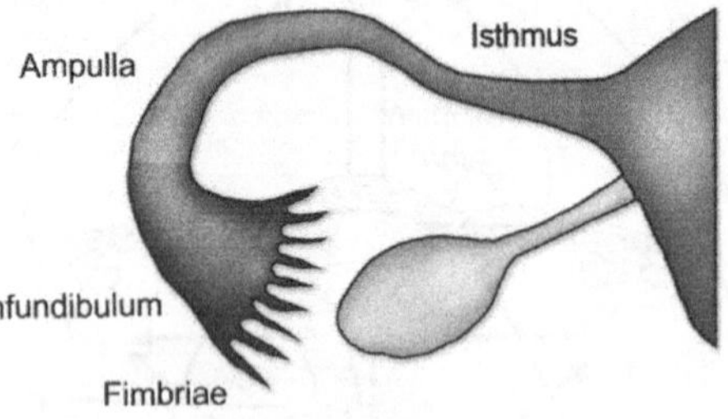

- **Blood supply:**
  - Uterine & ovarian artery
  - Venous drainage through pampiniform plexus into ovarian veins

- **Lined by: Ciliated** columnar epithelium
- **Length:** 10 cms

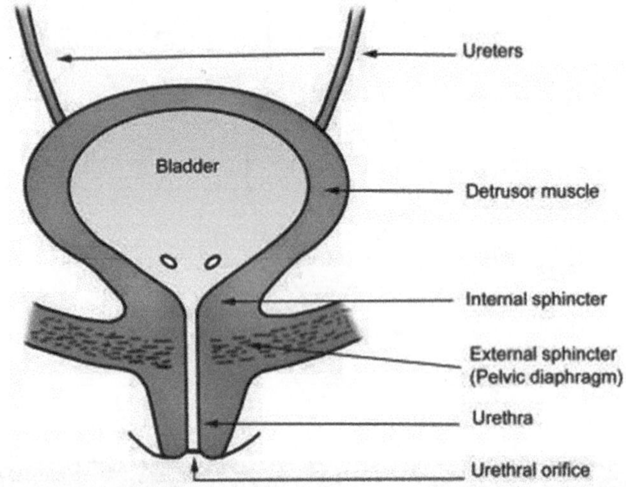

Female urethra

- **Length:** 4 cm (diameter: 6 mm)
- **Lining:** Transitional epithelium (**except** at the external urethral meatus where it becomes stratified squamous)
- Skene's gland (homologous to prostate) open into urethral posterior wall
- **Arterial supply:**
  - Proximal part by inferior vesical branch
  - Distal part by internal pudendal artery branch

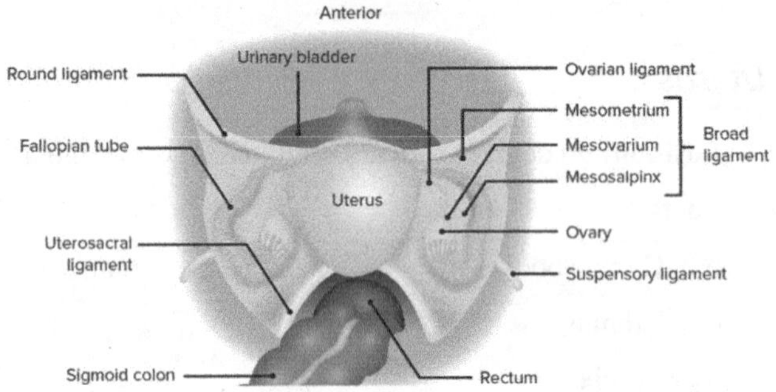

Ovary

- Attached to posterior leaf of the broad ligament by the mesovarium
- Ovarian fossa is related posteriorly to the ureter
- Cortex has follicular structures
- Medulla has hilus cells (like interstitial cells of testes)

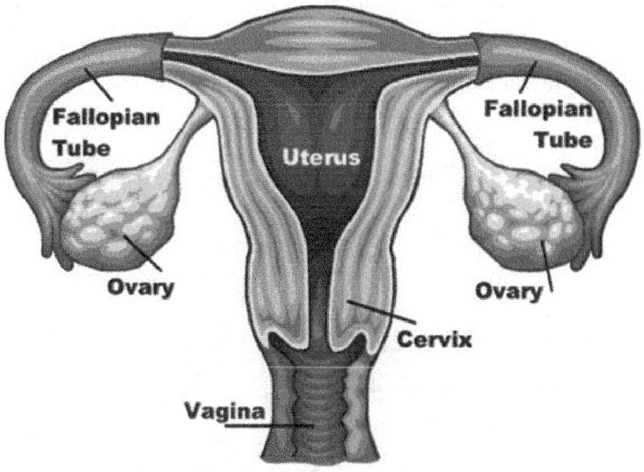

Vagina

- **4 fornices:**
  - o 2 lateral
  - o Anterior
  - o Posterior (deepest)
- For hormonal cytology (vaginal smears), the lateral wall of the upper third of the vagina is used as this part is **most** sensitive to the hormonal influence
- Epithelium is stratified squamous **without** any secreting glands
- pH is 4 – 5 (acidic) from puberty **till** menopause

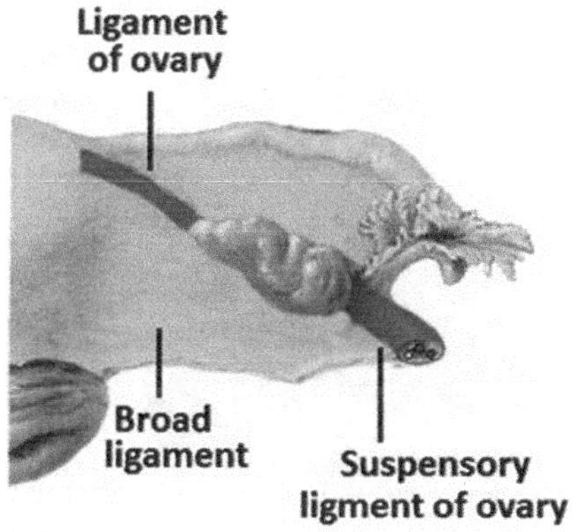

Broad ligament

- **4 parts:**
  - o Infundibulopelvic ligament
  - o Mesovarium
  - o Mesosalpinx
  - o Mesometrium
- Contains fallopian tube, round ligament, ovarian ligament, parametrium, nerves & lymphatics of uterus, tubes & ovaries

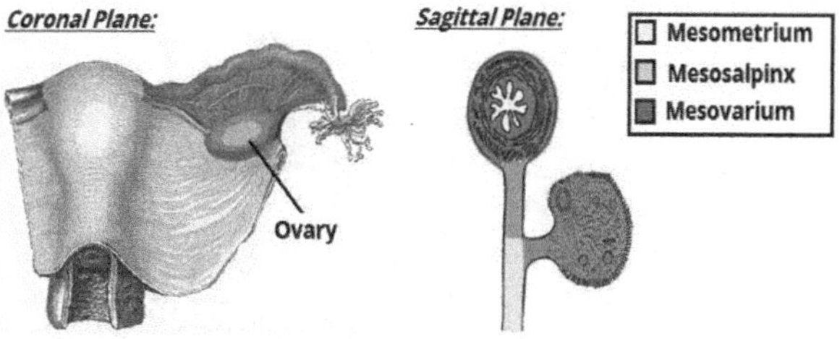

Round ligament

- 10-12 cm
- One end is attached to cornua of uterus and the other terminates in the anterior third of the labium majus

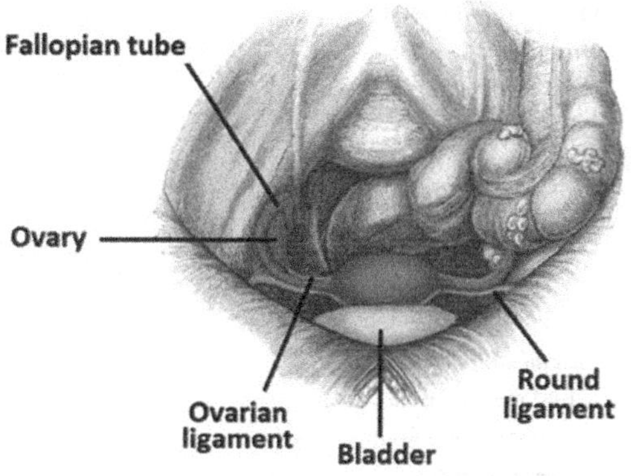

Perineal pouch/PP

- **Deep PP:** Formed by the inferior & superior layer of the urogenital diaphragm

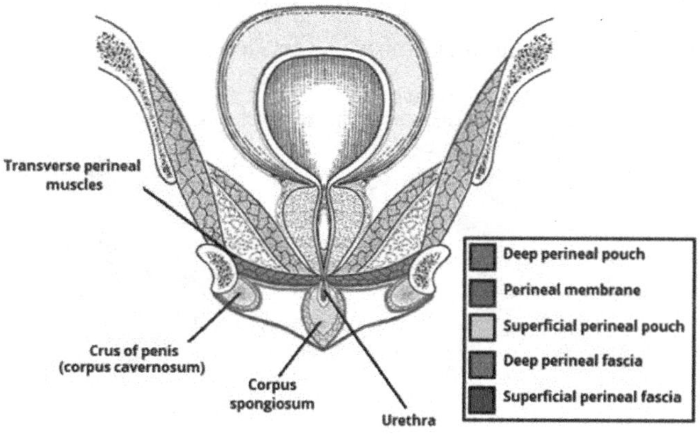

- **Superficial perineal pouch:** Formed by deep layer of the superficial perineal fascia and the inferior layer of the urogenital diaphragm

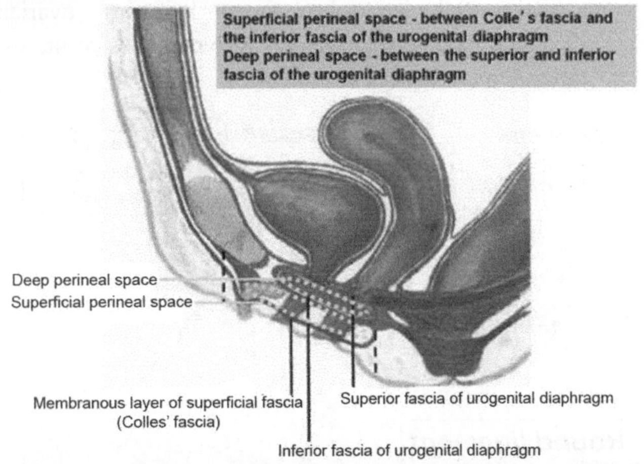

SUPPORT OF UTERUS

SUPPORTS OF UTERUS
PRIMARY SUPPORTS • **Fibromuscular supports:** (a) ***Muscular supports:*** 1. Pelvic diaphragm 2. Perineal body 3. Urogenital diaphragm (b) ***Ligamentary supports:*** 1. Pubocervical ligament 2. Transverse cervical ligament 3. Uterosacral ligament (c) ***Fascial support:*** 1. Endopelvic fascia 2. Vesicovaginal fascia 3. Rectovaginal fascia • **Uterine axis** • **Round ligamnet**

Relevant anatomy

- Important support structures of uterus are:
  - o The Cardinal/Transverse cervical ligament

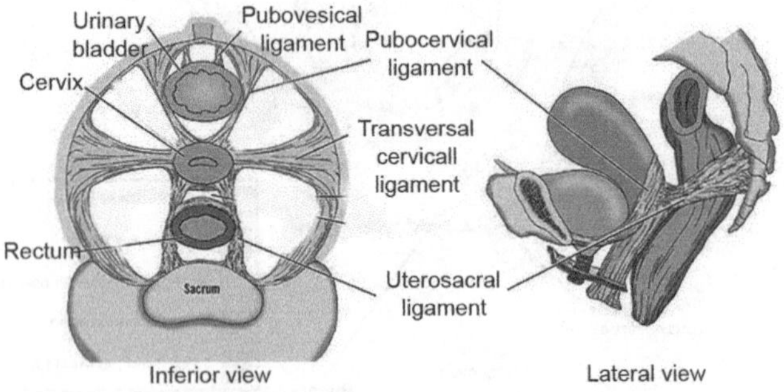

  - o Uterosacral ligament
  - o Pubocervical ligament
  - o Levator ani muscle (pubococcygeus, iliococcygeus, levator plate)

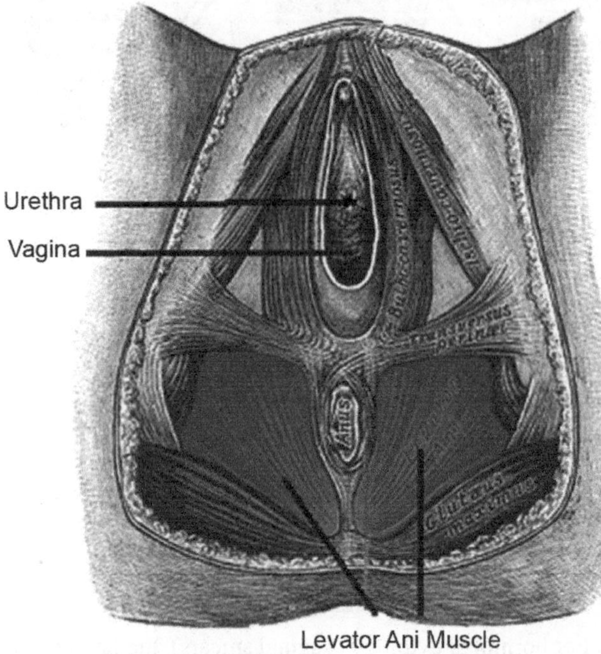

  - o Endopelvic fascia
  - o Perineal body

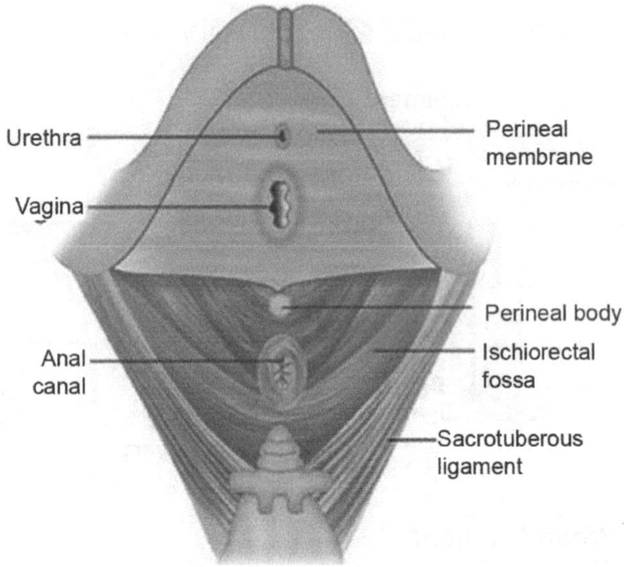

- The hammock like arrangements of the levator ani muscle, the condensed endopelvic fascia, especially the Mackenrodt's ligaments (transverse cervical/cardinal ligament) are the **cardinal** supports of the uterus

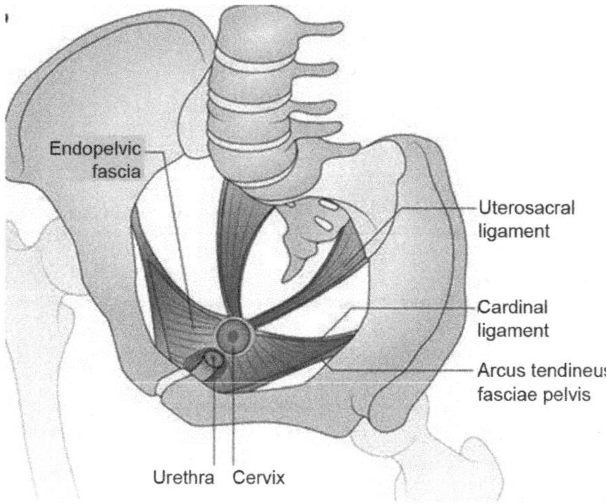

- The levator plate and the perineal body **maintains** the normal vaginal axis

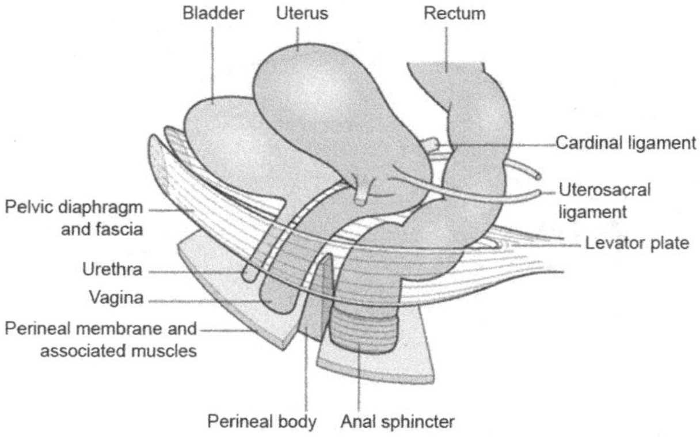

PHYSIOLOGY

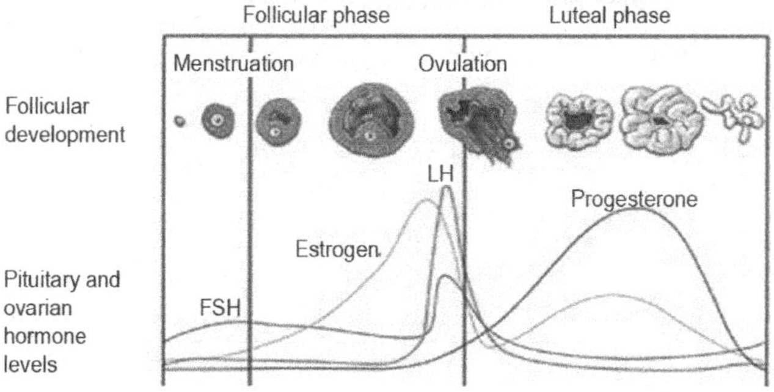

Ovulation

- **Best predictor of ovulation:** Pre-ovulatory rise in LH
- Sustained peak level of estradiol for about 24 hours beyond 200 pg/mL in late follicular phase results in LH surge (**positive** feedback effect)
- Ovulation occurs approximately **32-36** hours after the onset of LH surge and about **10-12** hours after the LH peak
- The mean duration of LH surge is about 24 hours

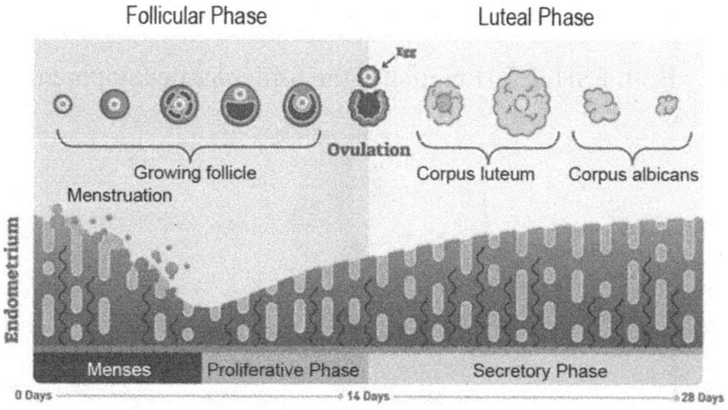

- After ovulation, the ruptured Graafian follicle becomes corpus luteum/CL
- Regression of CL starts on day **22-23** of infertile cycle
- LH hormone, with adequate number of LH receptors in the granulosa cells (as induced during folliculogenesis) with increased secretion of estradiol, is the **key** factor of adequate corpus luteum formation
- **Ovulatory period:** Corresponds to 14 days before next menstruation
- **LH stimulates:** Follicle rupture & ovulation

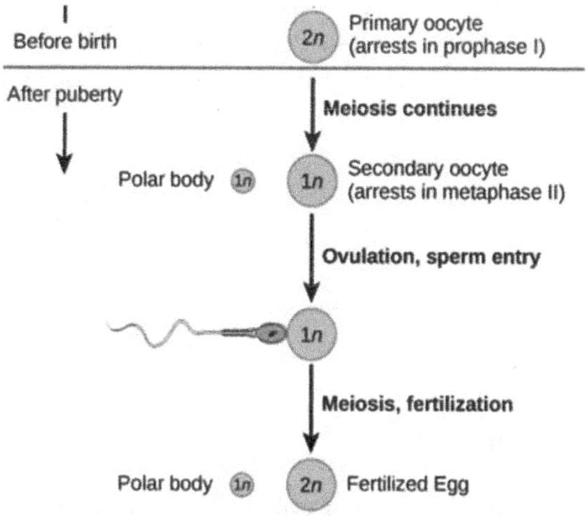

- Primary oocyte **undergoes** first meiotic division giving rise to secondary oocyte and one polar body just prior to ovulation

- The secondary oocyte completes the second meiotic division **only** after fertilization by a sperm in the fallopian tube
- **One follicle with highest antral concentration of estrogen & lowest androgen:** Estrogen ratio and the granulosa cells containing the maximum receptors for FSH becomes the **dominant** follicle
- Both FSH & LH regulates the follicular development

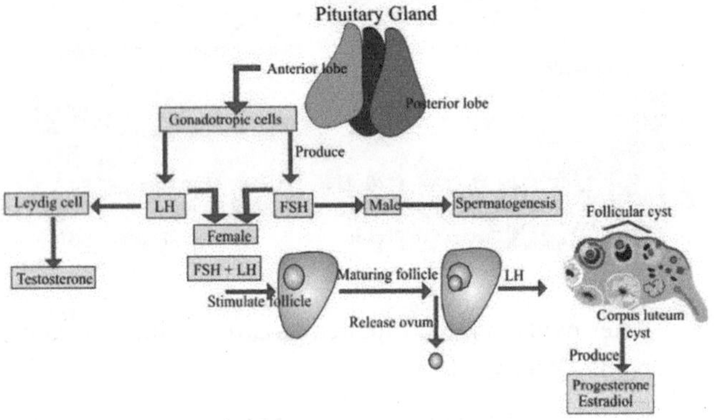

LH

- Stimulates (LH surge) the **completion** of first meiotic division
- Luteinization of granulosa cells
- Synthesis of progesterone & prostaglandins

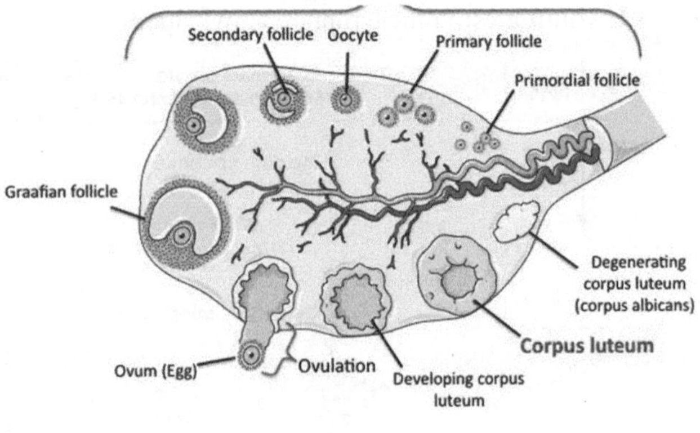

Corpus luteum

- **In normal menstrual cycle, progesterone is secreted by:** Corpus luteum
- Corpus luteum secretes estrogen & progesterone both

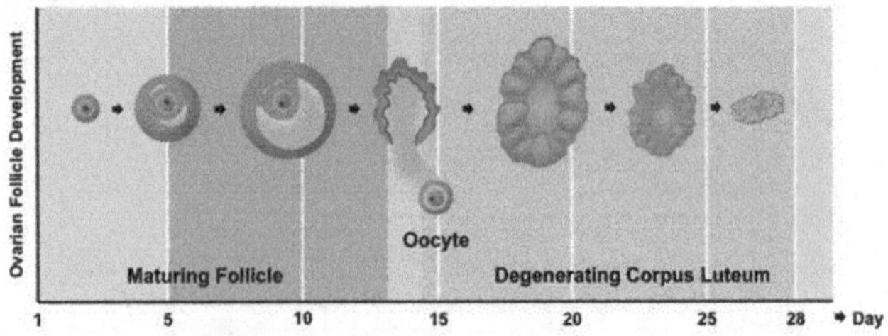

Follicular phase
- FSH causes follicle to mature and produce estrogen (inhibiting development of other follicles)

Ovulation
- An LH surge causes ovulation (follicle ruptures and releases a secondary oocyte)

Luteal phase
- Ruptured follicle forms a corpus luteum and secretes progesterone (and some estrogen)

Inhibin

- A peptide secreted by granulosa cells in response to FSH
- **Potent** inhibitor of FSH

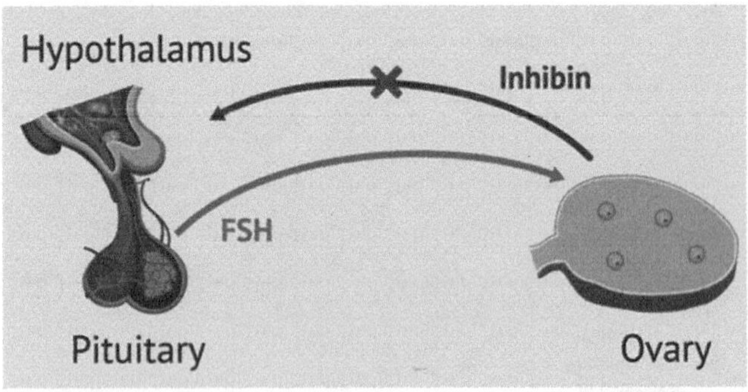

Menstruation

- **Amount of blood loss in menstruation:** Up to 80 ml (average 35 mL)
- **Average age of menarche:** 13 years
- **Average loss of iron in each menses:** 13 mg

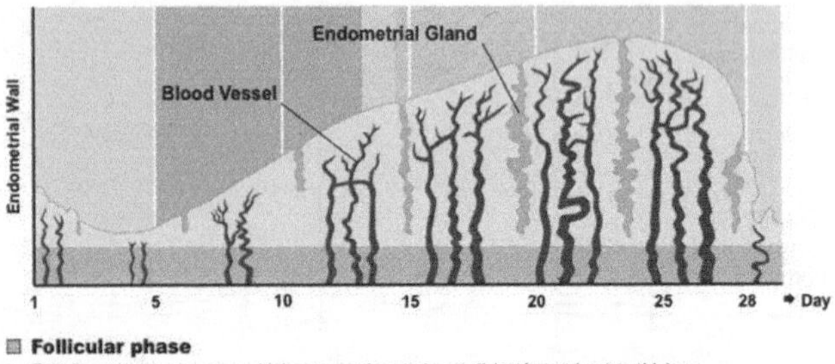

Follicular phase
- Follicles release estrogen which causes the uterine wall (endometrium) to thicken

Ovulation
- When the follicle ruptures and develops into a corpus luteum, progesterone is produced

Luteal phase
- Progesterone and estrogen are released from the corpus luteum and thicken the endometrium

Lactobacillus/Doderlein

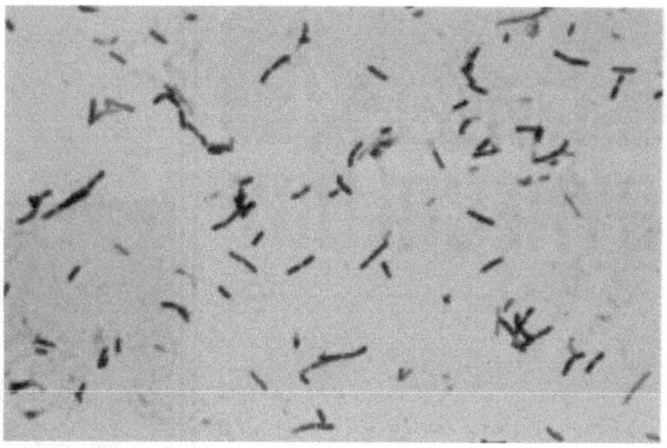

- Rod shaped gram-**positive** bacillus
- Appears at 3-4 days after birth & disappears after 10-14 days of birth
- Appears again at puberty & disappears after menopause
- Converts glycogen into lactic acid so that vaginal **pH** is maintained towards acidic side to prevent growth of pathogenic organisms
- **Protective bacterium in normal vagina:** Lactobacillus/ Doderlein

SECTION 4
GYNECOLOGY

Chapter 2

Genital Infections

BACTERIAL VAGINOSIS/BV

Bacterial vaginosis

- **Caused by:** Gardnerella/haemophilus vaginalis & anaerobic organisms (Bacteroides species, Peptococcus species, mobiluncus and Mycoplasma hominis)
- Marked **reduction** in lactobacilli
- **Features:**
  - Creamy (homogenous, greyish-white) and adherent vaginal discharge with **fishy** smell without evidence of inflammation

Bacterial Vaginosis Discharge

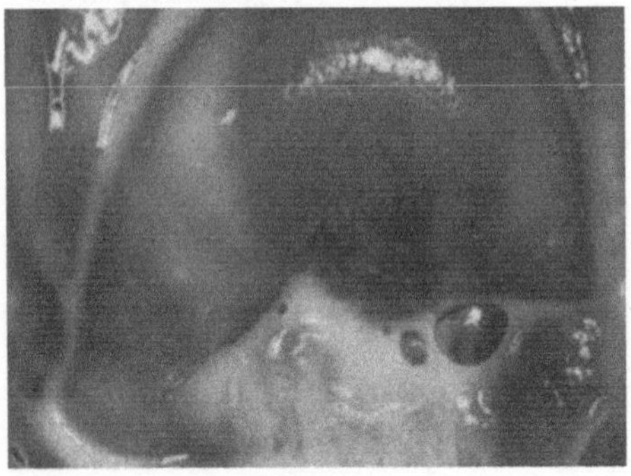

- **Amsel's four diagnostic criteria:**
  - Homogenous vaginal discharge
  - Vaginal pH >**4.5** (litmus paper test)
  - **Positive** Whiff test (Fishy/amine odor when a drop of discharge is mixed with 10% KOH solution)

Clue cells gram stain

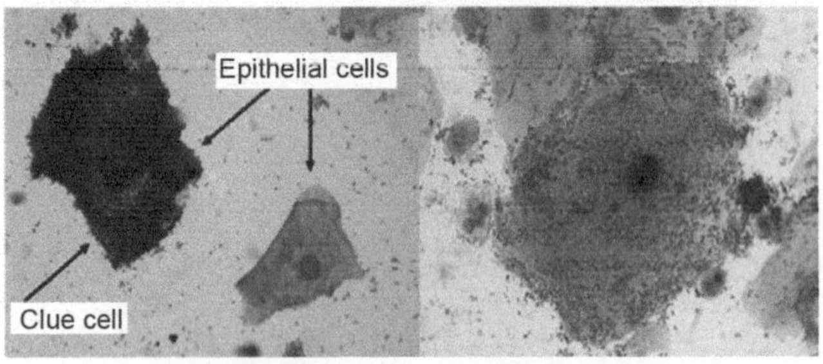

- **Presence of clue cells (>20% of cells):**
  - A smear of vaginal discharge is prepared with drops of normal saline & is seen under microscope
  - Vaginal epithelial cells are seen covered with coccobacilli & the cells appear as stippled or granular (clue **cells**)

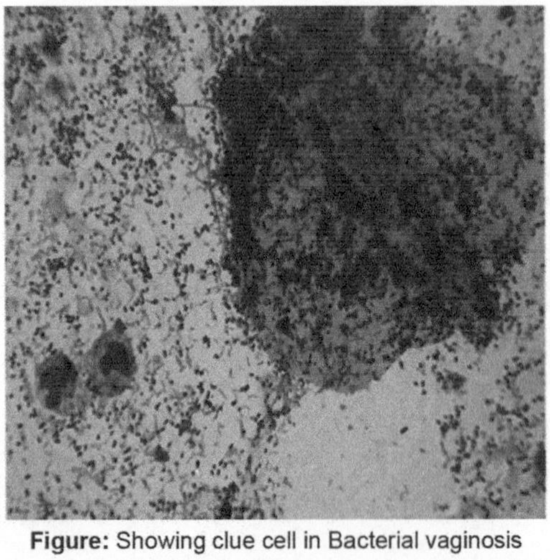

Figure: Showing clue cell in Bacterial vaginosis

- **Investigation:**
  - o **Gram-stained vaginal smear:** Presence of more Gardnerella or mobiluncus morphotypes with few or absent lactobacilli
- **Management:**
  - o Managed with oral metronidazole
  - o Clindamycin cream & metronidazole gel are recommended for vaginal application
  - o Treat the partner **simultaneously**
- **Clue cells in vagina, fishy odour, positive Whiff test signifies:** Infection with Hemophilus vaginalis (bacterial vaginosis)
- **ph more than 4.5, clue cells, amine odour:** Bacterial vaginosis

VULVOVAGINAL CANDIDIASIS/VVC

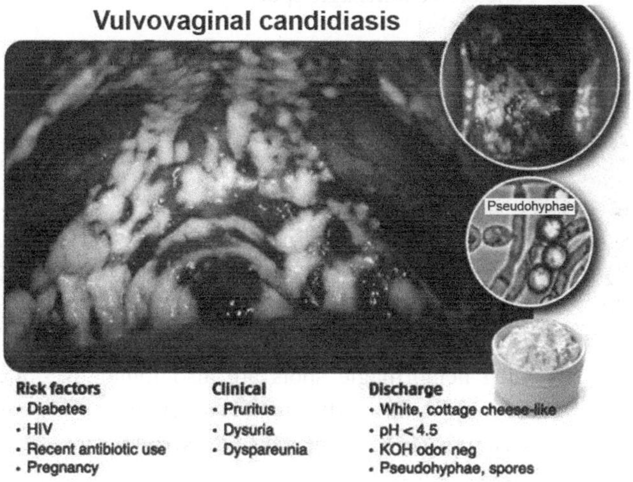

Candida vaginitis/moniliasis

- Candida albicans is a gram-positive yeast-like fungus
- **Predisposing conditions:** Diabetes, pregnancy, antibiotics, HIV

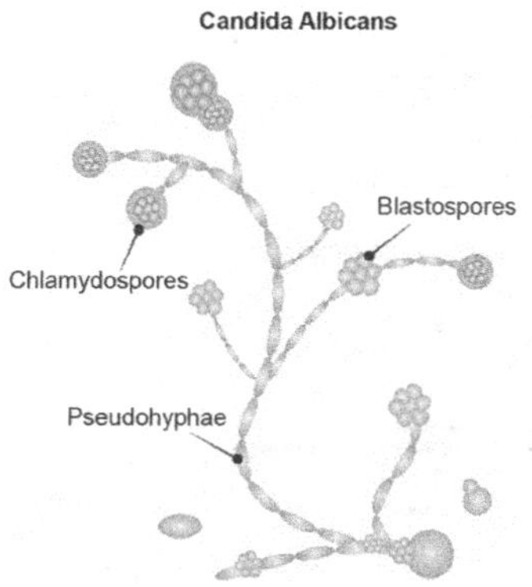

- **Features:**
  - o Vaginal discharge with intense vulvovaginal pruritis
  - o Pruritis is **out** of proportion to the discharge
  - o Discharge is thick, **curdy** white and in flakes (cottage cheese type) often adherent

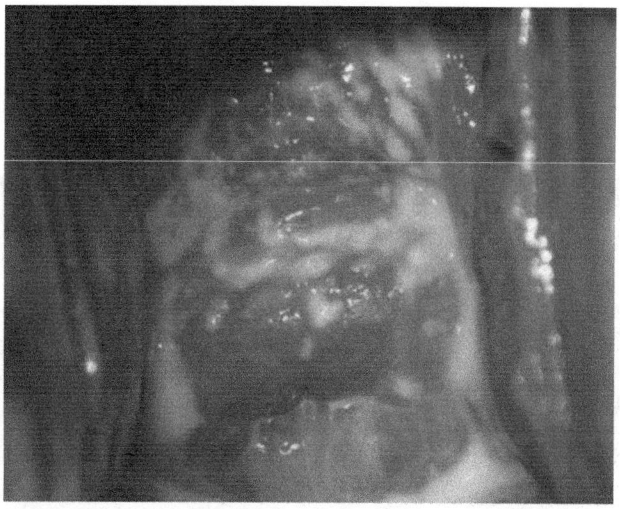

Figure: The speculum exam of a patient with vaginal candidiasis. There is thick white discharge without cervical inflammation

  - o Removal of white flakes reveals multiple oozing spots
- **Investigations:**
  - o Wet smear of vaginal discharge is prepared. KOH solution is added to lyse the other cells
  - o Filamentous form of mycelia, pseudohyphae can be seen under microscope

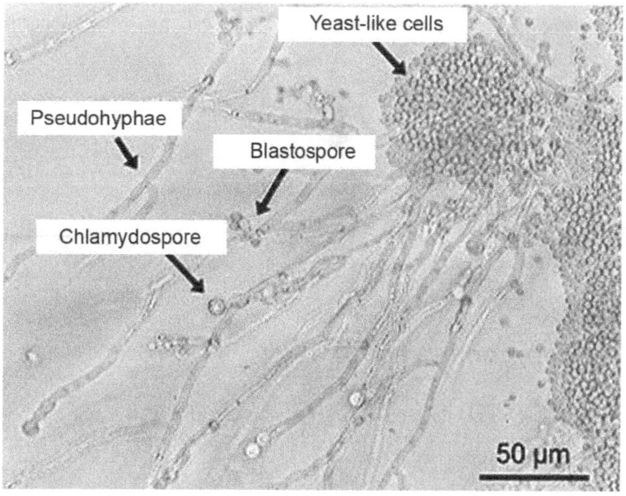

  - o Culture in Nickerson or Sabouraud's media become positive in 24-72 hours

- **Management:**
  - o Correction of predisposing conditions
  - o Local fungicidal preparations (cream/pessary) are used (nystatin, clotrimazole, miconazole)
  - o Single dose oral therapy with fluconazole/ itraconazole
  - o Treat the partner **simultaneously**
- **Intense Pruritis, vulvovaginitis, cheesy curdy discharge:** Candidiasis

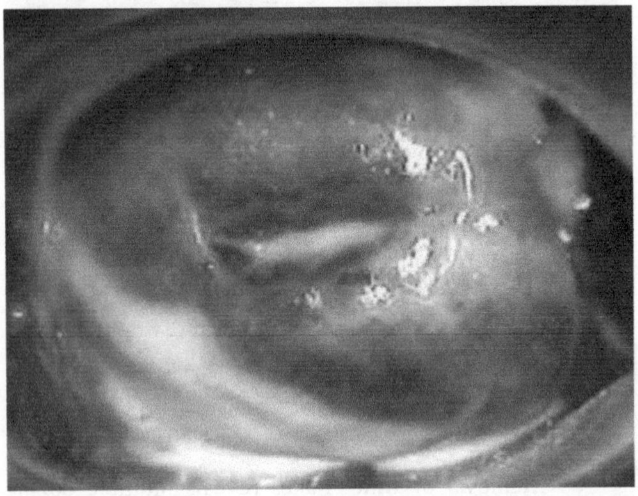

TRICHOMONAS VAGINITIS/TV

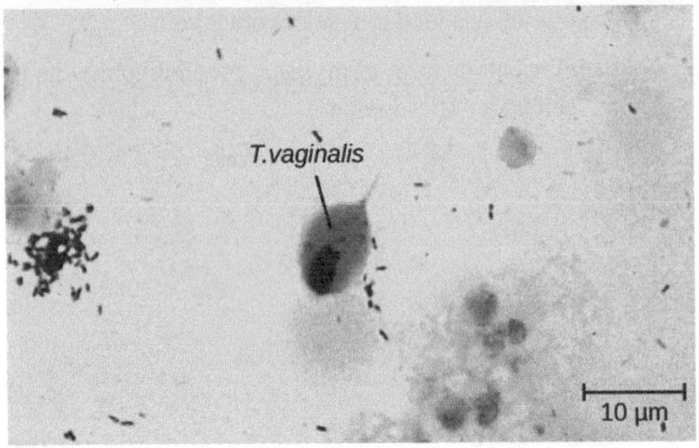

Trichomonas vaginitis

- **MC** (STD) cause of vaginitis in childbearing age
- **Features:**
  - o Sudden profuse and offensive vaginal discharge
  - o Irritation & itching
  - o Urinary symptoms (dysuria & frequency)

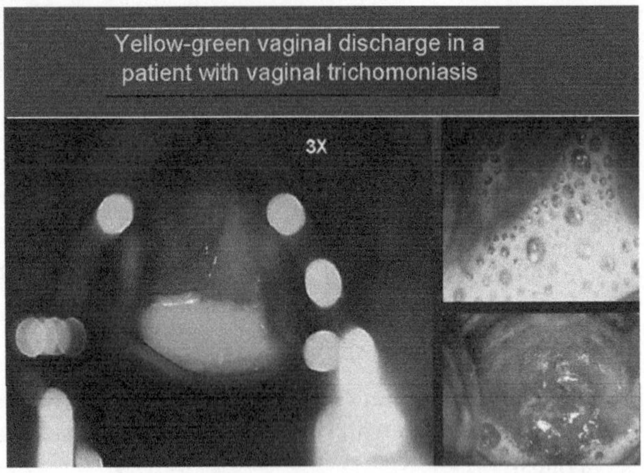

  - o Thin, **greenish**-yellow and frothy offensive discharge per vaginum
  - o Vulva is inflamed with evidence of pruritis
  - o Vaginal walls become red & inflamed with multiple punctate hemorrhagic spots

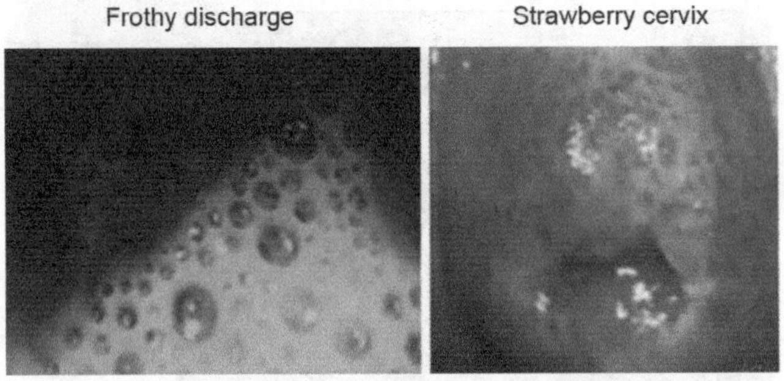

  - o Such hemorrhagic spots are also found over the mucosa of the portio vaginalis part of the cervix, giving rise to the appearance of '**strawberry**'
- **Investigation:**
  - o Identification of the trichomonas is done by hanging drop preparation

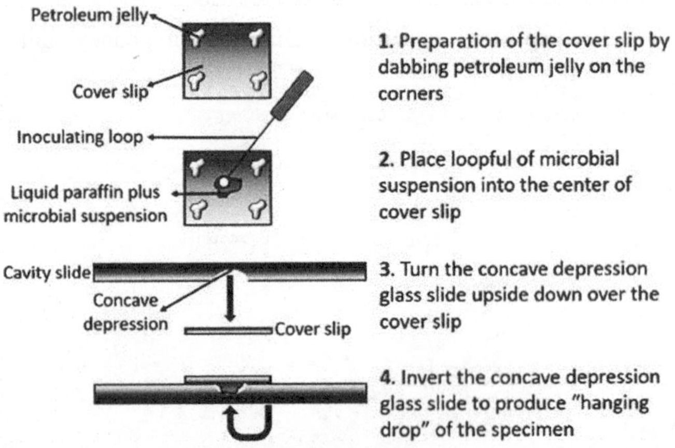

Figure: Procedure of hanging drop method

- o Culture of the discharge collected by swabs in Diamond's TYM or Feinberg Whittington medium
- **Management:**
  - o Managed by metronidazole
  - o **Husband** should be given the same treatment schedule
  - o Until the wife is cured, husband **should** use barrier contraceptive
- **Profuse, thin, creamy/slightly greenish, irritating frothy discharge & motile trophozoites (flagellate protozoa with motility):** Trichomonas vaginalis (pear shaped unicellular flagellate protozoa)

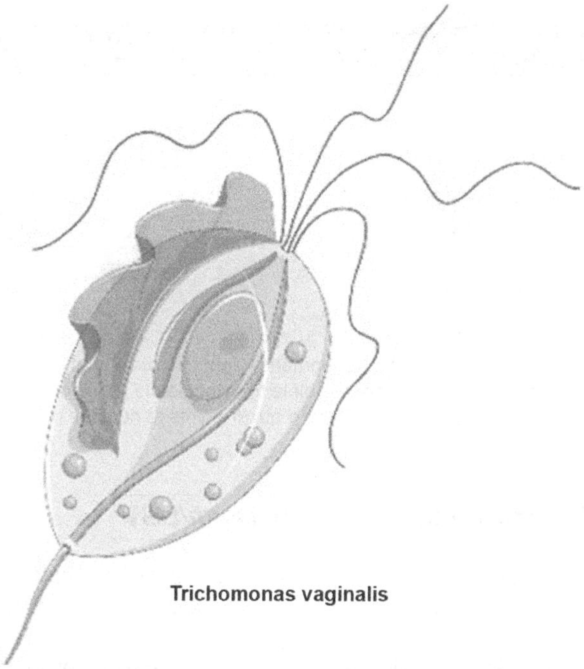

Trichomonas vaginalis

QUICK RECAP

Quick Recap

- **Bacterial vaginosis:**
  - o **Caused by:** Multibacterial
    - ♦ Hemophilus vaginalis
    - ♦ Gardnerella
    - ♦ Mobiluncus (corkscrew spinning anaerobe)
  - o **Clinical presentation:** White, **Milky**, homogenous & adherent discharge
  - o **Vaginal pH:** Alkaline (greater than 4.5)
  - o **Histological feature: Clue** cells
  - o **DOC:** Metronidazole
- **Vulvovaginal Candidiasis:**
  - o Profuse **curdy**, white discharge (cottage cheese appearance)
  - o Intense itching
- **Trichomonas vaginitis:**
  - o **Caused by:** Trichomonas vaginalis (flagellate parasite)
  - o **Clinical presentation:** Profuse, thin, frothy, **greenish** discharge (malodourous)
  - o **Appearance of vagina: Strawberry** vagina
  - o **DOC:** Metronidazole

	BV	VVC	TV
Symptoms	Asymptomatic	Vulvar pruritus and burning	Pruritus
Vaginal discharge	Gray, Fishy odor	White, Cottage cheese	Yellow, purulent, malodorous
Vaginal wall	Normal	Erythema, edema	Erythema
pH	>4.5 (4.7 to 5.7)	<4.5	>5
Whiff test	Positive	Negative	Negative
Microscopy	Clue cells	Budding yeast forms or mycelia	Trichomonads, leukocytes

GONORRHOEA

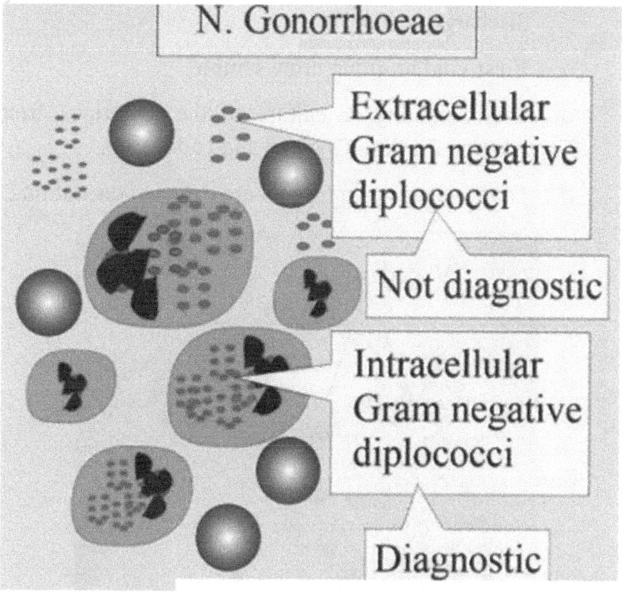

Gonorrhoea

- **Caused by**: N. gonorrhoeae, a gram-negative diplococcus
- **Principal** sites of involvement are endocervix, urethra, Skene's gland and Bartholin's gland (columnar and transitional epithelium)
- Squamous epithelium is resistant to gonococcal invasion, so vaginitis in adults is **not** possible
- **Features:**
  - o 50% cases are asymptomatic
  - o Urinary symptoms (dysuria)

Female Gonorrhoea

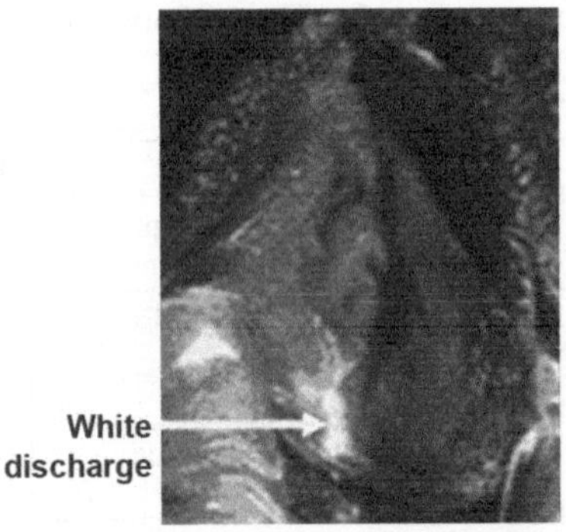

  - o Irritant vaginal mucopurulent discharge
  - o On squeezing the urethra and giving pressure on the Bartholin's glands, purulent exudate escapes
- **Investigations:**
  - o Nucleic acid amplification testing/NAAT (**very** sensitive & specific) of urine or endocervical discharge is done
  - o **First** void morning urine sample
  - o Gram staining & culture of the secretions from urethra, Bartholin's gland and endocervix
  - o Gram-negative diplococci are detected on staining

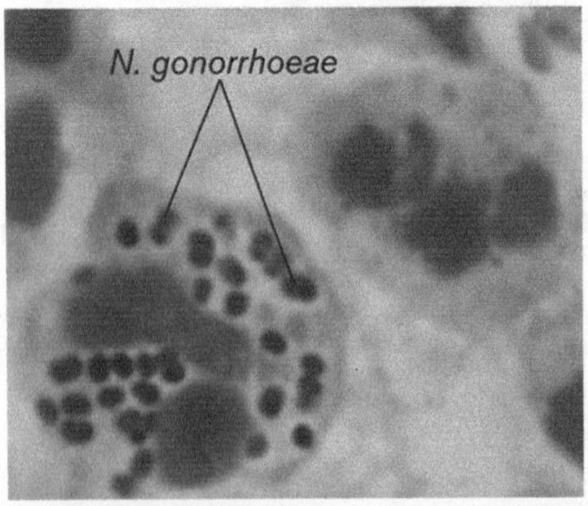

- **Culture:**
  - o Culture of the discharge in Thayer-Martin medium **confirms** the diagnosis
  - o Culture should be made 7 days after therapy
  - o Repeat culture should be made at monthly intervals following menses **for** three months
  - o If the reports are persistently negative, the patient is declared cured
- Managed by **single** dose regimen of ceftriaxone/ciprofloxacin/ofloxacin/cefixime/levofloxacin
- **Mucopurulent urethral discharge, gram-negative intracellular diplococci in PMN's:** N. Gonorrhoea

LYMPHOGRANULOMA VENEREUM

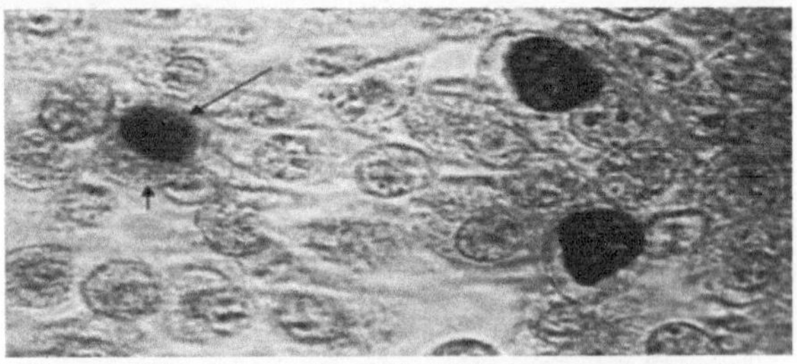

Figure: Chlamydia trachomatis–Light microscopy of cell culture. Long arrow points to cytoplasmic inclusion body of C.trachomatis; short arrow points to nucleus of cell

Lymphogranuloma venereum/LGV

- **Caused by:** L serotypes of Chlamydia trachomatis
- **Features:**
  - o **Initial** lesion is painless papule, pustule or ulcer in the vulva, urethra, rectum or the cervix
  - o Inguinal nodes are involved (**feels** rubbery)

Lymphogranuloma venereum, LGV lymphadenopathy

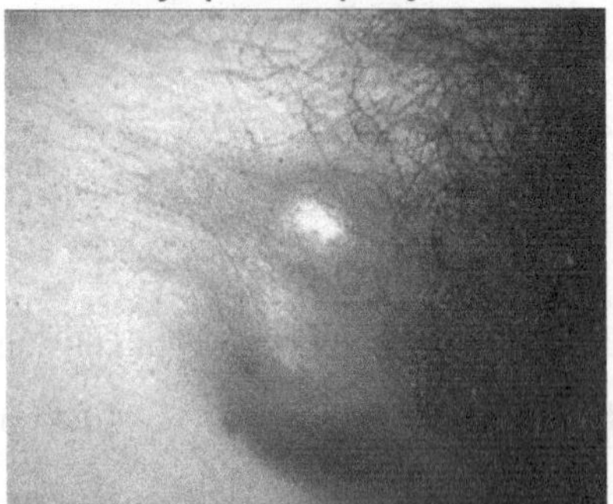

Mixed granulomatous and neutrophilic inflammation

- o Acute lymphangitis & lymphadenitis
- o Lymphatic obstruction leads to vulval elephantiasis
- o Glands become necrosed and abscess (**bubo**) forms
- o Bubo ruptures & multiple draining sinuses & fistula forms
- o **Classical** clinical sign is groove sign

LGV:

GROOVE SIGN

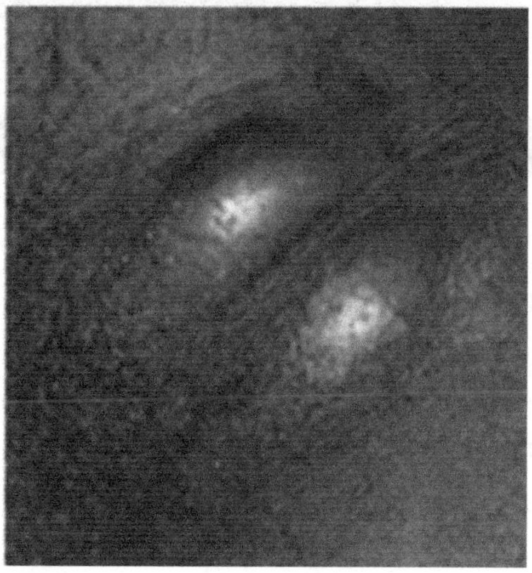

- **Diagnosis:**
  - o Culture & isolation (lymph node aspiration)
  - o Detection of LGV antigen in pus obtained from a bubo
  - o Detection of LGV antigen by ELISA
  - o LGV complement fixation test
  - o Intradermal Frei test (unreliable)
- Manage with Doxycycline/azithromycin/erythromycin
- Treat the **partner** as well
- Abscess should be aspirated (not excised)

Chlamydia inclusion bodies

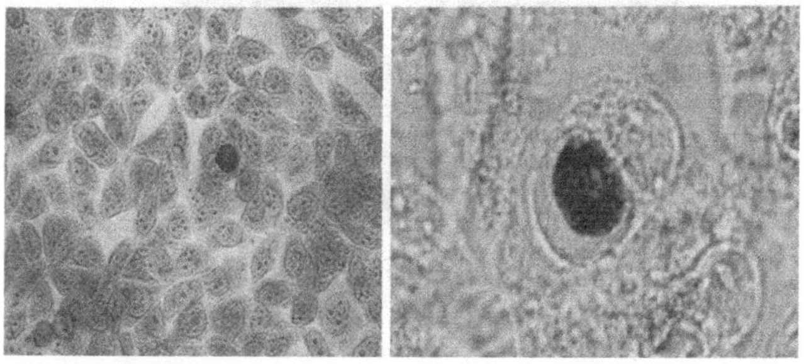

- **Culture (Feinberg-Whittington medium) & inclusion bodies in the smear from urethra & vaginal ulcer:** Chlamydia trachomatis

CHANCROID

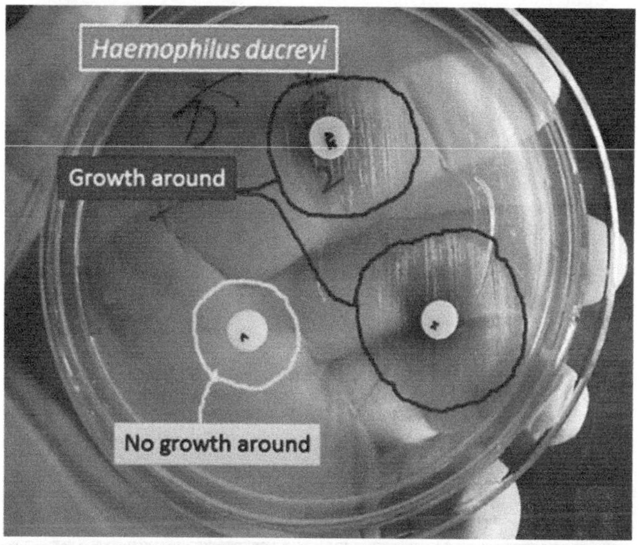

Chancroid/Soft sore

- **Caused by:** H. ducreyi (Gram-negative streptobacillus)

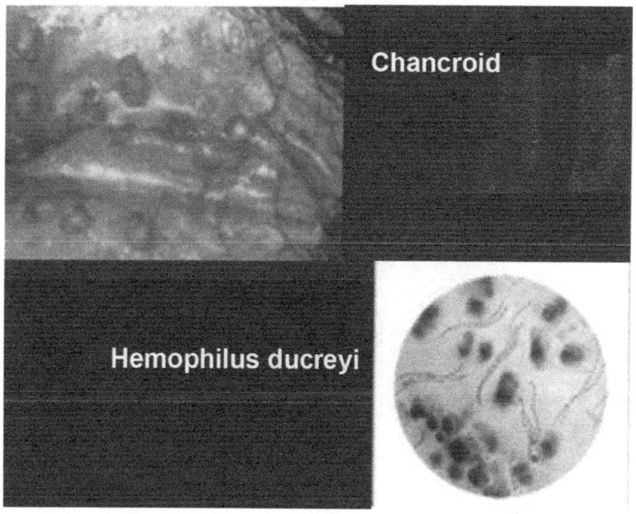

- **Presentation:**
  - o Genital ulcer (**painful**)
  - o Lesion start as multiple vesiculopustules over the vulva, vagina or cervix
  - o It then sloughs to form shallow ulcers
  - o Lesion is very tender (there may be cluster of ulcers)
  - o Inguinal adenitis (inguinal **buboes**)

- o Unilateral inguinal lymphadenitis may occur which may suppurate to form abscess (buboes)
- **Culture appearance:** School of fish/Shoal of fish appearance

Chancroid-gram stain of *H. ducreyi*

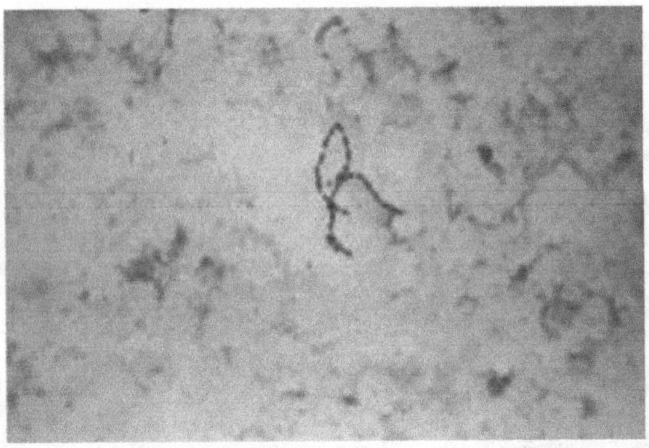

- It is **difficult** to grow the organism on culture medium
- **DOC:** Azithromycin/Ceftriaxone/Ciprofloxacin/Co-trimoxazole

SYPHILIS

Primary chancre on cervix

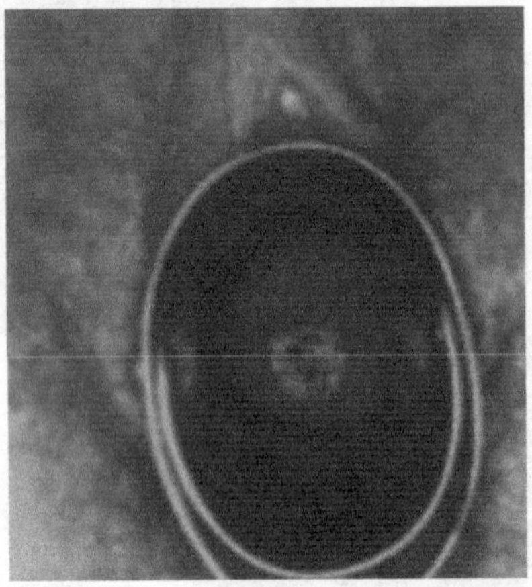

Syphilis

- **Caused by:** Treponema pallidum
- Hard chancre of primary syphilis is **painless** with an indurated base
- VDRL & TPHA tests are used for **screening** and FTA-abs is used for **confirmation**
- I/M Benzathine penicillin is used for treatment

Syphilitic chancre, Female abdomen

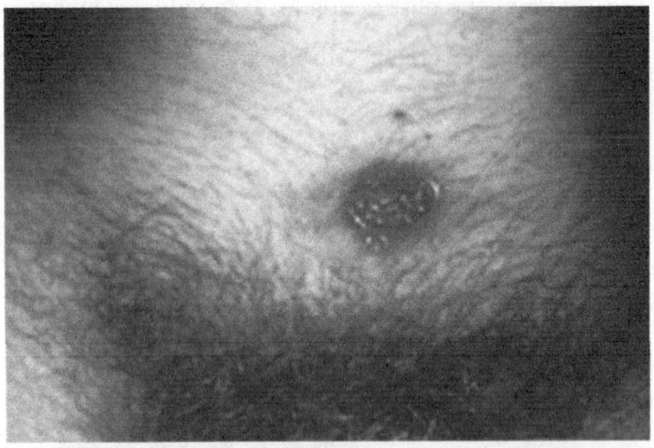

GENITAL TUBERCULOSIS

Genital TB

- **MC site of primary TB infection in body:**
  - o Lungs (50%)
  - o Lymph nodes (40%)
- **MC site of affection in genital TB:** Fallopian tubes
- Pelvic organs are affected secondarily, the **primary** site is predominantly in lung
- Spread is by hematogenous route
- Fallopian tubes are almost always affected **(100%)** bilaterally
- **Presentation:**
  - o Infertility presents in 70% of cases
  - o Menorrhagia may be the **early** symptom but more commonly, the patient presents with oligomenorrhoea/amenorrhoea

Beaded Appearance..

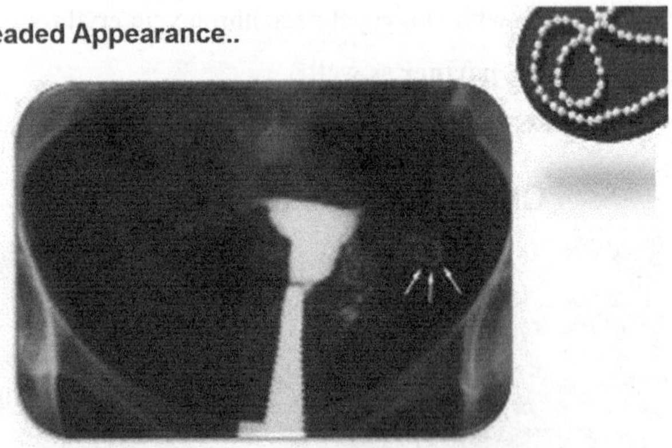

Figure: Multiple constrictions along the course of fallopian tube on HSG due to fibrotic strictures

- **Diagnosis is confirmed by:**
  - o Histological examination
  - o Culture in Lowenstein-Jensen media and guinea-pig inoculation
  - o Identification of bacteria by Ziehl-Neelsen's stain from the uterine curettage material
- PCR is **most** sensitive

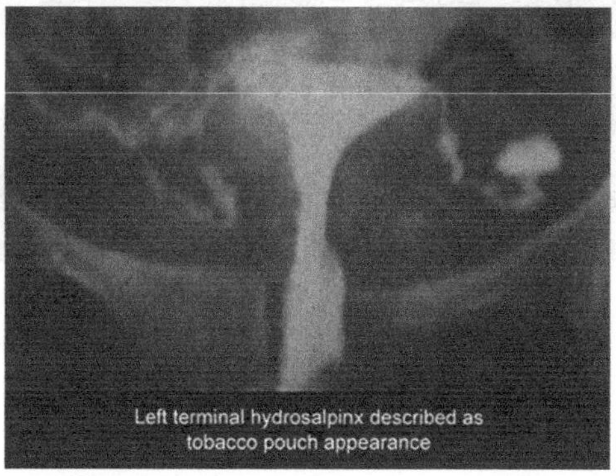

Left terminal hydrosalpinx described as tobacco pouch appearance

- **Hysterosalpingography:**
  - o In a proved case, HSG is **contraindicated** for the risk of reactivation of lesion
  - o **HSG done as a routine workup in the investigation of infertility may reveal:**
    - ♦ Rigid/lead pipe tubes
    - ♦ Tobacco **pouch** appearance with blocked fimbrial end

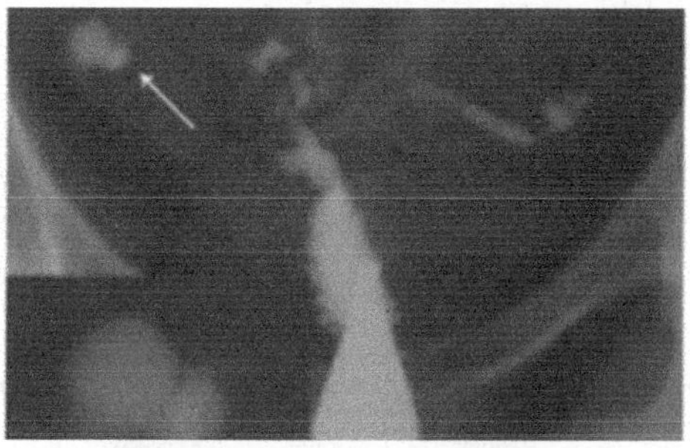

TOBACCO POUCH APPREANCE

Terminal hydrosalpinx with the conical narrowing is seen in the right tube (arrow). Eversion of the fimbria secondary to adhesions, with a patent orifice produces the tobacco pouch appearance in the left terminal

    - ♦ Bilateral cornual block
    - ♦ **Beaded** appearance of the tube with variable filling density

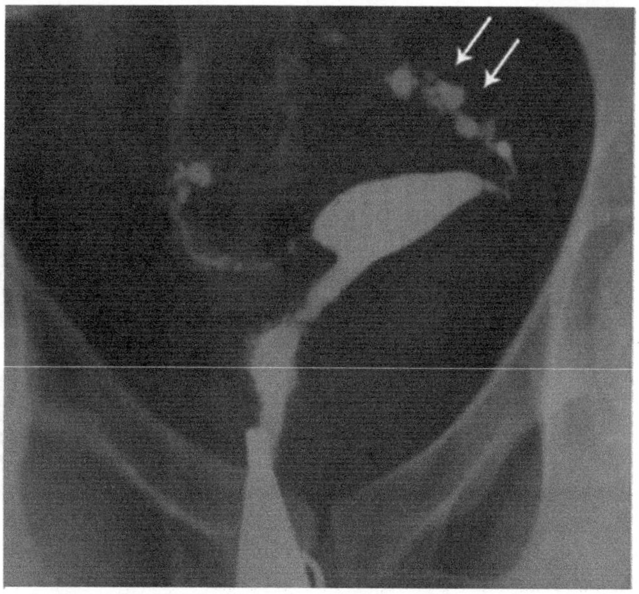

"Beaded tube". Multiple constrictions along the fallopian tube giving rise to a "beaded" appearance [arrows (32)]

- **Treatment:**
  - o **4 drugs ATT (RIPE):** Initial phase for 2 months
  - o **2 drugs ATT (RI):** Continuation phase for 4 months
- **Prognosis:**
  - o In terms of future reproduction, prognosis is most **unfavorable**
  - o Pregnancy rate is rare (5-10%)
  - o Ectopic pregnancy is more (40%)
  - o Pregnancy rarely goes up to full term

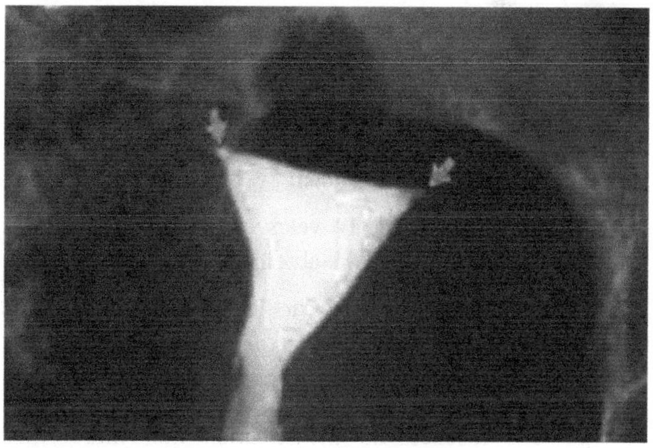

Bilateral cornual block

SECTION 4
GYNECOLOGY

Chapter 3

Menstrual Disorders

TERMINOLOGY

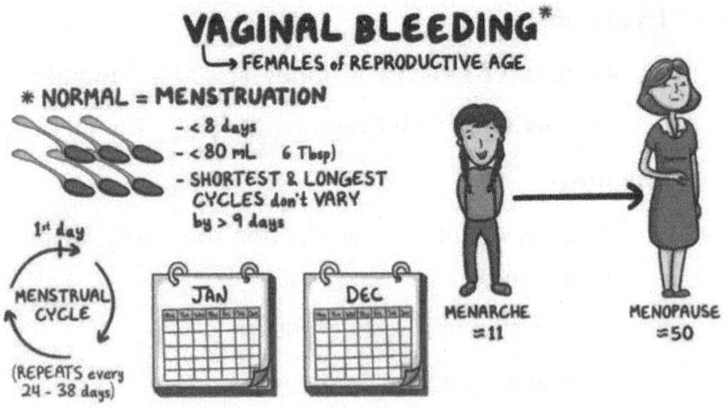

Some terms

- **Amenorrhoea:**
  - **Absence** of menstruation
  - **Primary amenorrhoea:**
    - In a girl of **14** years, thelarche, pubarche & menarche all are absent
    - In a girl of **16** years, thelarche, pubarche are present but no menarche
  - **Secondary amenorrhoea:**
    - Absence of menstruation for more than **6** months in a previously menstruating female, pregnancy being ruled out
- **Hypomenorrhoea:**
  - Periods are **scanty**
  - But regular

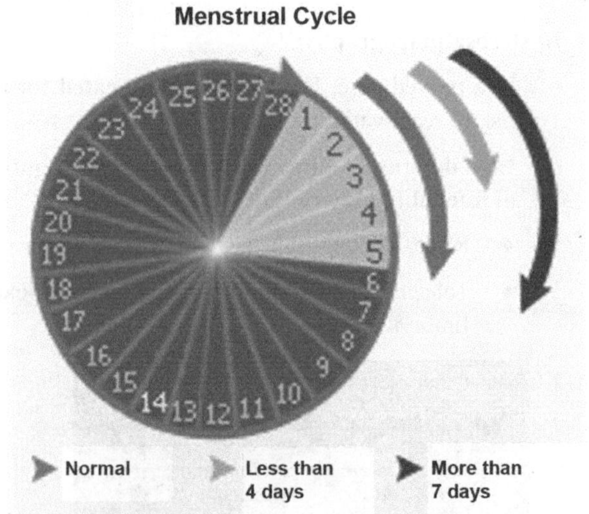

Definition	Interval	Frequency	Amount	Others
Polymenorrhea	Regular	**Increase**	Normal	< 21 days
Menorrhagia	Regular	Normal	**Excessive**	> 7 days > 80 ml
Oligomenorrhea	Regular	**Decrease**	Normal	> 35 days
Metrorrhagia	**Irregular**	Normal	Normal	————
Menometrorrhagia	**Irregular**	Normal	**Excessive**	Combination Meno + Metro

- **Polymenorrhoea:**
  - Frequent cycles
  - Menstrual cycle duration is **less** than 21 days

Polymenorrhea Menstrual Cycle

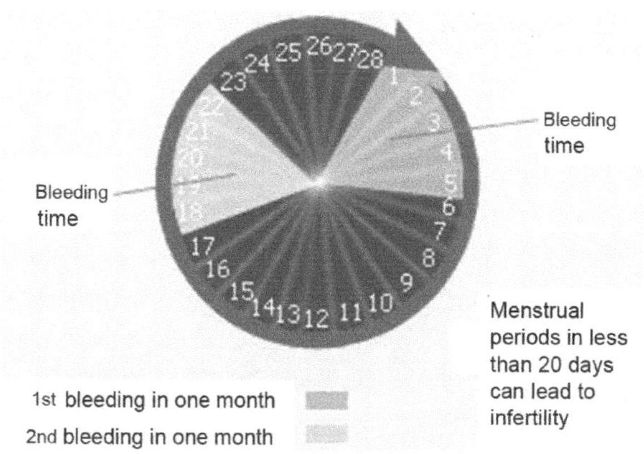

- **Menorrhagia:**
  - o Regular but **heavy** cycles
  - o Blood less is more than 80 ml
- **Oligomenorrhoea:**
  - o Duration of menstrual cycle is **more** than 35 days
- **Metrorrhagia:**
  - o **Irregularly** times episodes of bleeding
  - o Superimposed on normal cyclical bleeding
- **Precocious menstruation:**
  - o Menstruation starts **before** the age of 10 years
- **Precocious puberty:**
  - o Development of secondary sexual characters **before** the age of 8 years

ENDOMETRIOSIS

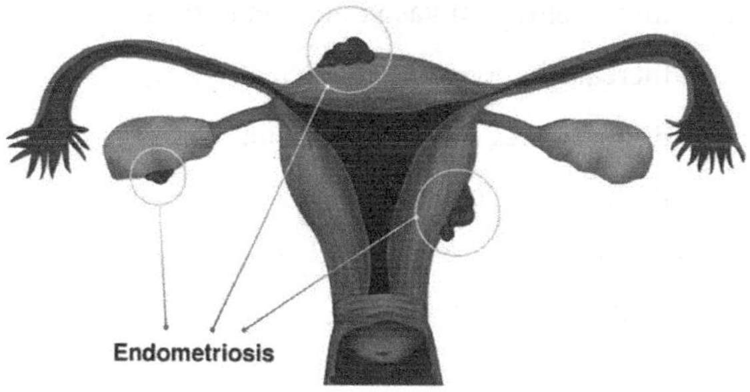

Pathology

- Presence of ectopic endometrial tissue **outside** the true cavity of the uterus
- Endometriosis **manifests** as islands of flame-shaped chocolate deposits or appear like powder burn marks
- It can cause extensive adhesions between the ovaries, back of the uterus and the pouch of Douglas, obliterating the same and causing dense rectal adhesions
- It may appear as a cystic ovarian enlargement or ovarian endometriomas (**chocolate** cyst)

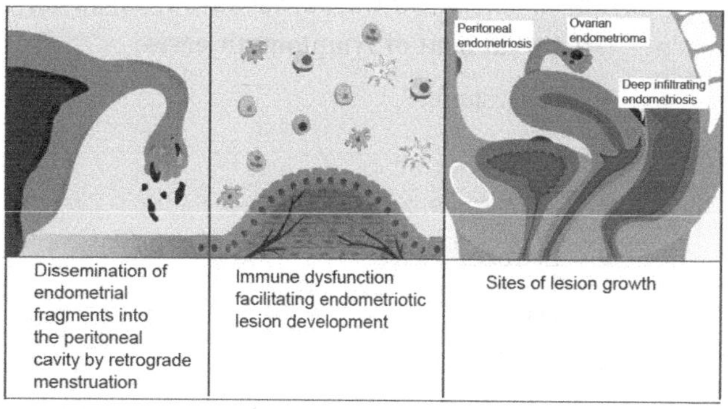

Features

- **MC accepted etiological theory:**
  - o Sampsons theory of retrograde menstruation (reflux of menstrual endometrium through the fallopian tubes and its subsequent implantation and growth on pelvic peritoneum and the surrounding structures)
  - o Other **Theories** of origin include coelomic metaplasia, vascular embolization and lymphatic permeation
- **MC presentation:**
  - o Dysmenorrhoea *(painful menstruation)*
  - o Pain begins before the onset of menstruation, builds up continuously until the flow begins, and thereafter it gradually declines
  - o Patient presents with pelvic pain, dyspareunia, menstrual disturbances and infertility
- **Associated feature:** Chocolate cysts

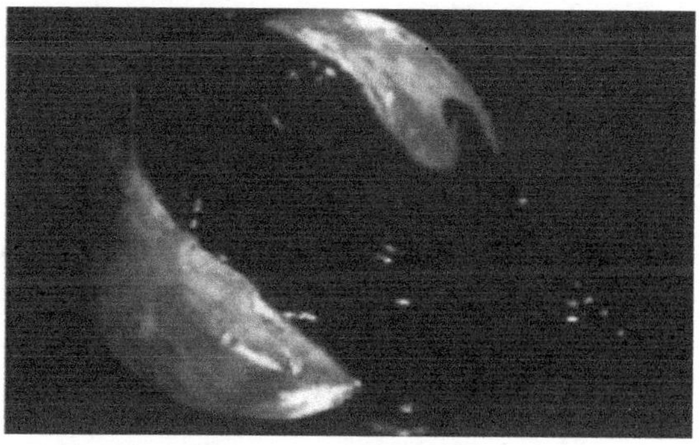

This is a section through an enlarged 12 cm ovary to demonstrate a cystic cavity filled with old blood typical for endometriosis with formation of an endometriotic, or "chocolate" cyst

- **Treatment:**
  - o **Medical** treatment consists of analgesics to control pain
  - o Cyclic hormonal therapy & GnRH analogues provide relief from pain & help regress
  - o **Drug treatment of symptomatic cases:**
    - ♦ Progesterone
    - ♦ OCPs
    - ♦ Androgens
    - ♦ Letrozol
    - ♦ Danazol
    - ♦ GnRH analogues
  - o For women desirous of childbearing, operative laparoscopy with electrocauterization/laser ablation of endometriosis, evacuation of large endometriomas with cautery, peeling of its lining and surgery to restore tubo-ovarian relationship help in improve fertility
  - o **Surgical procedures include:**
    - ♦ Laparotomy
    - ♦ Incision of chocolate cyst and removal of lining
    - ♦ Salpingo-oophorectomy
    - ♦ Hysterectomy & bilateral salpingo-oophorectomy
    - ♦ Excision of scar endometriosis

MENOPAUSE

Premature menopause

- When menstruation ceases **before** 40 years of age
- Delayed menopause is one when the menopause fails to occur even **beyond** 55 years

Menopause

- **Permanent** cessation of menstruation at the end of reproductive life due to ovarian follicular inactivity
- Average age being **50** years
- Genetically predetermined
- Estradiol level **falls** to the optimal 20 pg/ml when menopause sets in

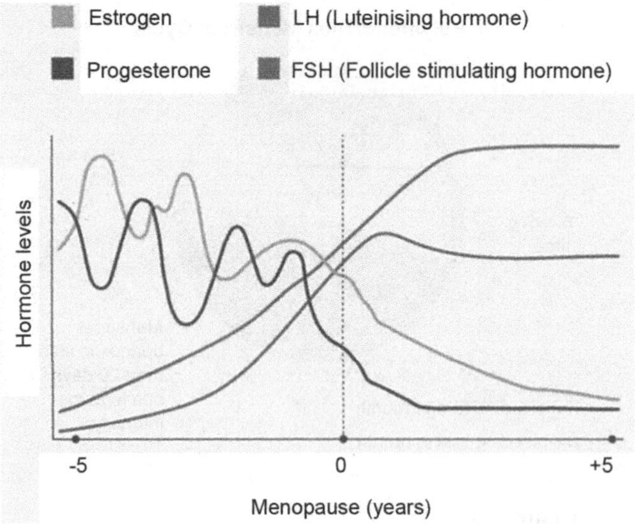

- Increased androgen secretion from the ovarian stroma & from adrenal
- **Diagnosis is by:**
  - o Classical symptom of '**hot** flush' (50%)
  - o Elevated FSH levels to >100 mIU/ml
  - o Serum estradiol level <20 pg/ml

Hormone replacement therapy

- For a woman with intact uterus, progestin (for last 12-14 days) **must** be combined with estrogen
- **Otherwise**, unopposed estrogen therapy will increase the risk of endometrial hyperplasia and adenocarcinoma
- Estrogen without a progestin is recommended for a post-menopausal woman who had hysterectomy
- **Benefits of HRT:**
  - o Improvement in vasomotor symptoms
  - o Increase in bone mineral density
  - o Reduced risk of vertebral & hip fractures
  - o Reduction in colorectal Ca
- **Risks of HRT:**
  - o **Endometrial** Ca
  - o Breast Ca
  - o Venous thromboembolism/VTE
  - o Coronary heart disease
- **Contraindications to HRT:**
  - o Undiagnosed genital tract bleeding

- o Estrogen dependent neoplasm
- o History of VTE
- o Acute liver diseases
- o Gallbladder diseases

AMENORRHOEA

Physiology & pathology

- **Physiological** before puberty, during pregnancy & lactation and following menopause
- **MC** cause of amenorrhoea in a woman of reproductive age is pregnancy
- Regular menstruation indicates cyclical ovarian function in response to intact Hypothalamo-Pituitary-Ovarian/ HPO axis
- Amenorrhoea/oligomenorrhoea indicates ovarian, endometrial and/or HPO axis dysfunction

Primary amenorrhoea

- Failure of menses in a girl by **16** years of age (regardless of the presence of secondary sexual characters)
- Failure of menses in a girl by **14** years of age (in the absence of secondary sexual characters)
- **Causes of primary amenorrhoea:**
  - o Mullerian agenesis
  - o Primary ovarian failure
  - o Turner syndrome
  - o Androgen insensitivity syndrome
  - o Adrenogenital syndrome
- **Common causes of primary amenorrhoea:**
  - o Gonadal failure
  - o Abnormal chromosomal pattern
  - o Development defect of genital tract
  - o Disturbed function of the HPO axis

Secondary amenorrhoea

- **MC pathological cause of secondary amenorrhea** (absence of menstruation for **6** months or more in a woman in whom normal menstruation has been established)
  - o **In India:** Endometrial **TB**
  - o **Worldwide:** Hypothalamic dysfunction
- **Other causes of secondary amenorrhoea:**
  - o PCOD
  - o Cushing's syndrome
  - o Sheehan's syndrome
  - o Hypothyroidism

DYSFUNCTIONAL UTERINE BLEEDING/DUB

Dysfunctional uterine bleeding

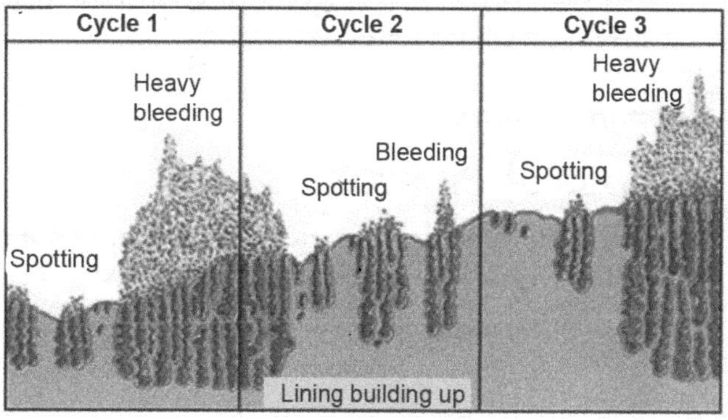

Definition

- DUB is defined as a state of **abnormal** uterine bleeding **without** any clinically detectable organic, systemic and iatrogenic cause (pelvic pathology, e.g., tumor, inflammation or pregnancy is excluded)
- Currently DUB is defined as a state of abnormal uterine bleeding following anovulation due to the dysfunction of hypothalamo-pituitary-ovarian axis (endocrine origin)

Classification of DUB	
Anovulatory (80%)	**Ovulatory (20%)**
Threshold bleeding of puberty menorrhagia	Irregular ripening
Metropathia haemorrhagia	Irregular shedding
Premenopausal DUB	IUCD insertion
	Following sterilization operation

Pathology

- **MC, endometrium in DUB is:**
  - o **In 60% cases:** Endometrium is normal
  - o **In 30%:** Endometrium is hyperplastic
  - o **In the remaining:** Irregular shedding, irregular ripening, or atrophic pattern

- **Irregular shedding:**
    - o Normally, regeneration of the endometrium is completed by 3rd day of menstruation
    - o In irregular shedding, desquamation is continued for a variable period with simultaneous failure of regeneration of endometrium
- **Irregular ripening:**
    - o There is **poor** formation and inadequate function of the corpus luteum
    - o Secretion of both estrogen & progesterone is **inadequate** to support the endometrial growth
    - o As such, light bleeding occurs and continues prior to the start of proper flow

Hormonal status

- **Increased** estrogen, **deficient** progesterone
- There is slow increase in secretion of estrogen but no negative feedback inhibition of FSH
- The net effect is gradual rise in the level of estrogen with concomitant phase of amenorrhoea for about 6-8 weeks

Metropathia hemorrhagica/cystic glandular hyperplasia/Schroeder's disease

- Specialized form of DUB
- Seen in 40-45 years (perimenopausal)
- Short period of amenorrhoea is **followed** by continuous bleeding per vaginum (a time period of 8 weeks between the LMP and the onset of continuous hemorrhage)
- **Microscopically:**
    - o There is intense cystic glandular hypertrophy, with marked disparity in sizes
    - o Some of the glands are small, others are large giving the appearance of "Swiss **Cheese**" pattern (small & large holes of Swiss cheese made in Switzerland)

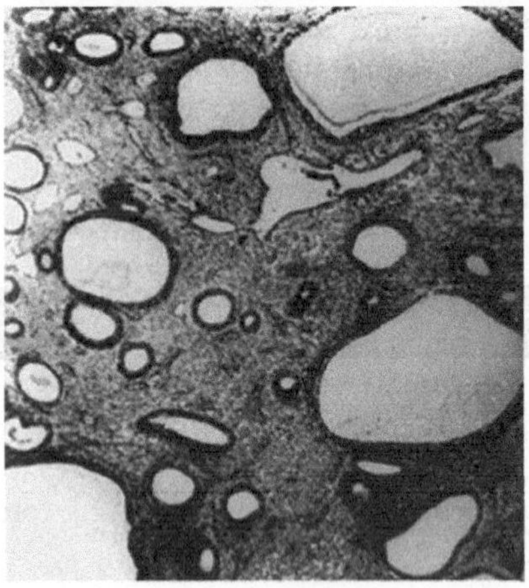

Mittelschmerz's syndrome/ovular pain

- Lower abdominal (hypogastrium/either iliac fossa) pain **cyclically** 2 weeks before menstruation (in mid menstrual period)
- The pain is located on one side and does **not** change from side to side according to which ovary is ovulating
- **Rarely** lasts >12 hours

ADENOMYOSIS

Physiology & pathology

- Presence of endometrium within the myometrium

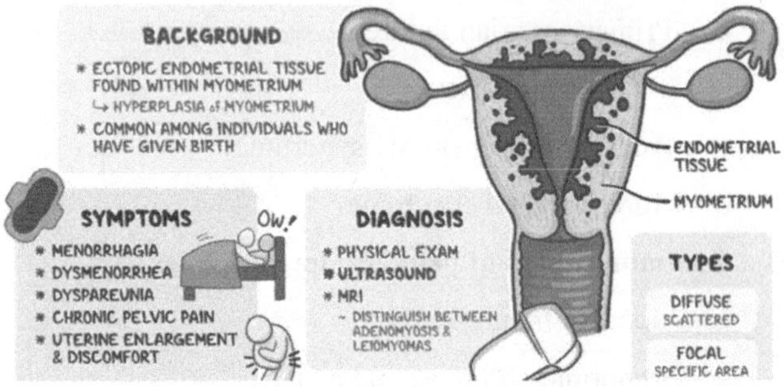

SECTION 4

GYNECOLOGY

Chapter 4

Genital Prolapse

SUPPORT OF UTERUS

SUPPORTS OF UTERUS
PRIMARY SUPPORTS
• **Fibromuscular supports**
(a) ***Muscular supports:***
1. Pelvic diaphragm
2. Perineal body
3. Urogenital diaphragm
(b) ***Ligamentary supports:***
1. Pubocervical ligament
2. Transverse cervical ligament
3. Uterosacral ligament
(c) ***Fascial support:***
1. Endopelvic fascia
2. Vesicovaginal fascia
3. Rectovaginal fascia
• **Uterine axis**
• **Round ligamnet**

Relevant anatomy

- Important support structures of uterus are:
  - o The Cardinal/Transverse cervical ligament

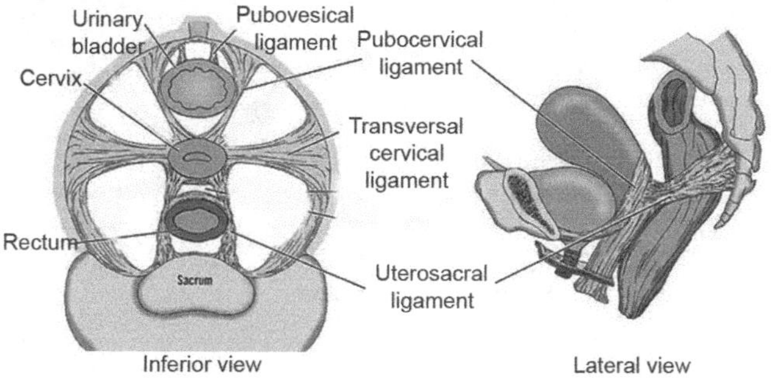

Inferior view Lateral view

  - o Uterosacral ligament
  - o Pubocervical ligament
  - o Levator ani muscle (pubococcygeus, iliococcygeus, levator plate)

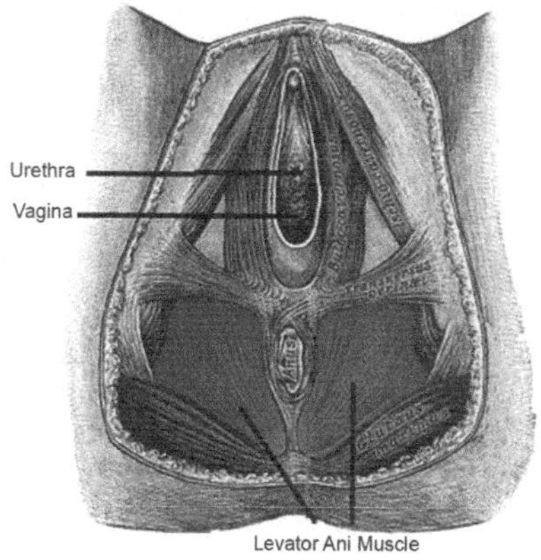

  - o Endopelvic fascia
  - o Perineal body

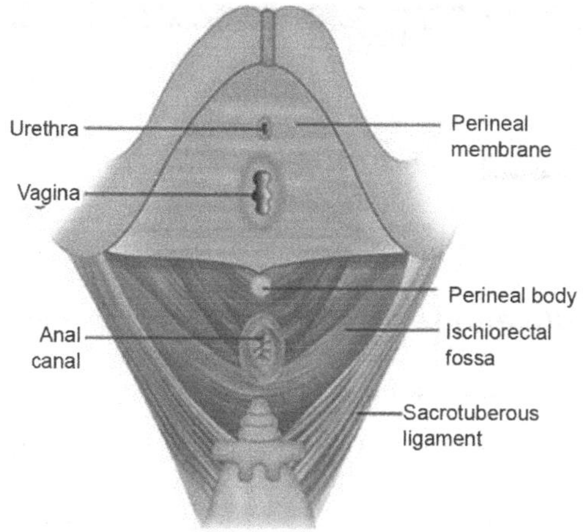

- The hammock like arrangements of the levator ani muscle, the condensed endopelvic fascia, especially the Mackenrodt's ligaments (transverse cervical/cardinal ligament) are the **cardinal** supports of the uterus

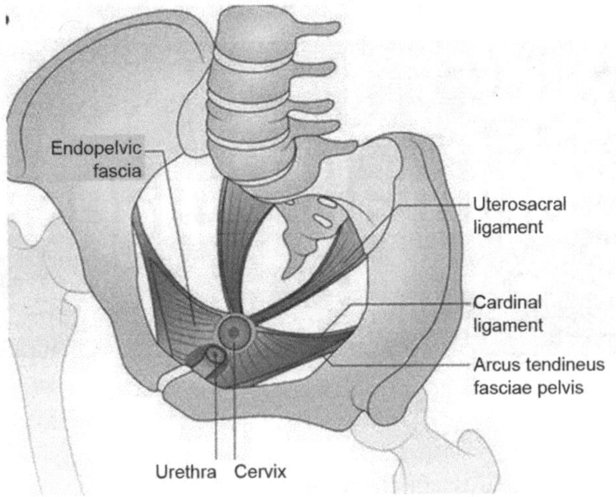

- The levator plate and the perineal body **maintains** the normal vaginal axis

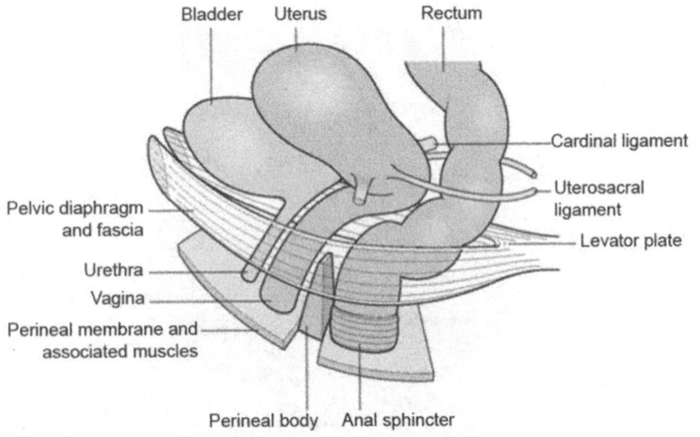

CLASSIFICATION

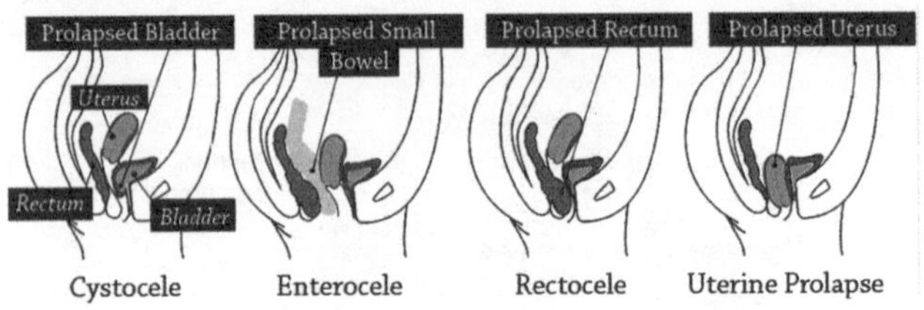

Classification

- **Anterior vaginal wall:**
  - o **Upper 2/3rd:** Cystocele
  - o **Lower 1/3rd:** Urethrocele
- **Posterior vaginal wall:**
  - o **Upper 1/3rd:** Enterocele
  - o **Lower 1/3rd:** Rectocele
- Uterine descent
- Procidentia

FEATURES

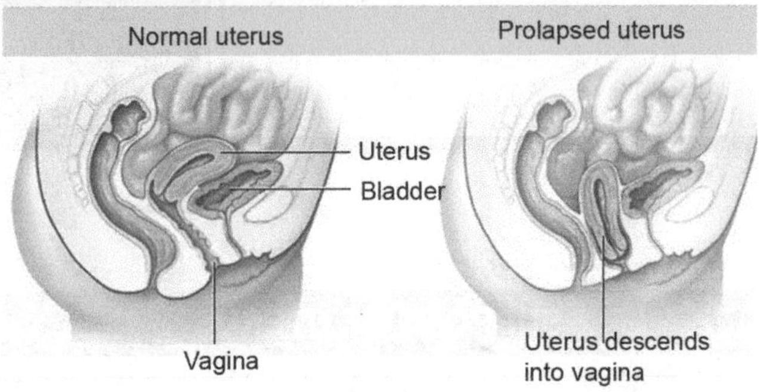

Features

- **Important** risk factors for prolapse is history of vaginal birth and the age of the woman
- Cystocele & urethrocele are **common** with gynecoid pelvis
- Urinary complaints in genital prolapse is difficulty in passing urine, incomplete evacuation, frequency, stress incontinence and rarely retention
- **Complications:** Decubitus ulcers (due to venous congestion) etc.

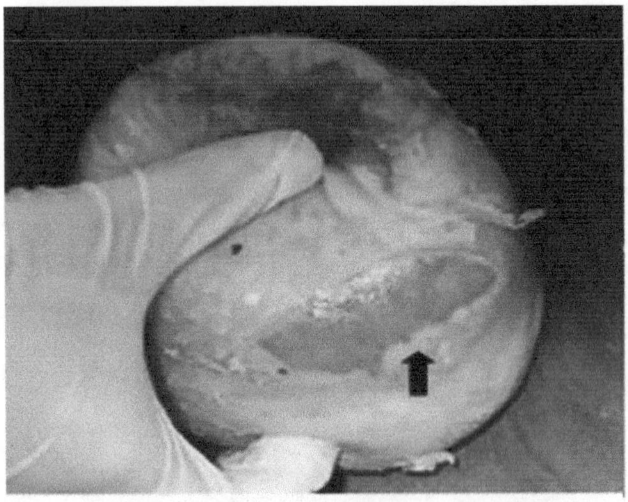

Figure: Decubitus ulcer

DEGREES OF UTERINE PROLAPSE

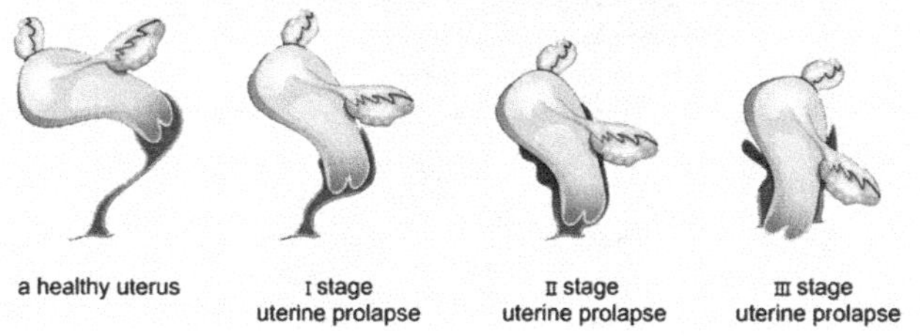

Degree of uterine prolapse

- **1st:** Uterus descends but external os remains in the vagina
- **2nd:** External os protrudes outside the vagina but uterine body remains inside
- **3rd:** Uterine body descends outside the vaginal introitus

MANAGEMENT

Management of prolapse

- Post-hysterectomy vault prolapses (0.1-10%) is usually accompanied by enterocele (70%)
- LeFort repair (**almost** obsolete)

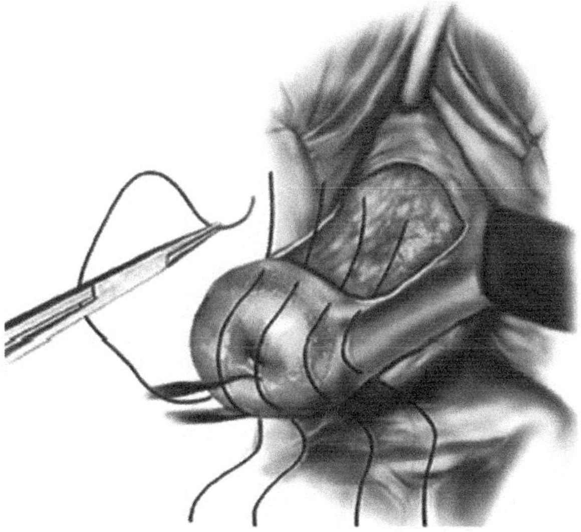

Figure: LeFort colpocleisis for prolapse repair

- **Colpocleisis:** Effective method for a woman who is no longer interested in coital function
- **In women < 40 years with complete family; wanting to retain menstrual & reproductive function:**

Manchester operation (Fothergill's operation)

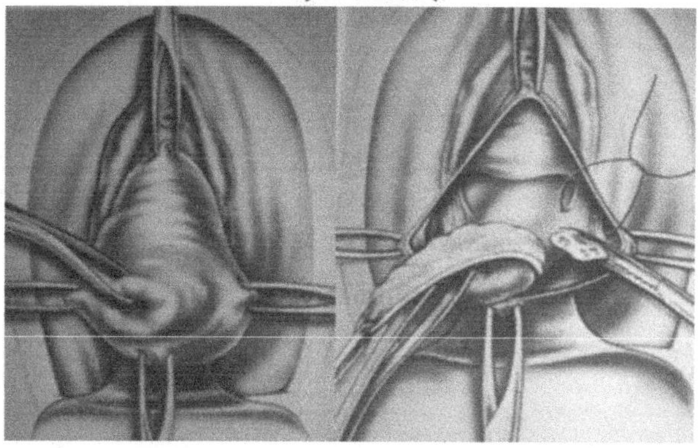

Fothergill's points–1 sub urethral, 2 on either side of the cervix 1 on posterior vaginal wall

- Fothergill's repair/Manchester operation
- **Steps:**
  - Dilatation & Curettage
  - Amputation of cervix
  - Plication of Mackenrodt's ligament in front of the cervix
  - Anterior colporrhaphy
  - Colpoperineorrhaphy

- **In young women, desirous of retaining their childbearing & menstrual functions:**
  - Cervicopexy (**Purandare's** operation)/Sling operation

Purandare's cervicopexy
• Fascial strips are anchored to the ant. aspect of isthmus
Advantages
• Easy to perform
• Dynamic support
• Minimum blood loss
Disadvantages
• Alters pelvic anatomy by obliterating U-V fold
• Vagina is being pulled forward so increased chances of enterocele formation

  - Cervicopexy is the method of repair for a patient with congenital or nulliparous prolapse
  - Perineal exercises

GENITAL PROLAPSE IN PREGNANCY

Management of genital prolapse in pregnancy

- **1st trimester:** Pessary

- o Pessary **cannot** cure prolapse
- o Relieves the symptoms of stretching the hiatus urogenitalis, thus preventing vaginal & uterine descent
- o Should be placed up to 18 weeks
- o Pessary treatment is indicated in early pregnancy, puerperium, patient unfit for surgery or while the patients are waiting for operation

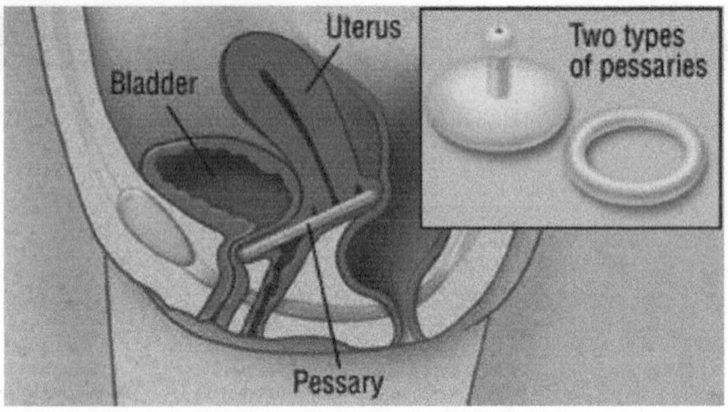

- **In 2nd trimester: Spontaneous** resolution

SECTION 4
GYNECOLOGY

Chapter 5

Genital Malignancies

OVARIAN CA

Pathology

- **Risk factors:**
  - Low parity
  - Decreased fertility
  - Delayed child bearing
  - PCOD
- **Protective factors:**
  - Multiparity
  - Pregnancy
  - OCPs
  - Lactation

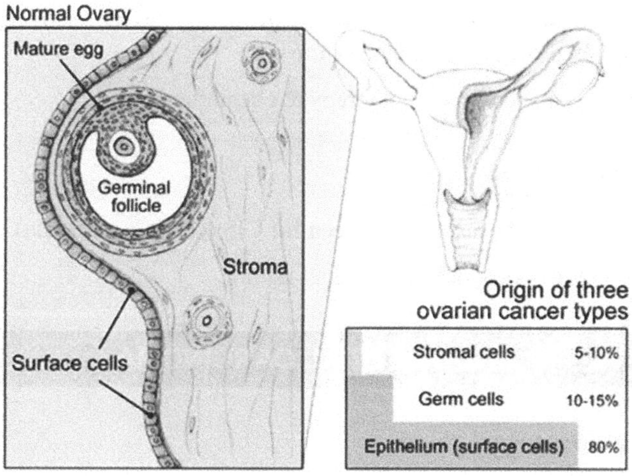

- **Classification:**
  - **Common epithelial ovarian tumours:**
    - Serous tumours
    - Mucinous tumours
    - Endometrioid tumours
    - Clear cell tumours
    - Brenner tumours
  - **Sex cord/Gonadal-stromal tumours:**
    - Granulosa cell tumours, theca cell tumours
    - Androblastomas:
      - Sertoli-Leydig cell tumours
    - Gynandroblastoma
  - **Germ cell tumours:**
    - Dysgerminoma
    - Endodermal sinus tumour
    - Embryonal cell Ca
    - Choriocarcinoma
    - Teratoma
  - Lipid cell tumours
  - Gonadoblastoma
  - Metastatic

CERVICAL CA

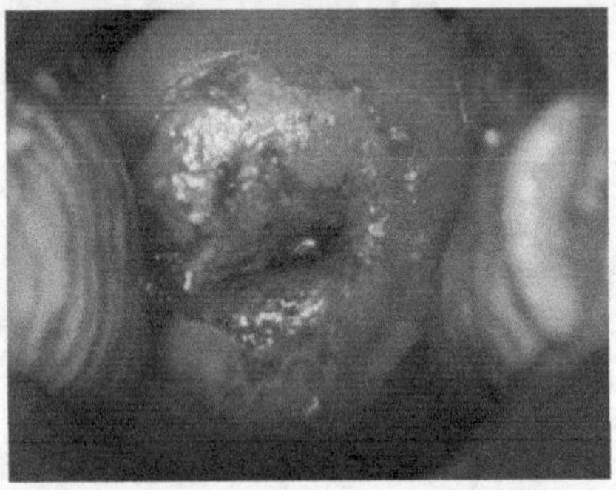

Pathology

- **Arises from:** Squamocolumnar junction
- **MC agent:** HPV 16
- **Other type of HPV which are associated with cervical Ca:** HPV 18, 31, 45, 51, 52 & 53
- **Other risk factors:**
  - o Early sexual intercourse
  - o Multiple sexual partners
- **Time taken for conversion of CIN to invasive Ca:** 10 years
- **MC histological type:** Squamous cell Ca
- Cellular grading of dysplasia is done by Bethesda system

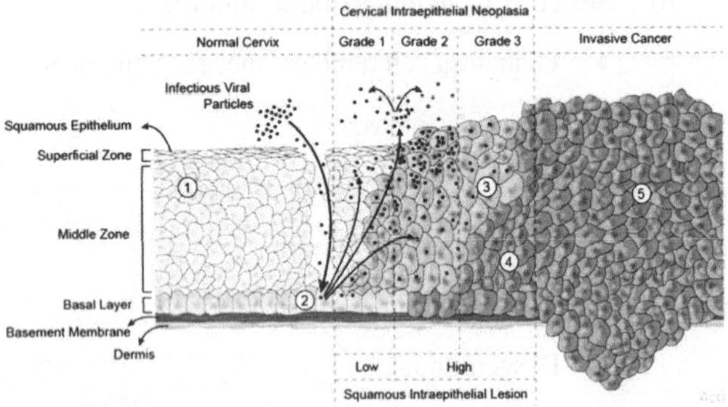

Features

- **Earliest symptom:** Post-coital bleeding
- **Other features:** Pelvic pain, cervical discharge

Lymph nodes affected

- Parametrial
- Obturator
- Hypogastric
- External iliac

Investigations

- **Cervical biopsy (punch/cone): Best** method for diagnosing
- Transvaginal Sonography, CT or MRI are useful investigation to assess the extent of neoplasm
- **Best method of screening:** Pap smear (Screens for cervical dysplasia)

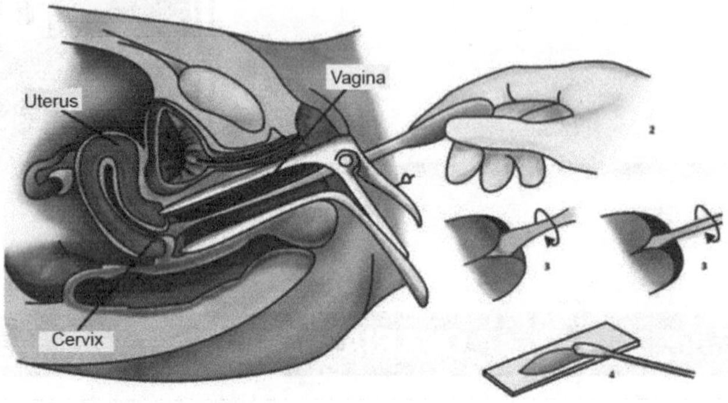

Management of stage II

- **IIA:** Involvement of upper 1/3rd of vagina
- **IIB:** Unilateral or bilateral invasion of the parametrium
- Extended hysterectomy, chemotherapy (Cisplatin) & intracavitary brachytherapy

Management of stage III

- **IIIA:** Disease extends up to lower 2/3rd of vagina
- **IIIB:** Unilateral or bilateral invasion of the parametrium and onto the pelvic side wall
- Unilateral/bilateral involvement of ureter causing hydronephrosis/renal failure
- Managed by Radiotherapy & chemotherapy

Prognosis

- **100% cure rates are seen in:** CIS (carcinoma in-situ)
- **MC cause of death:** Renal failure

ENDOMETRIAL CARCINOMA

Pathology

- **MC histological type:** Adenocarcinoma (up to 80%)
- **Most malignant type:** Clear cell Ca

- **MC hormonal cause of endometrial Ca:** Unopposed estrogen

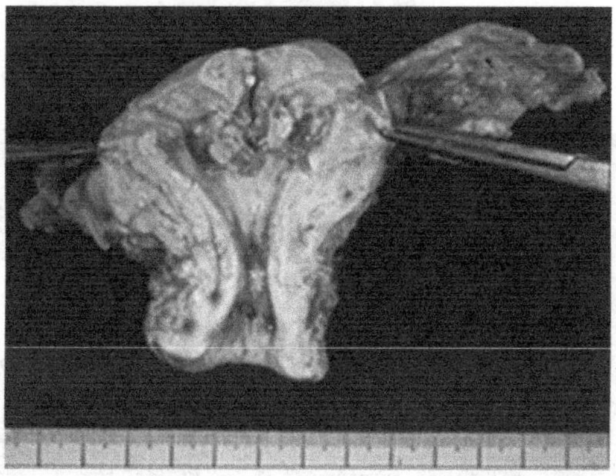

Predisposing factors

- Family history
- Obesity
- DM
- Tamoxifen therapy
- PCOD

Treatment of atypical endometrial hyperplasia

- Hysterectomy (Pan-hysterectomy in elderly)

OTHER TUMOURS

Triad of Meigs' syndrome

- Ascites
- Hydrothorax (right side)
- Benign tumour of ovary (fibroma)

Triad of Pseudo-Meigs' syndrome

- Ascites
- Hydrothorax (right side)
- Malignant ovarian tumour is included (instead of benign tumour)

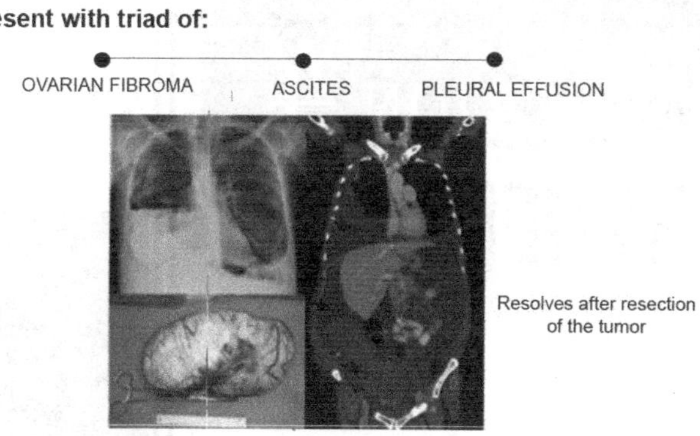

Figure: Meigs' syndrome

Masculinizing ovarian tumours

- Hilus cell tumour
- Sertoli cell tumour
- Leydig cell tumour

Feminizing cell tumour

- Theca cell tumour
- Granulosa cell tumour

Dysgerminoma

- **MC ovarian tumour (in < 20 years):** Dysgerminoma
- **Most radiosensitive ovarian tumour:** Dysgerminoma

Histological features & ovarian tumours

- **Rokitansky bodies:** Teratoma
- **Schiller Duval bodies:** Endodermal sinus tumour
- **Reinke's crystal:** Hilus cell tumour
- **Call Exner bodies:** Granulosa cell tumour

Ovarian tumours & markers

- **Placental alkaline phosphatase:** Dysgerminoma
- **LDH:** Dysgerminoma
- **Inhibin:** Granulosa cell tumour
- **CA 125:** Ovarian tumours

SECTION 4
GYNECOLOGY

Chapter 6

Fibroids

FIBROID/LEIOMYOMA

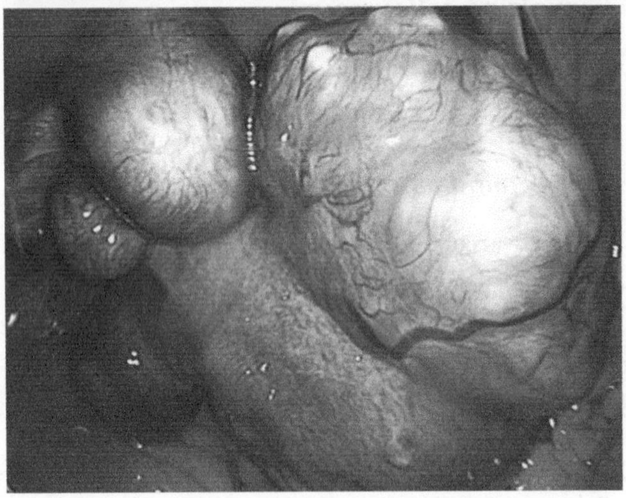

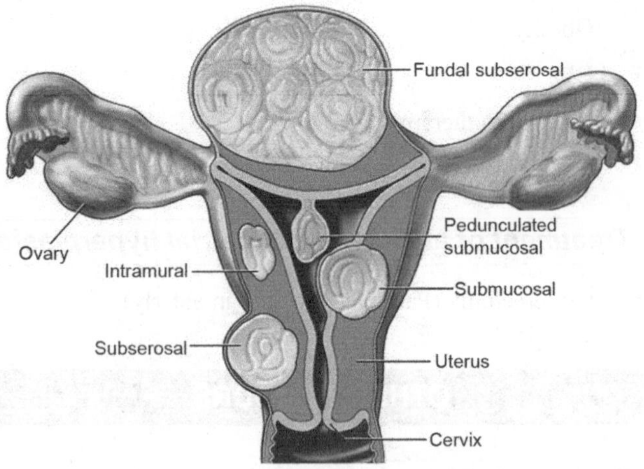

Pathology

- Benign uterine smooth muscle tumour
- Estrogen sensitive
- **Fibroids are associated with:**
  - o Nulliparity
  - o Family history
  - o Follicular ovarian cysts
  - o Endometriosis
  - o Endometrial hyperplasia
  - o Endometrial Ca
- **Types:**
  - o Intramural
  - o Submucosal
  - o Subserosal

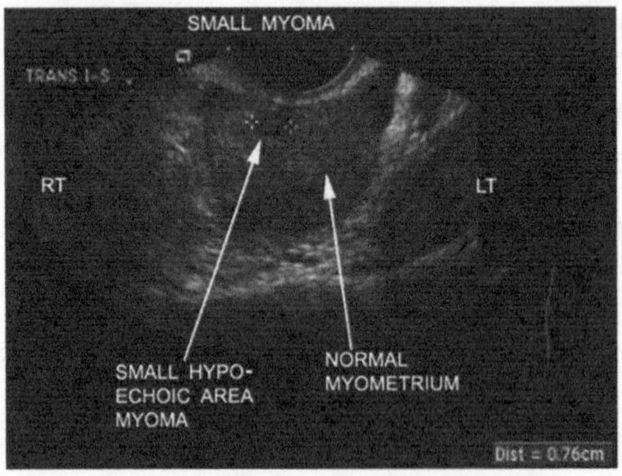

- **MC type of fibroid:** Intramural/interstitial (75%)
- **Most fibroid starts as:** Intramural/interstitial fibroids
- **MC to undergo malignant change (0.5%, rare before the age of 40):**
  - o Intramural
  - o Submucous
- **MC type of degeneration:** Hyaline (starts from the centre)
- **Treatment:**
  - o GnRH agonists to reduce the size of tumour
  - o Myomectomy for removal of symptomatic fibroids, in females who wish to retain fertility
  - o Hysterectomy in women with completed family

RED DEGENERATION OF FIBROID

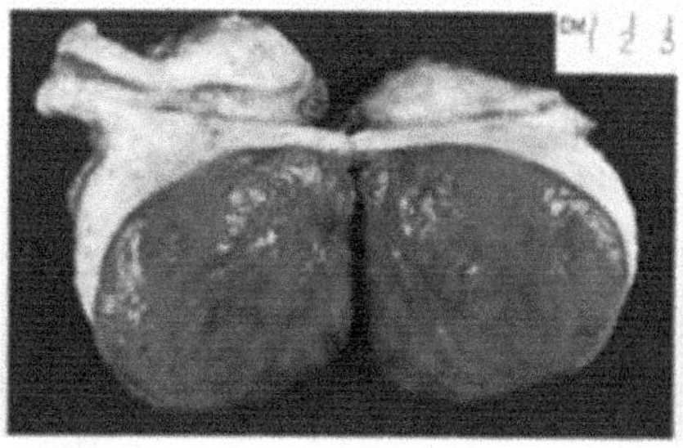

Red degeneration of fibroid

- Seen in 2nd half of pregnancy or puerperium
- Due to thrombosis of large veins of the tumour
- Infection has **no** role (this process is an aseptic one)
- Management is conservative (analgesics & sedatives)